Lupus

Editors

ALFRED H.J. KIM
ZAHI TOUMA

RHEUMATIC DISEASE CLINICS OF NORTH AMERICA

www.rheumatic.theclinics.com

Consulting Editor
MICHAEL H. WEISMAN

August 2021 • Volume 47 • Number 3

ELSEVIER

1600 John F. Kennedy Boulevard • Suite 1800 • Philadelphia, Pennsylvania, 19103-2899
http://www.theclinics.com

RHEUMATIC DISEASE CLINICS OF NORTH AMERICA Volume 47, Number 3
August 2021 ISSN 0889-857X, ISBN 13: 978-0-323-83556-5

Editor: Lauren Boyle
Developmental Editor: Karen Solomon

Rheumatic Disease Clinics of North America (ISSN 0889-857X) is published quarterly by Elsevier Inc., 360 Park Avenue South, New York, NY 10010-1710. Months of issue are February, May, August, and November. Business and editorial offices: 1600 John F. Kennedy Boulevard, Suite 1800, Philadelphia, PA 19103-2899. Periodicals postage paid at New York, NY and additional mailing offices. Subscription prices are USD 362.00 per year for US individuals, USD 1000.00 per year for US institutions, USD 100.00 per year for US students and residents, USD 427.00 per year for Canadian individuals, USD 1045.00 per year for Canadian institutions, USD 100.00 per year for Canadian students/residents, USD 465.00 per year for international individuals, USD 1045.00 per year for international institutions, and USD 230.00 per year for foreign students/residents. To receive student/ resident rate, orders must be accompanied by name of affiliated institution, date of term, and the *signature* of program/residency coordinator on institution letterhead. Orders will be billed at individual rate until proof of status received. Foreign air speed delivery is included in all *Clinics* subscription prices. All prices are subject to change without notice. **POSTMASTER:** Send address changes to *Rheumatic Disease Clinics of North America,* Elsevier Health Sciences Division, Subscription Customer Service, 3251 Riverport Lane, Maryland Heights, MO 63043. **Customer Service: 1-800-654-2452 (US and Canada). From outside of the US and Canada: 314-447-8871. Fax: 314-447-8029. For print support, e-mail: JournalsCustomerService-usa@elsevier.com. For online support, e-mail: JournalsOnlineSupport-usa@elsevier.com.**

Reprints. For copies of 100 or more of articles in this publication, please contact the Commercial Reprints Department, Elsevier Inc., 360 Park Avenue South, New York, New York, 10010-1710; Tel.: +1-212-633-3874, Fax: +1-212-633-3820, and E-mail: reprints@elsevier.com.

Rheumatic Disease Clinics of North America is covered in *MEDLINE/PubMed (Index Medicus), Current Contents/Clinical Medicine, Science Citation Index, ISI/BIOMED,* and *EMBASE/Excerpta Medica.*

Contributors

CONSULTING EDITOR

MICHAEL H. WEISMAN, MD
Adjunct Professor of Medicine, Stanford University, Distinguished Professor of Medicine Emeritus, David Geffen School of Medicine at UCLA, Professor of Medicine Emeritus, Cedars-Sinai Medical Center, Los Angeles, California, USA

EDITORS

ALFRED H.J. KIM, MD, PhD
Assistant Professor, Division of Rheumatology, Department of Medicine, Washington University School of Medicine, St Louis, Missouri, USA

ZAHI TOUMA, MD, PhD
Associate Professor, Division of Rheumatology, Department of Medicine, Toronto Western Hospital, Institute of Health Policy, Management and Evaluation, University of Toronto, Toronto, Ontario, Canada

AUTHORS

NARENDER ANNAPUREDDY, MD
Assistant Professor, Department of Medicine, Vanderbilt University, Nashville, Tennessee, USA

MARTIN ARINGER, MD
Professor of Medicine (Rheumatology), Division of Rheumatology, Department of Medicine III, University Medical Center, Faculty of Medicine Carl Gustav Carus at the TU Dresden, Dresden, Germany

SUSAN P. CANNY, MD, PhD
Fellow, Department of Pediatrics, University of Washington School of Medicine, Benaroya Research Institute, Seattle, Washington, USA

YASHAAR CHAICHIAN, MD
Clinical Assistant Professor, Division of Immunology and Rheumatology, Stanford University, Palo Alto, California, USA

ELIZA F. CHAKRAVARTY, MD, MS
Associate Member, Arthritis and Clinical Immunology, Oklahoma Medical Research Foundation, Oklahoma City, Oklahoma, USA

ANDREA FAVA, MD
Instructor of Medicine, Division of Rheumatology, Johns Hopkins University, Baltimore, Maryland, USA

RUTH FERNANDEZ-RUIZ, MD, MSCI
Colton Center for Autoimmunity, Division of Rheumatology, NYU Grossman School of Medicine, New York, New York, USA

SARFARAZ A. HASNI, MD, MSc
Director, Lupus Clinical Research, National Institute of Arthritis and Musculoskeletal and Skin Diseases, National Institutes of Health, Bethesda, Maryland, USA

ALBERTA Y. HOI, MBBS, FRACP, PhD
Associate Professor, Centre for Inflammatory Diseases, Monash University, Department of Rheumatology, Monash Health, Clayton, Victoria, Australia

SHAUN W. JACKSON, MBChB, MD
Assistant Professor, Department of Pediatrics, University of Washington School of Medicine, Seattle Children's Research Institute, Seattle, Washington, USA

SINDHU R. JOHNSON, MD, PhD
Associate Professor of Medicine, Division of Rheumatology, Department of Medicine, Toronto Western Hospital, Mount Sinai Hospital, Institute of Health Policy, Management and Evaluation, University of Toronto, Toronto, Ontario, Canada

MEENAKSHI JOLLY, MD
Professor, Department of Medicine, Rush University, Chicago, Illinois, USA

J. MICHELLE KAHLENBERG, MD, PhD
Department of Internal Medicine, Division of Rheumatology, Department of Dermatology, University of Michigan, Ann Arbor, Michigan, USA

MARIANA J. KAPLAN, MD
Systemic Autoimmunity Branch, Intramural Research Program, National Institute of Arthritis and Musculoskeletal and Skin Diseases, National Institutes of Health, Bethesda, Maryland, USA

STEPHANIE LAZAR, MD
Department of Internal Medicine, Division of Rheumatology, University of Michigan, Ann Arbor, Michigan, USA

YUDONG LIU, MD, PhD
Department of Clinical Laboratory, Peking University People's Hospital, Beijing, China

ERIC F. MORAND, MBBS, FRACP, PhD
Professor, Centre for Inflammatory Diseases, Monash University, Department of Rheumatology, Monash Health, Clayton, Victoria, Australia

AMANDA MOYER, MD
Departments of Medicine and Pediatrics, University of Oklahoma School of Medicine, Oklahoma City, Oklahoma, USA

TIMOTHY B. NIEWOLD, MD
Colton Center for Autoimmunity, NYU Grossman School of Medicine, New York, New York, USA

OMER PAMUK, MD
National Institute of Arthritis and Musculoskeletal and Skin Diseases, National Institutes of Health, Bethesda, Maryland, USA

JACQUELINE L. PAREDES, BA
Colton Center for Autoimmunity, NYU Grossman School of Medicine, New York, New York, USA

ANNA RADZISZEWSKA, BSc (hons), MSc
Department of Rheumatology, Division of Medicine, Rayne Building, University College London, Centre for Adolescent Rheumatology Versus Arthritis at UCL, UCLH, GOSH, London, United Kingdom

DEEPAK A. RAO, MD, PhD
Division of Rheumatology, Inflammation, Immunity, Assistant Professor, Department of Medicine, Brigham and Women's Hospital, Harvard Medical School, Boston, Massachusetts, USA

SOUMYA RAYCHAUDHURI, MD, PhD
Division of Rheumatology, Inflammation, Immunity, Professor, Department of Medicine, Harvard Medical School, Center for Data Sciences, Brigham and Women's Hospital, Boston, Massachusetts, USA; Program in Medical and Population Genetics, Broad Institute of MIT and Harvard, Cambridge, Massachusetts, USA; Centre for Genetics and Genomics Versus Arthritis, Centre for Musculoskeletal Research, Manchester Academic Health Science Centre, The University of Manchester, Manchester, United Kingdom

CHRISTOPHER REDMOND, MD
National Institute of Arthritis and Musculoskeletal and Skin Diseases, National Institutes of Health, Bethesda, Maryland, USA

SIRISHA SIROBHUSHANAM, PhD
Department of Internal Medicine, Division of Rheumatology, University of Michigan, Ann Arbor, Michigan, USA

TARANEH TOFIGHI, MD
Department of Medicine, University of Toronto, Toronto, Ontario, Canada

ZAHI TOUMA, MD, PhD
Associate Professor, Division of Rheumatology, Department of Medicine, Toronto Western Hospital, Institute of Health Policy, Management and Evaluation, University of Toronto, Toronto, Ontario, Canada

DANIEL J. WALLACE, MD, FACP, MACR
Clinical Professor of Medicine, Division of Rheumatology, Cedars-Sinai Medical Center, David Geffen School of Medicine, UCLA, Los Angeles, California, USA

CHRIS WINCUP, BSc (hons), MBBS, MRCP
Department of Rheumatology, Division of Medicine, Rayne Building, University College London, Centre for Adolescent Rheumatology Versus Arthritis at UCL, UCLH, GOSH, London, United Kingdom

Contents

Interferons in Systemic Lupus Erythematosus   297

Sirisha Sirobhushanam, Stephanie Lazar, and J. Michelle Kahlenberg

Skewing of type I interferon (IFN) production and responses is a hallmark of systemic lupus erythematosus (SLE). Genetic and environmental contributions to IFN production lead to aberrant innate and adaptive immune activation even before clinical development of disease. Basic and translational research in this arena continues to identify contributions of IFNs to disease pathogenesis, and several promising therapeutic options for targeting of type I IFNs and their signaling pathways are in development for treatment of SLE patients.

Neutrophil Dysregulation in the Pathogenesis of Systemic Lupus Erythematosus   317

Yudong Liu and Mariana J. Kaplan

The recent identifications of a subset of proinflammatory neutrophils, low-density granulocytes, and their ability to readily form neutrophil extracellular traps led to a resurgence of interest in neutrophil dysregulation in the pathogenesis of systemic lupus erythematosus (SLE). This article presents an overview on how neutrophil dysregulation modulates the innate and adaptive immune responses in SLE and their putative roles in disease pathogenesis. The therapeutic potential of targeting this pathogenic process in the treatment of SLE is also discussed.

The Power of Systems Biology: Insights on Lupus Nephritis from the Accelerating Medicines Partnership   335

Andrea Fava, Soumya Raychaudhuri, and Deepak A. Rao

The Accelerating Medicines Partnership (AMP) SLE Network united resources from academic centers, government, nonprofit, and industry to accelerate discovery in lupus nephritis (LN). The AMP SLE Network developed a set of protocols for high-throughput analyses to systematically study kidney tissue, urine, and blood in LN. This article summarizes approaches and results from phase 1 of AMP SLE Network effort, including single cell RNA-seq analysis of LN kidney biopsies, cellular and proteomic studies of LN urine, and mass cytometry immunophenotyping of blood cells. This work provides a framework to guide studies of the clinical implications of active cellular/molecular pathways in LN.

Patient-reported outcome (PRO) was identified as a core systemic lupus erythematosus (SLE) outcome in 1999. More than 20 years later, however, generic PRO measures evaluating impact in SLE are used mainly for research. Generic and disease-targeted PRO tools have unique advantages. Significant progress in identification of patient disease–relevant PRO concepts and development of new PRO tools for SLE has occurred over the past 20 years. Further research needs to focus on responsiveness and minimally important differences of existing, promising PRO tools to facilitate their use in SLE patient care and research.

T-cell dysregulation has been implicated in the loss of tolerance and over-activation of B cells in systemic lupus erythematosus (SLE). Recent studies have identified T-cell subsets and genetic, epigenetic, and environmental factors that contribute to pathogenic T-cell differentiation, as well as disease pathogenesis and clinical phenotypes in SLE. Many therapeutics targeting T-cell pathways are under development, and although many have not progressed in clinical trials, the recent approval of the calcineurin inhibitor voclosporin is encouraging. Further study of T-cell subsets and biomarkers of T-cell action may pave the way for specific targeting of pathogenic T-cell populations in SLE.

B cells exert a prominent contribution to the pathogenesis of systemic lupus erythematosus (SLE). Here, we review the immune mechanisms underlying autoreactive B cell activation in SLE, focusing on how B cell receptor and Toll-like receptor signals integrate to drive breaks in tolerance to nuclear antigens. In addition, we discuss autoantibody-dependent and autoantibody-independent B cell effector functions during lupus pathogenesis. Finally, we address efforts to target B cells therapeutically in human SLE. Despite initial disappointing clinical trials testing B cell depletion in lupus, more recent studies show promise, emphasizing how greater understanding of underlying immune mechanisms can yield clinical benefits.

The assessment of systemic lupus erythematosus (SLE) disease activity in clinical trials has been challenging. This is related to the wide spectrum of SLE manifestations and the heterogeneity of the disease trajectory. Currently, composite outcome measures are most commonly used as a primary endpoint while organ-specific measures are often used as secondary outcomes. In this article, we review the outcome measures and endpoints used in most recent clinical trials and explore potential avenues for further development of new measures and the refinement of existing tools.

Systemic lupus erythematosus (SLE) is an autoimmune disorder characterized by abnormalities within the innate and adaptive immune systems. Activation and proliferation of a wide array of immune cells require significant up-regulation in cellular energy metabolism, with the mitochondria playing an essential role in the initiation and maintenance of this response. This article highlights how abnormal mitochondrial function may occur in SLE and focuses on how energy metabolism, oxidative stress, and impaired mitochondrial repair play a role in the pathogenesis of the disease. How this may represent an appealing novel therapeutic target for future drug therapy in SLE also is discussed.

Systemic lupus erythematosus (SLE) is an autoimmune disease that primarily affects women of childbearing age. Pregnancy-related morbidity and mortality are well described in SLE; however, better management of disease activity throughout the disease course have minimized periods of disease activity and damage accrual, making pregnancy more feasible and desirable. A growing body of literature has defined risk factors for adverse pregnancy outcomes in patients with SLE, and coordinated medical and obstetric management has allowed most patients with SLE to safely achieve full-term pregnancies by timing pregnancy to maximal disease quiescence and use of pregnancy-compatible medications from preconception through lactation.

Large cohorts with diverse ethnic backgrounds and heterogenous clinical features have provided the real-life data about the safety and efficacy of various treatment regimens for systemic lupus erythematosus (SLE). There are multiple well-established regional, national, and international lupus cohorts that have made significant contributions to the understanding of SLE. Using social media for cohort-based studies can significantly increase the outreach in a short time period for studying rare diseases such as SLE. Lack of strict inclusion criteria allows study of a broad range of patients but selection bias and incomplete data are possible in long-term cohort studies.

Despite progress in the treatment of systemic lupus erythematosus (SLE), remission rates and health-related quality of life remain disappointingly low. The paucity of successful SLE clinical trials reminds us that we still have a long way to go. Nevertheless, there are clear signs of hope. We highlight results from recent studies of novel therapeutic strategies based on emerging insights into our understanding of SLE disease mechanisms. We also highlight several studies that inform optimal use of existing treatments to improve efficacy and/or limit toxicity. These developments suggest we may yet unlock the key toward more satisfactory treatment outcomes in SLE.

Since the European League Against Rheumatism/American College of Rheumatology 2019 classification criteria for systemic lupus erythematosus (SLE) were published, they were externally validated by groups worldwide. In particular, the new criteria worked well also in East Asian and pediatric cohorts. Antinuclear antibodies (ANA) as an entry criterion were critically discussed, but the group of ANA-negative patients is small (<5%) worldwide. Specificity of the criteria is dependent on correct attribution only of those criteria that are not better explained by other causes. Although the classification criteria should not be used for diagnosis, many novel aspects inform diagnostic considerations.

The recent updates on treatment recommendations for the management of systemic lupus erythematous have provided greater clarity in the way existing anti-inflammatory and immunomodulatory drugs are used, in treating disease activity, preventing flares, and reducing irreversible organ damage and toxicity arising from the treatments themselves. Novel therapies will provide more options in the armamentarium for treating this complex disease, but ongoing studies are needed to improve understanding of the optimal treatment algorithm to maintain quality of life and improve survival for patients.

RHEUMATIC DISEASE CLINICS
OF NORTH AMERICA

SERIES OF RELATED INTEREST

Medical Clinics of North America
https://www.medical.theclinics.com/
Neurologic Clinics
https://www.neurologic.theclinics.com/
Dermatologic Clinics
https://www.derm.theclinics.com/
Physical Medicine and Rehabilitation Clinics of North America
https://www.pmr.theclinics.com/

THE CLINICS ARE AVAILABLE ONLINE!
Access your subscription at:
www.theclinics.com

Foreword

Lupus

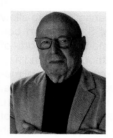

Michael H. Weisman, MD
Consulting Editor

Drs Kim and Touma have done a remarkable job in this issue keeping us informed about the latest information on diagnosis, treatment, pathobiologic mechanisms, and outlook for our lupus patients. Michelle Kahlenberg and her colleagues discuss the complexities of the relationships among the interferons themselves and between interferon signaling and lupus disease pathologic mechanisms. They correctly emphasize the genetic and environmental connections to the interferon story, leading us to be hopeful that further research in this area will permit greater understanding of the basic biology of lupus as well as the possibility for disease treatment and prevention. Liu and Kaplan, leaders in their respective fields, present an overview of the role of neutrophil dysregulation in lupus disease pathogenesis. Fava, Raychaudhuri, and Rao from the Accelerating Medicines Partnership (AMP) network describe advances in multiomic analyses of renal tissue, urine, and blood that provide insights into lupus pathogenesis; the hope is that these AMP studies will pave the way toward progress with larger clinically heterogeneous studies and subsequent therapeutic implications. Annapureddy and Jolly focus on the important area of generic and disease-targeted patient-reported outcome tools, emphasizing the need to further develop responsiveness and minimally important differences to place them in the working armamentarium for lupus care and research. Niewold and colleagues remind us of the importance of T-cell dysregulation implicated in the pathogenesis of systemic lupus erythematosus (SLE), pointing out the importance of further studying the role of T-cell subsets and their biomarkers as targets for therapeutic interventions. Canny and Jackson review for us the prominent contributory role of B cells to the pathogenesis of SLE, emphasizing how clinical benefit can result from a greater molecular understanding of how studying these immune mechanisms can yield clinical benefits.

Tofighi, Morand, and Touma discuss the challenges of how to address lupus disease activity in clinical trials; the selection of outcome measures (biological, clinical, patient reported, and so forth) are only pieces of the puzzle that can also be affected by patient

Rheum Dis Clin N Am 47 (2021) xiii–xiv
https://doi.org/10.1016/j.rdc.2021.06.002
0889-857X/21/© 2021 Published by Elsevier Inc.

rheumatic.theclinics.com

selection, concurrent care (especially corticosteroids), and the presence of irreversible damage. Wincup and Radziszewska teach us how abnormal mitochondrial function may occur in SLE and drill down on how energy metabolism, oxidative stress, and impaired mitochondrial repair play a role in the pathogenesis of the disease. Eliza Chakravarty, a world's expert in the field of reproductive health in SLE, gives us the latest information on how to define risk factors for adverse pregnancy outcomes in SLE; she makes a plea for coordinated medical and obstetrical management to allow the majority of SLE patients to have safe full-term pregnancies. Sarfaraz and colleagues at the NIH discuss in detail how well-documented and managed cohorts of SLE patients can effectively contribute to our understanding of pathogenesis and natural history of SLE; nevertheless, the contributions of patient registries and social media platforms for addressing similar issues can also provide valuable insights, particularly from real-world experience not captured by the cohort design. Chaichian and Wallace note the disappointing lack of progress in the treatment of SLE through the lens of failed clinical trials. Nevertheless, there is hope based upon targeted treatments focusing on more refined mechanisms as well as studies on the optimal use of existing strategies. Aringer and Johnson, experts in the field, discuss the conundrum of the relationship between classification criteria and the use of these criteria for diagnosis and management decisions, with a warning for us about focusing on uncommon clinical manifestations that are useful for diagnostic but not classification purposes. Finally, Hoi and Morand address the recent updates of treatment recommendations for SLE management, specifically highlighting for us the importance of focusing on treatment objectives to prevent flares, treat disease activity, and reduce the possibility of irreversible organ damage.

Michael H. Weisman, MD
Division of Rheumatology
Cedars-Sinai Medical Center
8700 Beverly Boulevard
Los Angeles, CA 90048, USA

E-mail address:
michael.weisman@cshs.org

Preface

Systemic Lupus Erythematosus: The Next Generation of Ideas and Scientists

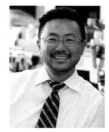 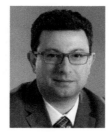

Alfred H.J. Kim, MD, PhD   Zahi Touma, MD, PhD
Editors

Systemic lupus erythematosus (SLE) remains one of the most challenging diseases to diagnose and treat. Yet, numerous recent advances have been made in the study and understanding of SLE, moving our collective understanding of SLE into a new realm. In this issue, the authors provide their expertise and reflect on these important advances.

Three themes are described in this issue: (1) a contemporaneous treatment of the clinical aspects of SLE, (2) new insights into the cellular and molecular mechanisms of SLE, and (3) an overview of the different research methodologies used to study SLE.

The first theme focuses on the clinical aspects of SLE. The authors describe advances in the classification, diagnosis, and treatment of SLE, along with an article addressing important considerations of SLE and pregnancy. The second theme explores new mechanisms that drive SLE pathophysiology, including innate immunity (interferons and neutrophils/NETosis), adaptive immunity (T and B cells), immunometabolism (mitochondrial dysfunction), and a tissue-level understanding of immune cell subsets and pathways from the Accelerating Medicines Partnerships SLE Network. The third theme dedicates several articles on the research methodologies critical to understanding SLE, including patient-reported outcomes, assembling SLE cohorts, and novel therapeutic trial designs.

It is important to highlight that most of these articles are authored from younger faculty who represent the next generation of SLE investigators. Based on the critical groundwork established by senior SLE investigators, these younger investigators

Rheum Dis Clin N Am 47 (2021) xv–xvi
https://doi.org/10.1016/j.rdc.2021.06.001
0889-857X/21/© 2021 Published by Elsevier Inc.

rheumatic.theclinics.com

have already made significant contributions to our understanding and study of SLE. Let's consider this issue to be the first opus of our new understanding of SLE.

Alfred H.J. Kim, MD, PhD
Division of Rheumatology
Department of Medicine
Washington University School of Medicine
St. Louis, MO, USA

Zahi Touma, MD, PhD
Division of Rheumatology
Department of Medicine
Toronto Western Hospital
University of Toronto
Toronto, ON, Canada

E-mail addresses:
akim@wustl.edu (A.H.J. Kim)
Zahi.Touma@uhn.ca (Z. Touma)

Interferons in Systemic Lupus Erythematosus

Sirisha Sirobhushanam, PhD[a,1], Stephanie Lazar, MD[a,1],
J. Michelle Kahlenberg, MD, PhD[b,c],*

KEYWORDS

- Interferon • Lupus • JAK • STAT

KEY POINTS

- Interferons are elevated in the blood and organs of patients with systemic lupus erythematosus (SLE).
- Genetic risk and environmental signals can drive interferon production.
- Interferons are important for disease pathogenesis in some, but maybe not all, manifestations of SLE.
- Targeting interferons and their signaling pathways is an exciting therapeutic avenue in SLE.

INTRODUCTION

The past 10 years has witnessed an acceleration in the understanding of the biology of systemic lupus erythematosus (SLE). One of the key discoveries that has prompted this work is the identification of the elevated type I interferon (IFN) signature in systemic lupus patients.[1] This review summarizes the biology of type I IFN signaling, the mechanisms of production, and the clinical impact of IFNs on disease.

DISCUSSION
Interferons, Their Subtypes, and Signaling Pathways

IFNs are important cytokines that mediate resistance to virus proliferation and thus maintain a powerful primary defense mechanism against pathogens. IFN signaling results in the coordinated expression of hundreds of genes to increase the expression of

[a] Department of Internal Medicine, Division of Rheumatology, University of Michigan, 5568 MSRB 2, 1150 West Medical Center Drive, Ann Arbor, MI 49109, USA; [b] Department of Internal Medicine, Division of Rheumatology, University of Michigan, 5570A MSRB 2, 1150 West Medical Center Drive, Ann Arbor, MI 49109, USA; [c] Department of Dermatology, University of Michigan, 5570A MSRB 2, 1150 West Medical Center Drive, Ann Arbor, MI 49109, USA
[1] Equal contribution.
* Corresponding author. Department of Internal Medicine, Division of Rheumatology, University of Michigan, 5570A MSRB 2, 1150 West Medical Center Drive, Ann Arbor, MI 49109.
E-mail address: mkahlenb@med.umich.edu
Twitter: @Kahlenberglab (J.M.K.)

Rheum Dis Clin N Am 47 (2021) 297–315
https://doi.org/10.1016/j.rdc.2021.04.001
0889-857X/21/© 2021 Elsevier Inc. All rights reserved.

major histocompatibility complex, cytokines, and chemokines to recruit immune cells, increase antigen presentation, and thus coordinate immune response.[2] Three subtypes of IFNs are known: the type I IFN family, comprising 13 subtypes of IFNα, IFNβ, IFNω, IFNκ, and IFNε; type II IFN, of which IFNγ is the only member; and type III IFNs, initially referred to as IFN-like cytokines, that include IFNλ1 (interleukin-29 [IL-29]), IFNλ2 (IL28A), IFNλ3 (IL28B), and IqFNλ4 (not expressed in all humans).[2–4]

Type I Interferons

Type I IFNs exhibit a conserved structure with 6 α-helices like other members of the class II cytokine family (interleukins: IL-10, IL-19, IL-20, IL-22, IL-24, and IL-26) and can potentially be produced by every cell type in the body.[5] Baseline expression of IFNβ and IFNκ maintains a basal activation via expression of STAT1 and IRF9 that permits rapid signal amplification when additional IFNs are detected.[6–8] Activation of pathogen recognition receptors (PRRs), such as toll-like receptors (TLRs; plasma membrane and endosomal), or cytoplasmic sensors, such as retinoic acid–inducible gene I (RIG-I) and melanoma differentiation associated protein 5 (MDA5), by pathogen and danger-associated molecular patterns, including nucleic acids (viral DNA or RNA or endogenous nucleic acids exposed because of damage) and bacterial macromolecules (lipopolysaccharides, peptidoglycan and flagellin), induce high IFN production.[9] This IFN activation is followed by a feed-forward IRF7-driven loop that accelerates IFN production in cells like plasmacytoid dendritic cells (pDCs) that are significant sources of type I IFNs.[10–15]

All type I IFNs signal through the heterodimeric IFNα receptor (IFNAR) 1 and 2 complex, which triggers Janus kinase 1 (JAK1) and Tyrosine kinase 2 (TYK2) activation and subsequent phosphorylation of signal transducers and activators of transcription (STAT) 1 and 2 (**Fig. 1**). STAT1 and STAT2 bind IFN-regulatory factor 9 (IRF-9) to form ISGF3, which translocates into the nucleus. ISGF3 binds to IFN-sensitive response elements (ISREs) containing the consensus sequence TTTCNNTTTC and induces the coordinated transcription of IFN-stimulated genes (ISGs), such as Mx1 and OAS.[9,16,17]

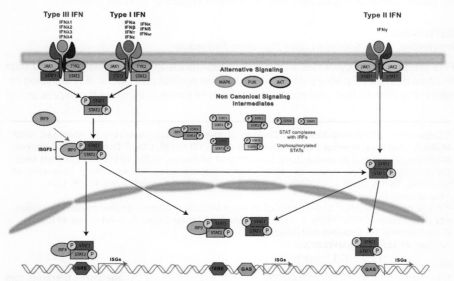

Fig. 1. IFN signaling pathways for type I, type II, and type III IFNs.

Type II Interferons

IFNγ, initially called macrophage activating factor, is mainly produced by immune cells, including natural killer (NK) cells, innate lymphoid cells, and cells of the adaptive immune system, namely T helper 1 cells and CD8+ cytotoxic T lymphocytes.[3] IFNγ is induced by PRR activation as well as certain cytokines (IL-12 and IL-18). IFNγ signals through the ubiquitous heterodimeric IFNγ receptor (IFNGR1 and 2) activating JAK1/JAK2 kinases followed by STAT1 phosphorylation and dimerization (see **Fig. 1**). STAT1 dimers bind to IFNγ activation sites (GAS) with the consensus sequence TTCNNNGGA and induce transcription of ISGs, affecting antiviral and antibacterial responses.[3,17,18]

Type III Interferons

Type III IFNs (IFNλs) are produced by pDCs, epithelial cells, and myeloid cells after PRR activation and cytosolic nucleic acid sensing.[3,19–21] The IFNλ receptor complex is composed of IFNλ-receptor 1 (IFNLR1) and IL-10R2 subunits. Although structurally different from type I IFNs, functionally, IFNλs are similar to type I IFNs and result in JAK1/TYK2- STAT1-STAT2 activation and transcription of ISGs (see **Fig. 1**). IFNλs can also be induced by type I IFNs potentially demonstrating the involvement of different IFNs at different stages of infection.[5,22,23] Interestingly, IFNLR1 is restricted to NK cells, pDCs, dendritic cells (DCs), and mucosal epithelial cells, suggesting a significant role in mucosal regulation. IFNLR is also highly expressed in macrophages, resulting in IFNλ-mediated functional enhancement while also promoting their secretion of chemokines and cytokines for NK cell function (cytotoxicity) and IFNγ production.[24]

Noncanonical Signaling by Interferons

Type I and II signaling pathways overlap significantly, and characteristic signatures are hard to differentiate.[2,3,25] ISREs as well as GAS sequences in the same genes allow for activation by type I and type II IFNs. In addition to the STAT1-STAT2 heterodimer that forms ISGF3, type I IFNs can induce STAT1 and STAT3 homodimers and heterodimers and STAT4, STAT5, and STAT6 activation in other cell types.[26] The activation of noncanonical STATs can lead to different transcriptional outcomes.[18,26] Type I IFN signaling can also occur through Rap1, Map kinases, and PI3- kinase pathways[27–30] (see **Fig. 1**).

Suppression of Interferons

IFN activation also induces signal regulatory genes, including suppressor of cytokine signaling, that compete with STATs, and ubiquitin carboxy-terminal hydrolase 18, that helps dissociate JAK1 from IFNAR2, thus reducing downstream signaling. Self-regulation by IFNs also occurs through activation of STAT3 homodimers that lead to anti-inflammatory responses.[2] Other IFN suppression mechanisms are internalization of the receptor complex, regulation by microRNAs (miR146a and miR155), and deactivation of the signaling intermediates by means of proteins, such as SH2 domain-containing protein tyrosine phosphatase 2.[18]

Sex Bias in Interferon Production and Activity

Sex bias is predominant in SLE with a significant skew toward women.[31] Loss of X-chromosome inactivation (XCI) of TLR7 and IRAK1 and estrogen-modulated increase in TLR8 are linked to elevated IFN production.[32–34] XCI is implicated in higher expression of CXorf21, which colocalizes with TLR7 in B cells, is linked to lower lysosomal pH, and is induced by IFNs.[35,36] In addition, increase in the transcription factor Vestigial like 3 in women results in altered IFN response gene expression, including

B-cell activating factor, IFNκ and CXCL13, all genes important in the pathogenesis of cutaneous and systemic lupus.[37]

Activation of Interferon Pathways in Systemic Lupus Erythematosus

IFNs are produced downstream of many sensors, which respond to pathogens, thus affecting immune response. Indeed, genetic polymorphisms in members of these response pathways are genetic risks for SLE.

Toll-like receptors

The lysosomal-localized TLR family is an important source of IFN production in SLE patients. Beyond response to bacteria and viruses, endogenous nucleic acids resulting from environmental insult or uptake of immune complexes containing nucleic acids trigger the production of IFNs. TLR7 (binds single-stranded RNA) and TLR9 (binds double-stranded DNA [dsDNA]) expression in B cells is critical for spontaneous germinal center development, contributing to autoantibody production. Increased expression of TLR7, secondary to genetic polymorphisms or escape of XCI, can lead to dose-dependent development of SLE in humans and mice.[32–34] Conventional DCs from lupus-prone mice show higher IL-10 and IL-27 (elevated in SLE patients) production upon TLR stimulation, and this is enhanced by IFN priming.[38] Hypersensitivity to TLR7 activation and low TRAF5 contribute to autoreactive naïve B-cell differentiation into plasma cells and establishes extrafollicular B-cell activation in SLE.[39] TLR7/8 activation also induces early IFNβ production followed by IFNα at later time points; in granulocytes, TLR8 but not TLR7 activates IFN production.[40]

Cytosolic sensors

Polymorphisms in genes associated with cytosolic nucleic acid detection, breakdown, and repair mechanisms, and IFN pathway (SAMHD1, RNASEH2ABC, ADAR1, IFIH1 [MDA5], ISG15, ACP5, TMEM173 stimulator of IFN genes [STING])[41] also confer risk for SLE. These risk variants contribute to intracellular nucleic acid accumulation and activation of cytosolic sensors leading to high IFN production.[42–46] The cyclic-GMP-AMP synthase (cGAS) and the cyclic-GMP-AMP receptor STING axis detects cytosolic microbial/self-nucleic acids to induce type I IFNs.[47] Higher expression of cGAS in peripheral blood mononuclear cells correlated with disease activity in SLE.[48] Genome instability owing to RNAseH2 (removes ribonucleotides incorporated into DNA) deficiency can also lead to an autoimmune phenotype by recruitment of cGAS.[49] Pores formed by voltage-dependent anion channel allow short DNA fragments from stressed mitochondria (reactive oxygen species [ROS] production) into the cytosol activating robust IFN production via cytosolic sensors, such as STING.[2,50,51] Cytosolic viral RNA sensors, such as RIG-I and MDA5 (encoded by *IFIH1*), that then recruit mitochondrial antiviral-signaling protein (MAVS) also drive IFN production. *IFIH1* mutations and MDA5 hyperactivation result in increased type I IFN production and possible SLE.[52–54] Mice harboring a gain-of-function mutation in IFIH1 developed lupus nephritis (LN) and dsDNA autoantibodies supporting a role for increased sensitivity to RNA complexes.[55,56]

Oxidation of nucleic acids may further promote IFN production. ROS induce MAVS aggregation,[57,58] and reducing mitochondrial ROS via oral mitochondrial antioxidants decreased MAVS oligomer formation and type I IFN levels in serum of MRL-lpr mice.[59] Inhibition of oxidized DNA repair results in higher autoantibody production (anti-dsDNA and anti-ribonuclear protein), increased total immunoglobulin G (IgG), and ISG expression in a pristane-induced lupus mouse model.[60] Furthermore, amplification of cytosolic nucleic acid signaling occurs through type I IFN-mediated inhibition of autophagy-related DNA degradation, thus increasing substrates for pathway activation.[61]

Role of Interferons in the Pathogenesis of Systemic Lupus Erythematosus

SLE is a complex, multiorgan system disease most commonly presenting with constitutional symptoms, oral ulcers, rash, and arthritis. Systemic organ involvement can be severe and includes LN, including glomerulonephritis, central and peripheral nervous system involvement, cardiac and lung manifestations, and autoimmune hepatitis, among others. Autoantibodies and deposition of immune complexes have been implicated in the pathogenesis of these disease manifestations; however, this alone is not sufficient to generate disease: T cells are now understood to also play a critical role. In addition, before development of autoantibodies, the innate immune system is abnormal and may be a precursor to adaptive immune system changes. Most notably, sustained high levels of IFN function as a central pathogenic mediator in early immune dysregulation bridging the link between innate and adaptive immunopathogenesis in a feed-forward mechanism.

Interferon-α Can Induce Systemic Lupus Erythematosus

The first suggestion that IFN may drive SLE pathogenesis was reported in 1969 after administration of IFN to genetically susceptible lupus-prone mice resulted in increased autoantibodies and end-organ damage.[62] These data points have been corroborated in human observational studies of patients undergoing recombinant IFNα treatment of viral, autoimmune, and malignant diseases.[63] A subset of susceptible individuals treated with IFNα have subsequently developed autoantibodies, a "lupus-like" syndrome, or infrequently, clinical lupus after treatment.[64]

In those treated for hepatitis C virus with interferons, patients with preexisting antinuclear antibody (ANA) positivity were found to have an increase in titer with IFNα exposure.[65] Further reports show patients treated for pancreatic or carcinoid tumors with IFNα resulted in development of dsDNA antibodies.[66] The SLE-like syndrome of patients undergoing IFN treatment includes myalgia, arthritis, oral ulcer, malar rash, lymphopenia, serositis, lymphadenopathy, fever, and renal disease, and these effects resolve when IFN treatment is discontinued.[67–69]

Murine models have also provided evidence that type I IFN exposure can drive SLE. Upregulation of IFNα in inducible IFNα transgenic mice not prone to autoimmunity is sufficient to produce lupus-like findings, including serum immune complexes, anti-dsDNA antibodies, immune-complex glomerulonephritis, alopecia, splenic-onion skin lesions, epidermal liquefaction, and a positive lupus band test of skin.[70] Treatment of mice with adenovirus that drives IFN expression also induces inflammatory cytokine upregulation and can promote renal immune complex deposition in non-lupus-prone mice.[71] Furthermore, IFNα adenovirus can drive increased autoantibody formation and refractoriness to treatment of LN in lupus-prone NZB/NZW$_{F1}$ mice.[72]

Heritable Risk Factors for Systemic Lupus Erythematosus Involve Interferon Pathways

SLE is a complex, heritable, polygenic disease likely resulting from alterations at several genetic loci linked to immune function.[43] Among families, high serum IFNα activity has been observed in both patients with SLE and healthy first-degree relatives independent of autoantibody profiles.[73] Genome-wide association studies have identified more than 40 loci linked to SLE susceptibility with a notable disproportionate number of IFN pathway-related genes, which function to regulate IFN production, signaling, function, and downstream effects.[74]

Many IFN pathway genes are under investigation, and several have been implicated in development of disease. *IRF5, IRF7, IRF8,* members of the IFN regulatory factor family, are transcription factors that regulate IFN-related pathways, and variants have been associated with risk to development of SLE.[75–77] Indeed, IRF5, an important mediator of IFN production induced by the TLR-MyD88 axis, is critical in murine lupus pathogenesis, and IRF5 genetic polymorphisms lead to higher IFN production in lupus patients.[43,50,78,79] Furthermore, nuclear localization (activation) is noted in SLE patient monocytes, and preclinical treatment with an IRF5 inhibitor improves murine lupus.[80] Impaired TRIM21-mediated proteasomal degradation of IRFs in SLE also contributes to amplified IFN responses, highlighting the impact of defective IFN regulatory mechanisms in SLE risk.[81]

Genetic polymorphisms in components of the IFN signaling pathway also confer risk for SLE. *STAT4* functions in cytokine signaling and participates in nonclassical IFN signaling; variants have been associated with dsDNA antibodies, younger age at disease onset, and history of nephritis.[74] Loss of STAT4 is associated with lower levels of IFNγ, higher mortality, and nephritis in lupus-prone mouse models.[82] Loss-of-function mutations in *STAT3* in patients result in higher ISG expression and higher neutrophil extracellular trap formation, supporting its negative regulatory function in SLE.[83] *TYK2* is a member of the JAK family of signaling molecules associated with the type I IFN receptor and is involved in cytokine signaling cascades; alterations at *TYK2* loci have been associated with SLE.[74]

Interestingly, SLE clinical manifestations and pathogenesis show differences based on ancestral background, and the genetics of IFN-related pathways may be a key factor.[84] IFNα production is higher in individuals from non-European ancestry.[73] Ko and colleagues[85] showed that IFN-pathway activation was dependent on circulating anti-RNA binding protein antibodies in African American patients but not in patients of European ancestry. Genetic differences in IFN pathway activation may prove important in order to determine likelihood of response for therapeutics targeting type I IFNs and their receptor.

Interferons Increase Before Onset of Disease

Both type I and type II IFNs, as well as specific autoantibodies (ANA, anti-dsDNA, anti-Ro, anti-La, anti-RNP, anti-smith), are found in SLE patients months to years before any disease manifestations[86,87] and likely form a key feedback loop that drives innate and adaptive immune system pathologic condition. Autoantibody positivity appears to follow or coincide with type II IFN dysregulation, whereas IFNα activity and elevation of B-lymphocyte stimulator (BLyS) occur more proximal to SLE classification.[86] Regression analysis of IFN levels in 248 patients by Oke and colleagues[88] shows that high IFN activity is associated with active SLE (active LN, high Systemic Lupus Erythematous Disease Activity Index [SLEDAI], anti-Sm, anti-dsDNA). When different IFN subtypes were evaluated, high IFNα was associated with mucocutaneous lupus (anti-Ro and anti-La), whereas IFNγ correlated with high SLEDAI scores and LN, and high IFNλ1 associated with antinucleosome antibodies and higher frequency of antiphospholipid antibodies. Only patients exhibiting both ANAs and an IFN signature progress to clinical SLE diagnosis and can help predict advancement to end-stage renal disease.[50,89]

Even before type I IFN elevation and autoantibody detection, an earlier perturbation in the immune system is elevation of type II IFN (IFNγ), found greater than 4 years before disease onset.[86] IFNγ is expressed by many cells of both the innate and the adaptive immune system, including NK cells, NK T cells, T cells, and B cells, and like other IFNs, signals via JAK-STAT pathway (see **Fig. 1**).[90]

IFNγ and IFNγ-related gene activity correlates with SLEDAI score and dsDNA antibody levels, further suggesting a key role in pathologic autoantibody production.[91] Furthermore, close interaction between type I and type II IFN has been demonstrated with IFNγ induction of type I IFN during viral infection[92] and a role for synergistic amplification of ISG expression with coexposure of IFNγ and IFNα.[93]

Patients with evidence of autoimmunity but without full criteria for diagnosis can be used to evaluate "early" changes related to IFNs. Patients with clinical incomplete lupus (ILE) who demonstrate features of SLE but do not meet classification criteria for the diagnosis, a subset of whom will progress to SLE, demonstrate elevated circulating type I IFN gene signatures that correlate with disease burden.[94] A subset of patients with positive ANA without clinical criteria for systemic autoimmune disease will show elevated IFNα levels and gene expression, correlating with specific autoantibody profiles, including anti-Ro and anti-La.[95,96] More recently, this increased IFN signature has also been demonstrated in the skin of ANA-positive patients without SLE.[97] In addition, IFN gene expression is correlated with markers of inflammation and disease activity, such as erythrocyte sedimentation rate and IgG levels, and negatively correlated with C4 levels and IgM levels, further demonstrating its role in immunoglobulin class switching and disease activity.[94,98] Ongoing trials are evaluating whether intervention via use of hydroxychloroquine, which can lower IFN signatures in ILE,[99] can prevent development of SLE.

Roles of Type I Interferons in Organ-Specific Inflammation

Beyond a global risk for SLE, research has identified specific effects of IFNs that contribute to specific organ involvement (summarized in **Fig. 2**).

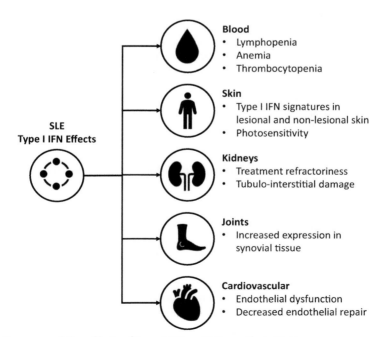

Fig. 2. Summary of the effects of type I IFN on SLE manifestations.

Blood and blood cells

Circulating type I IFN levels, as measured by response assays, have been shown to correlate with SLE disease activity.[100–102] Newer technologies have confirmed elevated circulating IFNα protein levels in SLE patients, ranging from 10 fg/mL to 10 pg/mL. Furthermore, type I IFN activity is functional in SLE serum, as serum from SLE patients can induce monocytes to differentiate into DCs via IFNα[103] and promotes endothelial dysfunction.[104]

IFN-pathway overactivation is closely tied to B-cell dysregulation, another salient feature in SLE pathogenesis. New-onset SLE-patient transitional B cells (Btr) have higher IL-6–producing capacity and increased survival via type I IFN signaling.[105] Btr cells have been identified previously as a source of IL-10 regulatory B cells; however, this is disrupted in SLE patients, and chronic stimulation by type I IFN has been a proposed mechanism.[106] Single-cell RNA-sequencing has also identified subsets of many circulating inflammatory cell populations that have been exposed to type I IFNs and consequently express increased inflammatory markers and correlate with disease activity measures in pediatric and adult lupus.[107]

In addition, there may be direct effects of type I IFNs on the bone marrow. IFNα administration suppresses bone marrow production resulting in leukopenia, anemia, and thrombocytopenia.[108] The contribution of type I IFNs to lymphopenia in SLE patients is further supported by phase 3 clinical trial data with anifrolumab, a monoclonal antibody to type I IFN receptor, which improves lymphocytopenia with blockade of type I IFN receptor.[109]

Skin

The pathogenesis of cutaneous lupus erythematous (CLE) is incompletely understood, but IFN-driven, cytotoxic inflammation likely plays a key role. Upregulation of type I IFN signatures is a hallmark of lesional SLE and CLE skin.[110] Myeloid cells, including pDCs, are recruited to CLE skin, which likely contributes to the IFN signature. In addition, epidermal production of IFNκ, a member of the type I IFN family, is increased in lesional and non-lesional SLE skin and contributes to inflammatory cytokine production and photosensitivity.[7,97,111,112] In addition, patients with subacute cutaneous lupus and discoid lupus demonstrate an increased IFN signature in blood that correlates with skin disease activity, suggesting IFN production in the skin may contribute to amplification of systemic disease.[113]

Further demonstrating the importance of IFN in the pathogenesis of CLE in vivo, skin disease improves with blockade of type I IFN and also with targeting of pDCs. Indeed phase 3 clinical trial data from anifrolumab, where cutaneous lupus erythematosus disease area and severity index (CLASI) activity score of greater than 10 at baseline improved more than 50% with treatment.[109] pDC-targeted therapies have shown success in early phase trials.[114]

Renal

Mouse and human studies have established a role for IFNs in the pathophysiology of LN. Murine models have shown that deficiency of the type I IFN receptor is protective in some models of nephritis and that systemically administered IFNα renders mice resistant to therapeutic intervention.[72,115] Renal tubular epithelial cells and infiltrating pDCs in kidney of patients with LN demonstrate a type I IFN signature, which is associated with local production of IFNα by the proximal tubular cells, suggesting an autocrine effect leading to tubulo-interstitial damage.[116] Indeed, tubular IFN signatures may also have prognostic implications.[117] Circulating IFNs may also be involved in pathogenesis as the IFN signature in infiltrating leukocytes in the kidney correlate with IFN signature in blood.[118] Furthermore, murine models and in vitro studies have shown systemic IFNα and IFNβ increase glomerular inflammation and proteinuria and decrease differentiation of renal progenitor cells to podocytes, promoting scar formation.[119]

The role for IFNγ is less studied but may also contribute to LN. Deficiency of IFNγ or blockade of its receptor prevents disease development.[120] IFNγ-positive cells are a prominent feature of kidney-infiltrating immune cells in LN and correlate with predominance of CD8$^+$ T-cell infiltrates on biopsy, suggesting this cell population as the source for IFNγ and a role in pathogenesis of LN.[121] Human monoclonal antibodies to IFNγ, AMG 811, were tested in a phase 1b randomizedcontrolled trial in patients with LN; however, no effect in SELENA-SLEDAI, proteinuria, C3, C4, or anti-dsDNA was noted.[122] It is hoped that further research will determine whether the presence of renal IFNγ is pathologic or a result of inflammation itself.

Joints

Synovial tissue of SLE patients with arthritis has shown downregulation of genes involved in extracellular matrix homeostasis and increased expression of type I IFNs, distinctly different from rheumatoid arthritis and osteoarthritis.[123] Recent analysis suggests that IFNγ signatures may more strongly correlate with lupus arthritis versus other manifestations, such as the skin, which is dominated by a type I IFN signature.[88] Further research into the role of IFNs in lupus arthritis is needed.

Cardiovascular Disease

Cardiovascular risk is elevated in SLE patients. IFNs have been shown to impact endothelial cell function and overall cardiovascular risk in SLE patients,[124] and this has been extensively reviewed.[125] The presence of increased neutrophil NETosis and the IFNs produced by low-density granulocytes likely contribute as well.[126] Indeed, recent data from systemic blockade of type I IFN signaling have shown improvement in markers of cardiovascular risk,[127] suggesting that IFN blockade may have positive impacts on cardiovascular function and risk for ischemic events.

Clinical Applications

Targeting the type I interferon receptor

Anifrolumab is a monoclonal antibody against subunit 1 of the type I IFN receptor, which antagonizes effects of all type I IFNs, including IFNα, IFNβ, IFNω, AND IFNκ.[128] A phase 2b randomized controlled trial (MUSE trial) showed a higher percentage of subjects in the anifrolumab treatment group met the primary endpoint of SLE responder index (SRI-4) compared with placebo with sustained reduction in corticosteroid use at week 24. The treatment arm also showed improvement in SRI-4, modified SRI-6, BICLA, BILAG-2004 at week 52, as well as improvement in CLASI score and tender and swollen joint counts.[129]

Given the success of the MUSE trial, 2 phase 3 randomized controlled clinical trials, TULIP-1 and TULIP-2, were performed to evaluate the efficacy and safety of anifrolumab in moderate to severe SLE patients receiving standard-of-care therapy. TULIP-1 was a multicenter, multinational, double-blind, parallel-group trial with subjects stratified by disease activity and IFN-signature (high vs low). The study failed to meet its primary endpoint with percentage of subjects achieving SRI-4 response at week 52 similar in both treatment and placebo groups. Given the discrepancy in results from the MUSE trial, a reanalysis was performed. Patients who used nonsteroidal anti-inflammatory drugs s during the trial and initially classified as nonresponders were reclassified. After this alteration, improvement in CLASI score, decrease in tender and swollen joint count, and a higher percentage of patients achieving BICLA response were noted in the anifrolumab group at week 52, although the primary end point was still not met.[130]

With improvement in the BICLA response but not SRI-4 in TULIP-1, TULIP-2 sought to evaluate efficacy of anifrolumab in moderate to severe SLE patients with the primary endpoint of BICLA response. Similarly, TULIP-2 was a multicenter, multinational, double-blind, parallel-group trial with subjects stratified by disease activity and IFN signature (high vs low). The primary end point was met with improved BICLA response in the treatment group compared with placebo at week 52. In addition, anifrolumab treatment arm showed reduced corticosteroid use, improved CLASI score, and higher percentage of patients with improved swollen and tender joint count.[109] Long-term extension and LN trials are ongoing with anifrolumab.

Anti-interferon antibodies

Two monoclonal antibodies targeting specifically IFNα, sifalimumab and rontalizumab, have been studied in phase 2 clinical trials. Sifalimumab met its primary endpoint with a higher percentage of patients achieving SRI-4 in the treatment group. Patients also showed improvement in the CLASI score, Physician's Global Assessment, BILAG, and reduction in tender and swollen joint counts with administration of sifalimumab.[131] Rontalizumab failed to meet its primary endpoint of reduction in BILAG-2004 or secondary endpoint of reduction in SRI; it is no longer being developed.[132] Subgroup analysis from this phase 2 trial showed patients with low IFN signature had higher SRI response, lower steroid use, and reduction in the SELENA-SLEDAI flare index with rontalizumab treatment.[132] Phase 3 studies of anifrolumab were pursued over sifalimumab, as it targets a broader range of type I IFN and more subunits of IFNα, possibly making it more efficacious.

Recent results of a phase 1, randomized, double-blinded, placebo-controlled trial of JNJ-55920839, a monoclonal antibody that neutralizes most IFNα subunits and IFNω, showed it is safe and well tolerated in healthy participants and those with mild to moderate SLE and elevated type I IFN signature.[133]

Of note, all of the above treatments, including anifrolumab, sifalimumab, rontalizumab, and JNJ-55920839, showed elevated rates of herpes zoster (HZV) infections in the treatment group compared with placebo.[109,129,131-133] Mitigation strategies on how to prevent HZV or other viral infections with IFN-targeting therapies, such as vaccination, should be considered and further studied.

Janus kinase inhibitors/tyrosine kinase 2 blockade

The JAK-STAT pathway mediates intracellular signaling from a variety of type I/II cytokine receptors, including type I IFN, IFNγ, IL-6, and IL-2.[134] This pathway has been implicated in SLE pathogenesis through IFN regulatory factor-related gene expression.[135] Several JAK-inhibitor small molecules are currently under development for treatment of a variety of autoimmune diseases, including SLE. Murine models have shown modulation of this pathway with JAK inhibition leads to decreased anti-dsDNA antibodies, decreased proteinuria, and improved nephritis and skin disease.[136-138] Other murine models have shown lesional keratinocytes and dermal immune cells strongly express phospho-JAK1 and blockade of JAK1 decreases expression of proinflammatory mediators, including BLyS and CXCL2, as well as skin lesions.[139]

Baricitinib, a JAK1/2 inhibitor that has been approved for rheumatoid arthritis, underwent a phase 2 placebo-controlled trial for treatment of nonrenal SLE with active skin or joint disease.[140] This study found the proportion of patients achieving resolution of arthritis or rash was significantly higher in the baricitinib 4-mg daily group compared with placebo, as defined by the SLEDAI-2K (P = .04).[140] Currently, there are 2 phase 3 randomized controlled studies of baricitinib in nonrenal SLE (NCT03616912, NCT03616964). In the future, new applications for JAK inhibitors in lupus may provide an additional therapeutic treatment option for SLE, primarily skin and joint disease.

Role as a biomarker

Many IFN-regulated chemokines have demonstrated correlation with SLE disease activity, showing promise for future biomarkers. Given the importance of preventing renal damage with early diagnosis of LN, there is a search to replace invasive renal biopsy with noninvasive biomarkers. Recent interest in urine proteomics has led to the discovery that urine chemokines mirror inflammatory cell infiltrates driven primarily by IFNγ.[121] Three IFN-inducible chemokines, CXCL10 (IP-10), CCL2 (MCP-1), and CCL19 (MIP-3B), have shown correlation with SLE disease activity, and CXCL10 is consistently the strongest predictor.[141,142] A recent meta-analysis showed serum CXCL10 levels correlated with SLE disease activity, and urine CXCL10 level detected active LN.[143]

SUMMARY

IFN signaling, particularly for type I IFNs, is elevated in SLE patients and contributes to many aspects of disease. Murine models have shown the benefits of IFN blockade, and now tools to block IFN function in patients are becoming available to simultaneously treat disease manifestations and to further understand the biology of IFNs in SLE.

CLINICS CARE POINTS

- Type I and type II interferons are elevated many years before disease onset; this offers opportunity for prevention.
- Type I interferons contribute to many aspects of systemic lupus erythematosus, including bone marrow suppression, skin disease, arthritis, lupus nephritis, and cardiovascular disease.
- A wide range of drugs are being explored to block interferon signaling and will offer new tools for mechanistic understanding and treatment of systemic lupus erythematosus.

DISCLOSURE

Dr J.M. Kahlenberg has participated in consulting and advisory boards for AstraZeneca, Admirex Pharmaceuticals, Aurinia Pharmaceuticals, Boehringer Ingelheim, Bristol Meyers Squibb, Eli Lilly, Provention Bio, and Ventus Therapeutics. Dr J.M. Kahlenberg receives grant funding from Q32 Bio and Bristol Myers Squibb. S. Sirobhushanam is supported by a postdoctoral translational science program grant from the Michigan Institute for Clinical and Health Services Research under NIH grant UL1TR002240. S. Lazar has received partial support for her training from the U.S. Veterans Administration. Dr J.M. Kahlenberg is supported by the National Institute of Arthritis and Musculoskeletal and Skin Diseases of the National Institutes of Health under awards R01-AR071384, K24-AR076975, and P30-AR075043, the Lupus Research Alliance, the Doris Duke Charitable Foundation under a physician scientist development award, and the A. Alfred Taubman Medical Research Institute and the Parfet Emerging Scholar Award.

REFERENCES

1. Crow MK, Wohlgemuth J. Microarray analysis of gene expression in lupus. Arthritis Res Ther 2003;5(6):279–87.
2. Barrat FJ, Crow MK, Ivashkiv LB. Interferon target-gene expression and epigenomic signatures in health and disease. Nat Immunol 2019;20(12):1574–83.
3. Ivashkiv LB. IFNgamma: signalling, epigenetics and roles in immunity, metabolism, disease and cancer immunotherapy. Nat Rev Immunol 2018;18(9): 545–58.
4. Lee S, Baldridge MT. Interferon-lambda: a potent regulator of intestinal viral infections. Front Immunol 2017;8:749.
5. Chyuan IT, Tzeng HT, Chen JY. Signaling pathways of type I and type III interferons and targeted therapies in systemic lupus erythematosus. Cells 2019; 8(9):963.
6. Gough DJ, Messina NL, Clarke CJ, et al. Constitutive type I interferon modulates homeostatic balance through tonic signaling. Immunity 2012;36(2):166–74.
7. Sarkar MK, Hile GA, Tsoi LC, et al. Photosensitivity and type I IFN responses in cutaneous lupus are driven by epidermal-derived interferon kappa. Ann Rheum Dis 2018;77(11):1653–64.
8. Schneider WM, Chevillotte MD, Rice CM. Interferon-stimulated genes: a complex web of host defenses. Annu Rev Immunol 2014;32:513–45.
9. Ivashkiv LB, Donlin LT. Regulation of type I interferon responses. Nat Rev Immunol 2014;14(1):36–49.
10. Honda K, Takaoka A, Taniguchi T. Type I interferon [corrected] gene induction by the interferon regulatory factor family of transcription factors. Immunity 2006;25(3):349–60.
11. Liu YJ. IPC: professional type 1 interferon-producing cells and plasmacytoid dendritic cell precursors. Annu Rev Immunol 2005;23:275–306.
12. Ning S, Pagano JS, Barber GN. IRF7: activation, regulation, modification and function. Genes Immun 2011;12(6):399–414.
13. Petro TM. IFN regulatory factor 3 in health and disease. J Immunol 2020;205(8): 1981–9.
14. Siegal FP, Kadowaki N, Shodell M, et al. The nature of the principal type 1 interferon-producing cells in human blood-annotated. Science 1999; 284(5421):1835–7.
15. Tamura T, Yanai H, Savitsky D, et al. The IRF family transcription factors in immunity and oncogenesis. Annu Rev Immunol 2008;26:535–84.
16. Schoggins JW. Interferon-stimulated genes: what do they all do? Annu Rev Virol 2019;6(1):567–84.
17. Stark GR, Darnell JE Jr. The JAK-STAT pathway at twenty. Immunity 2012;36(4): 503–14.
18. Ivashkiv LB. Cross-regulation of signaling by ITAM-associated receptors. Nat Immunol 2009;10(4):340–7.
19. Jewell NA, Cline T, Mertz SE, et al. Lambda interferon is the predominant interferon induced by influenza A virus infection in vivo. J Virol 2010;84(21): 11515–22.
20. Pott J, Mahlakoiv T, Mordstein M, et al. IFN-lambda determines the intestinal epithelial antiviral host defense. Proc Natl Acad Sci U S A 2011;108(19):7944–9.
21. Pandey S, Kawai T, Akira S. Microbial sensing by toll-like receptors and intracellular nucleic acid sensors. Cold Spring Harb Perspect Biol 2014;7(1):a016246.

22. Ank N, West H, Bartholdy C, et al. Lambda interferon (IFN-lambda), a type III IFN, is induced by viruses and IFNs and displays potent antiviral activity against select virus infections in vivo. J Virol 2006;80(9):4501–9.

23. Sui H, Zhou M, Imamichi H, et al. STING is an essential mediator of the Ku70-mediated production of IFN-lambda1 in response to exogenous DNA. Sci Signal 2017;10(488):1–11.

24. Read SA, Wijaya R, Ramezani-Moghadam M, et al. Macrophage coordination of the interferon lambda immune response. Front Immunol 2019;10:2674.

25. Banchereau R, Cepika AM, Banchereau J, et al. Understanding human autoimmunity and autoinflammation through transcriptomics. Annu Rev Immunol 2017; 35:337–70.

26. van Boxel-Dezaire AH, Rani MR, Stark GR. Complex modulation of cell type-specific signaling in response to type I interferons. Immunity 2006;25(3):361–72.

27. Lee AJ, Ashkar AA. The dual nature of type I and type II interferons. Front Immunol 2018;9:2061.

28. Uddin S, Lekmine F, Sharma N, et al. The Rac1/p38 mitogen-activated protein kinase pathway is required for interferon alpha-dependent transcriptional activation but not serine phosphorylation of Stat proteins. J Biol Chem 2000; 275(36):27634–40.

29. Uddin S, Majchrzak B, Woodson J, et al. Activation of the p38 mitogen-activated protein kinase by type I interferons. J Biol Chem 1999;274(42):30127–31.

30. Uddin S, Yenush L, Sun XJ, et al. Interferon-alpha engages the insulin receptor substrate-1 to associate with the phosphatidylinositol 3'-kinase. J Biol Chem 1995;270(27):15938–41.

31. Billi AC, Kahlenberg JM, Gudjonsson JE. Sex bias in autoimmunity. Curr Opin Rheumatol 2019;31(1):53–61.

32. Lyn-Cook BD, Xie C, Oates J, et al. Increased expression of Toll-like receptors (TLRs) 7 and 9 and other cytokines in systemic lupus erythematosus (SLE) patients: ethnic differences and potential new targets for therapeutic drugs. Mol Immunol 2014;61(1):38–43.

33. Souyris M, Cenac C, Azar P, et al. TLR7 escapes X chromosome inactivation in immune cells. Sci Immunol 2018;3(19):eaap8855.

34. Wang T, Marken J, Chen J, et al. High TLR7 expression drives the expansion of CD19(+)CD24(hi)CD38(hi) transitional B cells and autoantibody production in SLE Patients. Front Immunol 2019;10:1243.

35. Harris VM, Harley ITW, Kurien BT, et al. Lysosomal pH is regulated in a sex dependent manner in immune cells expressing CXorf21. Front Immunol 2019; 10:578.

36. Odhams CA, Roberts AL, Vester SK, et al. Interferon inducible X-linked gene CXorf21 may contribute to sexual dimorphism in systemic lupus erythematosus. Nat Commun 2019;10(1):2164.

37. Billi AC, Gharaee-Kermani M, Fullmer J, et al. The female-biased factor VGLL3 drives cutaneous and systemic autoimmunity. JCI Insight 2019;4(8):e127291.

38. Lee MH, Gallo PM, Hooper KM, et al. The cytokine network type I IFN-IL-27-IL-10 is augmented in murine and human lupus. J Leukoc Biol 2019;106(4): 967–75.

39. Jenks SA, Cashman KS, Zumaquero E, et al. Distinct effector B cells induced by unregulated toll-like receptor 7 contribute to pathogenic responses in systemic lupus erythematosus. Immunity 2018;49(4):725–739 e726.

40. Bender AT, Tzvetkov E, Pereira A, et al. TLR7 and TLR8 differentially activate the IRF and NF-kappaB pathways in specific cell types to promote inflammation. Immunohorizons 2020;4(2):93–107.

41. Costa-Reis P, Sullivan KE. Monogenic lupus: it's all new! Curr Opin Immunol 2017;49:87–95.

42. Almlof JC, Nystedt S, Leonard D, et al. Whole-genome sequencing identifies complex contributions to genetic risk by variants in genes causing monogenic systemic lupus erythematosus. Hum Genet 2019;138(2):141–50.

43. Langefeld CD, Ainsworth HC, Cunninghame Graham DS, et al. Transancestral mapping and genetic load in systemic lupus erythematosus. Nat Commun 2017;8:16021.

44. Liu W, Li M, Wang Z, et al. IFN-gamma mediates the development of systemic lupus erythematosus. Biomed Res Int 2020;2020:7176515.

45. Tsokos GC, Lo MS, Costa Reis P, et al. New insights into the immunopathogenesis of systemic lupus erythematosus. Nat Rev Rheumatol 2016;12(12):716–30.

46. Yin Q, Wu LC, Zheng L, et al. Comprehensive assessment of the association between genes on JAK-STAT pathway (IFIH1, TYK2, IL-10) and systemic lupus erythematosus: a meta-analysis. Arch Dermatol Res 2018;310(9):711–28.

47. Hopfner KP, Hornung V. Molecular mechanisms and cellular functions of cGAS-STING signalling. Nat Rev Mol Cell Biol 2020;21(9):501–21.

48. An J, Durcan L, Karr RM, et al. Expression of cyclic GMP-AMP synthase in patients with systemic lupus erythematosus. Arthritis Rheum 2017;69(4):800–7.

49. Li T, Chen ZJ. The cGAS-cGAMP-STING pathway connects DNA damage to inflammation, senescence, and cancer. J Exp Med 2018;215(5):1287–99.

50. Crow MK, Olferiev M, Kirou KA. Type I interferons in autoimmune disease. Annu Rev Pathol 2019;14:369–93.

51. Crow MK. Mitochondrial DNA promotes autoimmunity. Science 2019;366(6472):1445–6.

52. Buers I, Nitschke Y, Rutsch F. Novel interferonopathies associated with mutations in RIG-I like receptors. Cytokine Growth Factor Rev 2016;29:101–7.

53. Cunninghame Graham DS, Morris DL, Bhangale TR, et al. Association of NCF2, IKZF1, IRF8, IFIH1, and TYK2 with systemic lupus erythematosus. PLoS Genet 2011;7(10):e1002341.

54. Wang C, Ahlford A, Laxman N, et al. Contribution of IKBKE and IFIH1 gene variants to SLE susceptibility. Genes Immun 2013;14(4):217–22.

55. Funabiki M, Kato H, Miyachi Y, et al. Autoimmune disorders associated with gain of function of the intracellular sensor MDA5. Immunity 2014;40(2):199–212.

56. Gorman JA, Hundhausen C, Errett JS, et al. The A946T variant of the RNA sensor IFIH1 mediates an interferon program that limits viral infection but increases the risk for autoimmunity. Nat Immunol 2017;18(7):744–52.

57. Shao WH, Shu DH, Zhen Y, et al. Prion-like aggregation of mitochondrial antiviral signaling protein in lupus patients is associated with increased levels of type I interferon. Arthritis Rheumatol 2016;68(11):2697–707.

58. Buskiewicz IA, Montgomery T, Yasewicz EC, et al. Reactive oxygen species induce virus-independent MAVS oligomerization in systemic lupus erythematosus. Sci Signal 2016;9(456):ra115.

59. Fortner KA, Blanco LP, Buskiewicz I, et al. Targeting mitochondrial oxidative stress with MitoQ reduces NET formation and kidney disease in lupus-prone MRL-lpr mice. Lupus Sci Med 2020;7(1):e000387.

60. Tumurkhuu G, Chen S, Montano EN, et al. Oxidative DNA damage accelerates skin inflammation in pristane-induced lupus model. Front Immunol 2020;11: 554725.
61. Gkirtzimanaki K, Kabrani E, Nikoleri D, et al. IFNalpha impairs autophagic degradation of mtDNA promoting autoreactivity of SLE monocytes in a STING-dependent fashion. Cell Rep 2018;25(4):921–33.e925.
62. Steinberg AD, Baron S, Talal N. The pathogenesis of autoimmunity in New Zealand mice, I. Induction of antinucleic acid antibodies by polyinosinic-polycytidylic acid. Proc Natl Acad Sci U S A 1969;63(4):1102–7.
63. Gota C, Calabrese L. Induction of clinical autoimmune disease by therapeutic interferon-alpha. Autoimmunity 2003;36(8):511–8.
64. Niewold TB. Interferon alpha-induced lupus: proof of principle. J Clin Rheumatol 2008;14(3):131–2.
65. Okanoue T, Sakamoto S, Itoh Y, et al. Side effects of high-dose interferon therapy for chronic hepatitis C. J Hepatol 1996;25(3):283–91.
66. Kälkner KM, Rönnblom L, Karlsson Parra AK, et al. Antibodies against double-stranded DNA and development of polymyositis during treatment with interferon. QJM 1998;91(6):393–9.
67. Rönnblom LE, Alm GV, Oberg KE. Possible induction of systemic lupus erythematosus by interferon-alpha treatment in a patient with a malignant carcinoid tumour. J Intern Med 1990;227(3):207–10.
68. Niewold TB, Swedler WI. Systemic lupus erythematosus arising during interferon-alpha therapy for cryoglobulinemic vasculitis associated with hepatitis C. Clin Rheumatol 2005;24(2):178–81.
69. Wilson LE, Widman D, Dikman SH, et al. Autoimmune disease complicating antiviral therapy for hepatitis C virus infection. Semin Arthritis Rheum 2002;32(3): 163–73.
70. Akiyama C, Tsumiyama K, Uchimura C, et al. Conditional upregulation of IFN-α alone is sufficient to induce systemic lupus erythematosus. J Immunol 2019; 203(4):835–43.
71. Fairhurst AM, Mathian A, Connolly JE, et al. Systemic IFN-alpha drives kidney nephritis in B6.Sle123 mice. Eur J Immunol 2008;38(7):1948–60.
72. Liu Z, Bethunaickan R, Huang W, et al. IFN-α confers resistance of systemic lupus erythematosus nephritis to therapy in NZB/W F1 mice. J Immunol 2011; 187(3):1506–13.
73. Niewold TB, Hua J, Lehman TJ, et al. High serum IFN-alpha activity is a heritable risk factor for systemic lupus erythematosus. Genes Immun 2007;8(6):492–502.
74. Ghodke-Puranik Y, Niewold TB. Genetics of the type I interferon pathway in systemic lupus erythematosus. Int J Clin Rheumtol 2013;8(6). https://doi.org/10.2217/ijr.13.58.
75. Graham RR, Kozyrev SV, Baechler EC, et al. A common haplotype of interferon regulatory factor 5 (IRF5) regulates splicing and expression and is associated with increased risk of systemic lupus erythematosus. Nat Genet 2006;38(5): 550–5.
76. Harley JB, Alarcón-Riquelme ME, Criswell LA, et al. Genome-wide association scan in women with systemic lupus erythematosus identifies susceptibility variants in ITGAM, PXK, KIAA1542 and other loci. Nat Genet 2008;40(2):204–10.
77. Lessard CJ, Adrianto I, Ice JA, et al. Identification of IRF8, TMEM39A, and IKZF3-ZPBP2 as susceptibility loci for systemic lupus erythematosus in a large-scale multiracial replication study. Am J Hum Genet 2012;90(4):648–60.

78. Catalina MD, Owen KA, Labonte AC, et al. The pathogenesis of systemic lupus erythematosus: harnessing big data to understand the molecular basis of lupus. J Autoimmun 2020;110:102359.

79. Farh KK, Marson A, Zhu J, et al. Genetic and epigenetic fine mapping of causal autoimmune disease variants. Nature 2015;518(7539):337–43.

80. Song S, De S, Nelson V, et al. Inhibition of IRF5 hyperactivation protects from lupus onset and severity. J Clin Invest 2020;130(12):6700–17.

81. Kamiyama R, Yoshimi R, Takeno M, et al. Dysfunction of TRIM21 in interferon signature of systemic lupus erythematosus. Mod Rheumatol 2018;28(6): 993–1003.

82. Goropevsek A, Holcar M, Avcin T. The role of STAT signaling pathways in the pathogenesis of systemic lupus erythematosus. Clin Rev Allergy Immunol 2017;52(2):164–81.

83. Goel RR, Nakabo S, Dizon BLP, et al. Lupus-like autoimmunity and increased interferon response in patients with STAT3-deficient hyper-IgE syndrome. J Allergy Clin Immunol 2021;147(2):746–9.e9.

84. Goulielmos GN, Zervou MI, Vazgiourakis VM, et al. The genetics and molecular pathogenesis of systemic lupus erythematosus (SLE) in populations of different ancestry. Gene 2018;668:59–72.

85. Ko K, Koldobskaya Y, Rosenzweig E, et al. Activation of the interferon pathway is dependent upon autoantibodies in African-American SLE patients, but not in European-American SLE patients. Front Immunol 2013;4:309.

86. Munroe ME, Lu R, Zhao YD, et al. Altered type II interferon precedes autoantibody accrual and elevated type I interferon activity prior to systemic lupus erythematosus classification. Ann Rheum Dis 2016;75(11):2014–21.

87. Arbuckle MR, McClain MT, Rubertone MV, et al. Development of autoantibodies before the clinical onset of systemic lupus erythematosus. N Engl J Med 2003; 349(16):1526–33.

88. Oke V, Gunnarsson I, Dorschner J, et al. High levels of circulating interferons type I, type II and type III associate with distinct clinical features of active systemic lupus erythematosus. Arthritis Res Ther 2019;21(1):107.

89. Md Yusof MY, Psarras A, El-Sherbiny YM, et al. Prediction of autoimmune connective tissue disease in an at-risk cohort: prognostic value of a novel two-score system for interferon status. Ann Rheum Dis 2018;77(10):1432–9.

90. Castro F, Cardoso AP, Gonçalves RM, et al. Interferon-gamma at the crossroads of tumor immune surveillance or evasion. Front Immunol 2018;9:847.

91. Liu M, Liu J, Hao S, et al. Higher activation of the interferon-gamma signaling pathway in systemic lupus erythematosus patients with a high type I IFN score: relation to disease activity. Clin Rheumatol 2018;37(10):2675–84.

92. Barkhouse DA, Garcia SA, Bongiorno EK, et al. Expression of interferon gamma by a recombinant rabies virus strongly attenuates the pathogenicity of the virus via induction of type I interferon. J Virol 2015;89(1):312–22.

93. Levy DE, Lew DJ, Decker T, et al. Synergistic interaction between interferon-alpha and interferon-gamma through induced synthesis of one subunit of the transcription factor ISGF3. EMBO J 1990;9(4):1105–11.

94. Li QZ, Zhou J, Lian Y, et al. Interferon signature gene expression is correlated with autoantibody profiles in patients with incomplete lupus syndromes. Clin Exp Immunol 2010;159(3):281–91.

95. Weckerle CE, Franek BS, Kelly JA, et al. Network analysis of associations between serum interferon-α activity, autoantibodies, and clinical features in systemic lupus erythematosus. Arthritis Rheum 2011;63(4):1044–53.

96. Wither J, Johnson SR, Liu T, et al. Presence of an interferon signature in individuals who are anti-nuclear antibody positive lacking a systemic autoimmune rheumatic disease diagnosis. Arthritis Res Ther 2017;19(1):41.

97. Psarras A, Alase A, Antanaviciute A, et al. Functionally impaired plasmacytoid dendritic cells and non-haematopoietic sources of type I interferon characterize human autoimmunity. Nat Commun 2020;11(1):6149.

98. Lambers WM, de Leeuw K, Doornbos-van der Meer B, et al. Interferon score is increased in incomplete systemic lupus erythematosus and correlates with myxovirus-resistance protein A in blood and skin. Arthritis Res Ther 2019; 21(1):260.

99. Olsen NJ, McAloose C, Carter J, et al. Clinical and immunologic profiles in incomplete lupus erythematosus and improvement with hydroxychloroquine treatment. Autoimmune Dis 2016;2016:8791629.

100. Hooks JJ, Moutsopoulos HM, Geis SA, et al. Immune interferon in the circulation of patients with autoimmune disease. N Engl J Med 1979;301(1):5–8.

101. Rönnblom L, Alm GV, Eloranta ML. The type I interferon system in the development of lupus. Semin Immunol 2011;23(2):113–21.

102. Crow MK, Kirou KA. Interferon-alpha in systemic lupus erythematosus. Curr Opin Rheumatol 2004;16(5):541–7.

103. Blanco P, Palucka AK, Gill M, et al. Induction of dendritic cell differentiation by IFN-alpha in systemic lupus erythematosus. Science 2001;294(5546):1540–3.

104. Kahlenberg JM, Thacker SG, Berthier CC, et al. Inflammasome activation of IL-18 results in endothelial progenitor cell dysfunction in systemic lupus erythematosus. J Immunol 2011;187(11):6143–56.

105. Liu M, Guo Q, Wu C, et al. Type I interferons promote the survival and proinflammatory properties of transitional B cells in systemic lupus erythematosus patients. Cell Mol Immunol 2019;16(4):367–79.

106. Menon M, Blair PA, Isenberg DA, et al. A regulatory feedback between plasmacytoid dendritic cells and regulatory b cells is aberrant in systemic lupus erythematosus. Immunity 2016;44(3):683–97.

107. Nehar-Belaid D, Hong S, Marches R, et al. Mapping systemic lupus erythematosus heterogeneity at the single-cell level. Nat Immunol 2020;21(9):1094–106.

108. Peck-Radosavljevic M, Wichlas M, Homoncik-Kraml M, et al. Rapid suppression of hematopoiesis by standard or pegylated interferon-alpha. Gastroenterology 2002;123(1):141–51.

109. Morand EF, Furie R, Tanaka Y, et al. Trial of anifrolumab in active systemic lupus erythematosus. N Engl J Med 2020;382(3):211–21.

110. Berthier CC, Tsoi LC, Reed TJ, et al. Molecular profiling of cutaneous lupus lesions identifies subgroups distinct from clinical phenotypes. J Clin Med 2019; 8(8):1244.

111. Stannard JN, Reed TJ, Myers E, et al. Lupus skin is primed for IL-6 inflammatory responses through a keratinocyte-mediated autocrine type I interferon loop. J Invest Dermatol 2017;137(1):115–22.

112. Zahn S, Graef M, Patsinakidis N, et al. Ultraviolet light protection by a sunscreen prevents interferon-driven skin inflammation in cutaneous lupus erythematosus. Exp Dermatol 2014;23(7):516–8.

113. Braunstein I, Klein R, Okawa J, et al. The interferon-regulated gene signature is elevated in subacute cutaneous lupus erythematosus and discoid lupus erythematosus and correlates with the cutaneous lupus area and severity index score. Br J Dermatol 2012;166(5):971–5.

114. Furie R, Werth VP, Merola JF, et al. Monoclonal antibody targeting BDCA2 ameliorates skin lesions in systemic lupus erythematosus. J Clin Invest 2019;129(3): 1359–71.
115. Nacionales DC, Kelly-Scumpia KM, Lee PY, et al. Deficiency of the type I interferon receptor protects mice from experimental lupus. Arthritis Rheum 2007; 56(11):3770–83.
116. Castellano G, Cafiero C, Divella C, et al. Local synthesis of interferon-alpha in lupus nephritis is associated with type I interferons signature and LMP7 induction in renal tubular epithelial cells. Arthritis Res Ther 2015;17:72.
117. Der E, Ranabothu S, Suryawanshi H, et al. Single cell RNA sequencing to dissect the molecular heterogeneity in lupus nephritis. JCI Insight 2017;2(9): e93009.
118. Arazi A, Rao DA, Berthier CC, et al. The immune cell landscape in kidneys of patients with lupus nephritis. Nat Immunol 2019;20(7):902–14.
119. Migliorini A, Angelotti ML, Mulay SR, et al. The antiviral cytokines IFN-α and IFN-β modulate parietal epithelial cells and promote podocyte loss: implications for IFN toxicity, viral glomerulonephritis, and glomerular regeneration. Am J Pathol 2013;183(2):431–40.
120. Adamichou C, Georgakis S, Bertsias G. Cytokine targets in lupus nephritis: current and future prospects. Clin Immunol 2019;206:42–52.
121. Fava A, Buyon J, Mohan C, et al. Integrated urine proteomics and renal single-cell genomics identify an IFN-γ response gradient in lupus nephritis. JCI Insight 2020;5(12):e138345.
122. Boedigheimer MJ, Martin DA, Amoura Z, et al. Safety, pharmacokinetics and pharmacodynamics of AMG 811, an anti-interferon-γ monoclonal antibody, in SLE subjects without or with lupus nephritis. Lupus Sci Med 2017;4(1):e000226.
123. Nzeusseu Toukap A, Galant C, Theate I, et al. Identification of distinct gene expression profiles in the synovium of patients with systemic lupus erythematosus. Arthritis Rheum 2007;56(5):1579–88.
124. Somers EC, Zhao W, Lewis EE, et al. Type I interferons are associated with subclinical markers of cardiovascular disease in patients with systemic lupus erythematosus. PLoS One 2012;7(5):e37000.
125. Liu Y, Kaplan MJ. Cardiovascular disease in systemic lupus erythematosus: an update. Curr Opin Rheumatol 2018;30(5):441–8.
126. Bashant KR, Aponte AM, Randazzo D, et al. Proteomic, biomechanical and functional analyses define neutrophil heterogeneity in systemic lupus erythematosus. Ann Rheum Dis 2021;80(2):209–18.
127. Casey KA, Smith MA, Sinibaldi D, et al. Modulation of cardiometabolic disease markers by type I interferon inhibition in systemic lupus erythematosus. Arthritis Rheumatol 2021;73(3):459–71.
128. Yu T, Enioutina EY, Brunner HI, et al. Clinical pharmacokinetics and pharmacodynamics of biologic therapeutics for treatment of systemic lupus erythematosus. Clin Pharmacokinet 2017;56(2):107–25.
129. Furie R, Khamashta M, Merrill JT, et al. Anifrolumab, an anti-interferon-α receptor monoclonal antibody, in moderate-to-severe systemic lupus erythematosus. Arthritis Rheumatol 2017;69(2):376–86.
130. Furie RA, Morand EF, Bruce IN, et al. Type I interferon inhibitor anifrolumab in active systemic lupus erythematosus (TULIP-1): a randomised, controlled, phase 3 trial. Lancet Rheumatol 2019;1(4):e208–19.
131. Khamashta M, Merrill JT, Werth VP, et al. Sifalimumab, an anti-interferon-α monoclonal antibody, in moderate to severe systemic lupus erythematosus: a

randomised, double-blind, placebo-controlled study. Ann Rheum Dis 2016; 75(11):1909–16.

132. Kalunian KC, Merrill JT, Maciuca R, et al. A phase II study of the efficacy and safety of rontalizumab (rhuMAb interferon-α) in patients with systemic lupus erythematosus (ROSE). Ann Rheum Dis 2016;75(1):196–202.

133. Jordan J, Benson J, Chatham WW, et al. First-in-human study of JNJ-55920839 in healthy volunteers and patients with systemic lupus erythematosus: a randomised placebo-controlled phase 1 trial. Lancet Rheumatol 2020;2(10):e613–22.

134. Villarino AV, Kanno Y, O'Shea JJ. Mechanisms and consequences of Jak-STAT signaling in the immune system. Nat Immunol 2017;18(4):374–84.

135. Kawasaki M, Fujishiro M, Yamaguchi A, et al. Possible role of the JAK/STAT pathways in the regulation of T cell-interferon related genes in systemic lupus erythematosus. Lupus 2011;20(12):1231–9.

136. Ikeda K, Hayakawa K, Fujishiro M, et al. JAK inhibitor has the amelioration effect in lupus-prone mice: the involvement of IFN signature gene downregulation. BMC Immunol 2017;18(1):41.

137. Wang S, Yang N, Zhang L, et al. Jak/STAT signaling is involved in the inflammatory infiltration of the kidneys in MRL/lpr mice. Lupus 2010;19(10):1171–80.

138. Furumoto Y, Smith CK, Blanco L, et al. Tofacitinib ameliorates murine lupus and its associated vascular dysfunction. Arthritis Rheumatol 2017;69(1):148–60.

139. Fetter T, Smith P, Guel T, et al. Selective Janus kinase 1 inhibition is a promising therapeutic approach for lupus erythematosus skin lesions. Front Immunol 2020; 11:344.

140. Wallace DJ, Furie RA, Tanaka Y, et al. Baricitinib for systemic lupus erythematosus: a double-blind, randomised, placebo-controlled, phase 2 trial. Lancet 2018;392(10143):222–31.

141. Bauer JW, Baechler EC, Petri M, et al. Elevated serum levels of interferon-regulated chemokines are biomarkers for active human systemic lupus erythematosus. PLoS Med 2006;3(12):e491.

142. Bauer JW, Petri M, Batliwalla FM, et al. Interferon-regulated chemokines as biomarkers of systemic lupus erythematosus disease activity: a validation study. Arthritis Rheum 2009;60(10):3098–107.

143. Puapatanakul P, Chansritrakul S, Susantitaphong P, et al. Interferon-inducible protein 10 and disease activity in systemic lupus erythematosus and lupus nephritis: a systematic review and meta-analysis. Int J Mol Sci 2019;20(19): 4954.

Neutrophil Dysregulation in the Pathogenesis of Systemic Lupus Erythematosus

Yudong Liu, MD, PhD[a], Mariana J. Kaplan, MD[b],*

KEYWORDS

- Systemic lupus erythematosus • Neutrophils • Low-density granulocytes
- Immune dysregulation • Organ damage • Type I interferons

KEY POINTS

- Neutrophil dysfunction driven by low-density granulocytes and aberrant neutrophil extracellular trap formation/clearance is implicated in systemic lupus erythematosus (SLE) pathogenesis. Lupus neutrophils can modulate disease through various aspects that include bidirectional interactions with different components of the innate and adaptive immune arms, modification and externalization of autoantigens, and direct induction of organ and vascular damage.
- Although several neutrophil-associated biomarkers exhibit promising diagnostic potential, further prospective studies will help to understand whether some of these biomarkers can provide clinicians with a precision-medicine approach to complex clinical problems, thus improving the clinical decision-making process.
- Correcting neutrophil dysfunction may provide additional efficacy to the current treatment regimen, but continued preclinical and clinical studies are needed to determine how to translate these findings into clinical practice.

INTRODUCTION

Systemic lupus erythematosus (SLE) is a systemic autoimmune disorder that predominantly affects women and is characterized by a loss of immune tolerance to a wide variety of autoantigens, dysregulated innate and adaptive immune responses, and a

Funding: Y. Liu was supported by funds from National Natural Science Foundation of China, grant no. 81971521, and Peking University People's Hospital Research and Development Fund, grant no. RDY2019-14. M.J. Kaplan was supported by the Intramural Research Program at NIAMS/NIH, ZIAAR041199.
[a] Department of Clinical Laboratory, Peking University People's Hospital, 11 Xizhimen South Street, Xicheng District, Beijing 100044, China; [b] Systemic Autoimmunity Branch, Intramural Research Program, National Institute of Arthritis and Musculoskeletal and Skin Diseases, National Institutes of Health, 10 Center Drive, 12N248C, Bethesda, MD 20892-1930, USA
* Corresponding author.
E-mail address: mariana.kaplan@nih.gov

characteristic type I interferon (IFN-I) gene signature.[1,2] SLE affects multiple organs and systems, including the brain, the kidney, the skin and the vasculature. Over the last decade, significant progress has been made toward understanding how aberrant immune responses contribute to organ inflammation and damage in SLE. The wide spectrum of clinical manifestations in SLE suggests the involvement of multiple pathogenic processes. The identification of a subset of lupus proinflammatory neutrophils, low-density granulocytes (LDGs), has led to a resurgence of interest in the role of neutrophils as shapers of immune dysregulation and as inducers of organ damage.[3,4] This article provides an overview of how neutrophil dysregulation and aberrant neutrophil extracellular trap (NET) formation may contribute to the pathogenesis of SLE. It also discusses the therapeutic potential of targeting these neutrophil-relevant pathways in the treatment of SLE.

Neutrophils and Low-Density Granulocytes Modulate Immune Responses in Systemic Lupus Erythematosus

Neutrophils are equipped with the ability to engage in a diverse arsenal of antimicrobial mechanisms, including phagocytosis, generation of reactive oxygen species (ROS), degranulation, and formation of NETs.[5] Neutrophils also play an important role in bridging the innate and adaptive immune arms through the release of a broad repertoire of immune and proinflammatory mediators with pleiotropic functions. For example, by producing tumor necrosis factor (TNF)-α, activated neutrophils promote maturation of dendritic cell (DCs) that in turn promote T-cell proliferation and polarization to helper T (Th) 1 cells.[6] In addition, neutrophils crosstalk with Th17 cells through chemokine-dependent reciprocal interactions, which involve CCL2 and CCL20 production by neutrophils and CXCL8 production by Th17 cells.[7] Further, splenic neutrophils can induce immunoglobulin class switching, somatic hypermutation, and antibody production by activating marginal zone (MZ) B cells through a mechanism that involves the cytokines B cell–activating factor (BAFF), FR-related apoptosis-inducing ligand and IL-21.[8]

In SLE, neutrophil dysregulation is characterized by impaired phagocytic capabilities,[9] reduced ability to recognize and remove dead cells through the C1q/calreticulin/cluster of differentiation (CD) 91–mediated apoptotic pathway,[10] and various abnormalities in metabolic pathways.[11] SLE genetic risk variants in *ITGAM* (encoding for CD11b, the α-subunit of Mac-1)[12] can alter Mac-1 function on neutrophils, resulting in impairment of both Mac-1–mediated neutrophil phagocytosis via Fc receptors and Mac-1–mediated firm adhesion.[13] Genetic variants in *NCF1* (encoding the p47[phox] subunit of the phagocyte NADPH [nicotinamide adenine dinucleotide phosphate, reduced form] oxidase [NOX2]), which is significantly associated with SLE risk, can cause dysregulated oxidative pathways in myeloid cells.[14] Similarly, lupus-associated causal mutations in neutrophil cytosolic factor 2 (*NCF2*) also lead to dysregulated ROS production in neutrophils, implicating alterations in immunometabolism in the pathogenesis of SLE.[15]

IFN-I plays a central role in the pathogenesis of SLE,[16–18] and lupus neutrophils have been reported to produce bioactive IFNα on stimulation with purified chromatin, independent of toll-like receptor (TLR) 9 stimulation[19] as well as other type I IFNs in response to various TLRs. Considering circulating neutrophils are much more abundant than plasmacytoid DCs (pDCs), neutrophils may represent an important source of type I IFNs in SLE. In addition to circulating neutrophils, bone marrow resident lupus neutrophils also contribute to IFN production and the secretion of cytokines that may promote abnormal B-cell development in the bone marrow (BM) in patients with SLE.[20]

Low-density granulocytes

LDGs represent a distinct proinflammatory neutrophil subset present in the peripheral blood mononuclear layer (PBMC) layer following a gradient separation of SLE peripheral blood. The increased levels of LDGs in SLE associate with the IFN gene signature, disease severity, and vascular injury.[21–24] Furthermore, LDGs secrete higher levels of interleukin (IL)-6, IL-8, TNF-α, and IFN-I than their normal-density granulocyte (NDG) counterparts.[24] Further, compared with NDGs, lupus LDGs express higher levels of degranulation markers (CD63 and CD107a) and reduced levels of intracellular arginase-1, indicating that these cells are phenotypically activated.[21] Although some degranulation markers are increased, electron microscopy data do not support that LDGs represent degranulated cells.[25] Lupus LDGs promote proinflammatory cytokine production by CD4+ T cells, including IFN-γ, TNF-α, and lymphotoxin-α,[21] which is different from polymorphonuclear myeloid-derived suppressor cells (PMN-MDSCs), an immunosuppressive myeloid subset sharing similar surface markers to LDGs.[26] Of interest, a different study has reported that lupus cells expressing markers of PMN-MDSCs induce Th17 responses and promote organ damage in an arginase-1–dependent manner.[27] Although both studies suggest that LDGs and PMN-MDSCs play a pathogenic role in SLE, the discrepancies between the two studies indicate a clear need for further detailed immunophenotypic and functional comparisons between bona fide LDGs and PMN-MDSCs in the context of different stages of lupus progression, as well as a requirement of reaching a consensus on isolating techniques and phenotypic characterization of neutrophil subsets.

At the transcriptional level, lupus LDGs are distinct from healthy control or autologous lupus NDGs.[28] Furthermore, there is significant transcriptional heterogeneity within lupus LDGs, with the identification of at least 2 subsets, the intermediate-mature CD10$^+$ LDGs and the immature CD10$^-$ LDGs.[29] CD10$^+$ LDGs, which represent most of the lupus LDGs, show several pathogenic features, including enhanced NET formation with oxidized nucleic acid release, and promotion of endothelial dysfunction, thereby accounting for the most significant associations with organ damage.[29] In contrast, the CD10$^-$ LDG subset, which is impaired in several canonical neutrophil functions, represents a transcriptionally active LDG population that upregulates genes related to cell cycle progression and has decreased transcription of immune response genes compared with other neutrophils.[29] Of interest, the CD10$^+$ subset shows the highest expression of type I IFN-stimulated genes (ISGs) compared with other myeloid and nonmyeloid subsets in the lupus mononuclear cell fraction, suggesting that they significantly contribute to the characteristic lupus type I IFN signature.[29] It will be important to determine whether these various LDG subsets are present in other autoimmune diseases associated with increased levels of LDGs, and their putative pathogenic roles.[30–32]

Lupus LDGs are also distinct from healthy control or autologous lupus NDGs at the epigenetic level. DNA methylome analysis shows that lupus neutrophils showed an overall hypomethylated status compared with control neutrophils.[33] Further assay for transposase-accessible chromatin (ATAC)-seq analysis revealed that CD10$^-$ LDGs have enhanced chromatin accessibility compared with CD10$^+$ LDGs, autologous NDGs, and healthy control NDGs, suggesting that CD10$^-$ LDGs are a transcriptionally active subset of neutrophils.[29]

A study using a multifaceted analysis of proteomics, biomechanical profiles, and trafficking, comparing SLE LDGs and NDGs and resting or stimulated healthy control NDGs, confirmed that LDGs represent a distinct neutrophil subset rather than expansion of immature/primed neutrophils present in healthy people.[34] SLE LDGs show distinct protein cargo, including enhanced levels of IFN-inducible proteins and modulation of proteins involved in the actin cytoskeleton. This protein cargo is coupled to the finding that the biomechanical properties of lupus LDGs are distinct from autologous lupus NDGs or resting and stimulated healthy control neutrophils. Furthermore, these distinct biomechanical properties may affect LDG's ability to travel through the vasculature, interact with the endothelium, and enhance their trapping in the small vessels of various organs, such as the lung.[34]

A key feature of LDGs is their enhanced ability to form NETs and damage the vasculature.[11,28,35,36] NET formation dysregulation and its implications in SLE pathogenesis are discussed next.

Neutrophil extracellular traps and modulation of autoimmune responses in systemic lupus erythematosus

NETs are extracellular weblike structures composed of decondensed chromatin bound to neutrophil-derived proteins, particularly those present in granules.[37] NET formation is primarily considered a mechanism of neutrophil cell death triggered by complex and still incompletely characterized intracellular pathways.[38] NETs are triggered by a variety of microbial and sterile inflammatory stimuli and, physiologically, their function seems to be related to trapping of microbes and promotion of coagulation.[39] ROS generation (through the NOX machinery, the mitochondria or myeloperoxidase [MPO]) seems to be a shared feature required for most types of NET formation.[39] During many forms of NET formation, peptidylarginine deiminase (PAD) 4, an enzyme primarily expressed in neutrophils, converts positively charged histone arginine residues to more neutrally charged citrulline residues on histone tails, promoting chromatin decondensation in the nucleus.[40] Neutrophil elastase and MPO translocate into the nucleus and further promote chromatin cleavage, nuclear membrane dissolution, and expulsion of chromatin into the cytosol.[39]

Certain genetic polymorphisms associated with SLE risk may be linked to neutrophil dysregulation, characterized by enhanced NET formation. For example, neutrophils with genetic variants in *TNFAIP3* (A20) deubiquitinase (DUB) domain showed an upregulated expression of *PADI4*, resulting in enhanced protein citrullination and NET formation.[41] Patients with SLE with these variants showed increased NET formation and increased frequency of autoantibodies to citrullinated epitopes.[41] Further, genetic variants in protein tyrosine phosphatase nonreceptor type 22 (*PTPN22*) disrupt its interaction with PAD4, which leads to enhanced citrullination and NET formation.[42] Similarly, interferon regulatory factor (IRF)-5 genetic risk variants drive myeloid-specific IRF5 hyperactivation in SLE, leading to enhanced NET formation.[43] A recent study reported that neutrophils from patients with *STAT3* loss-of-function mutations formed more spontaneous NETs than neutrophils from matched healthy controls, which may contribute to the SLE-like autoimmunity with predominant renal involvement observed in some of these patients.[44]

Lupus neutrophils, in particular LDGs, have an increased propensity to form NETs compared with neutrophils from healthy donors.[11,28,35,36] In addition, compared with plasma from healthy controls, lupus plasma induces more NET formation in healthy control neutrophils and there is evidence that SLE autoantibodies, immune complexes (particularly RNP/anti-RNP), and complement activation products can induce NET formation.[11,22,45] In particular, lupus RNP/anti-RNP complexes can stimulate healthy control neutrophils to synthesize more mitochondrial ROS and form NETs that carry higher levels of oxidized mitochondrial DNA.[11] Further, a significant proportion of patients with lupus show impairments in NET clearance, which may in part be caused by genetic or induced impairments in the function of intracellular and extracellular DNases.[46] The enhanced half-life of NETs in blood and tissues in SLE can have significant immunomodulatory consequences.

NETs show critical roles in the activation, regulation, and effector functions of the innate and adaptive immune systems through a variety of diverse mechanisms (**Fig. 1**). For example, NETs can stimulate macrophages to release IL-1β and IL-18 by promoting NLRP3 inflammasome activation through a P2X7 receptor–mediated mechanism.[47] In turn, these cytokines can further promote NET synthesis.[47] Thus, enhanced NET formation in patients with lupus can lead to increased inflammasome activation in macrophages, creating a feed-forward inflammatory loop that amplifies inflammatory pathways. Lupus NETs can also activate pDCs to synthesize IFN-I through activation of endosomal TLRs.[35,36] Of interest, the significantly enhanced ability of LDGs to generate NETs[24] depends on their enhanced synthesis of mitochondrial ROS.[11] These NETs generated through enhanced mitochondrial ROS are enriched in oxidized nucleic acids, including genomic and mitochondrial DNA, which endows them with heightened immunostimulatory potential compared with NETs generated by other stimuli.[11] Indeed, LDG NETs have an enhanced ability to stimulate target cells to upregulate proinflammatory cytokines and ISGs. Importantly, oxidized nucleic acids generated during NET formation have extended half-life, because they are more resistant to degradation by nucleases, and can signal through the cyclic GMP-AMP synthase-stimulator of interferon genes (cGAS-STING) pathway for enhanced IFN-I production.[11,48] This phenomenon may be relevant for both extracellular NET-bound nucleic acids but also for NET-bound nucleic acids internalized by target cells.[49] In addition, NETs can directly prime T cells by reducing their activation threshold to specific antigens and even to suboptimal stimuli.[50] Of interest, a recent study showed that lupus NETs trigger polyclonal B-cell activation via TLR9 and expand self-reactive memory B cells for anti-NET autoantibody production in SLE.[51] In addition, NETs can promote the transition of endothelial cells toward a mesenchymal phenotype, a process in which endothelial cells lose their endothelial-specific markers and gain a mesenchymal phenotype.[52] Further, active SLE NETs can also activate fibroblasts and induce expression of CCN2, a matricellular protein implicated in fibrosis, collagen production, and proliferation/migration rates.[53] Overall,

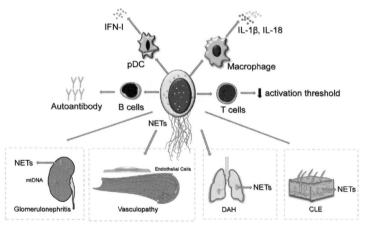

Fig. 1. NETs in the pathogenesis of SLE. NETs can induce IFN-I production by pDCs, and proinflammatory cytokine production (ie, IL-1β and IL-18) by macrophages. NETs can activate memory B cells, promoting autoantibody production, and can directly prime T cells by reducing their activation threshold to specific antigens. NETs are implicated in kidney damage, vasculopathy, cutaneous lupus erythematosus (CLE) and diffuse alveolar hemorrhage (DAH). mtDNA, mitochondrial DNA.

these observations indicate that NETs have pleiotropic immunostimulatory and profibrotic effects in the context of SLE that may promote immune dysregulation and contribute to tissue damage.

Recent work has revealed that gasdermin D (GSDMD), a pore-forming protein activated during pyroptosis, is implicated in some forms of NET formation.[54,55] Counterintuitively, loss of GSDMD resulted in enhanced mortality and exacerbated lupus clinical phenotype, including more severe renal and pulmonary inflammation, and increased levels of autoantibody production, in a TLR-7–induced lupus model.[56] Notably, NET formation in lupus GSDMD-deficient mice was not impaired in this model, suggesting that GSDMD's role in a variety of cell death mechanisms, particularly in SLE, may be context dependent.[56]

Neutrophils and NETs in Lupus Nephritis

Lupus nephritis (LN) represents one of the most common organ manifestations in SLE.[57] Gradual enrichment of neutrophil transcripts in the blood transcriptome has been reported in patients with SLE during progression to active renal disease, indicating an association between neutrophils and kidney involvement.[58] Another modular repertoire analysis using microarray data found that a neutrophil signature was associated with LN and could stratify LN risk and monitor treatment response,[59] further supporting an involvement of neutrophils in LN. A recent study found that SLE serum can induce an inflammatory response by human glomerular endothelial cells that enhances neutrophil migration and adhesion, which may contribute to the development of LN.[60] In a subgroup of Caucasian patients with SLE, percentages of CD10$^+$ LDGs negatively correlated with renal function, whereas percentages of CD10$^-$ LDGs correlated with proteinuria, suggesting that the two LDGs subsets may associate with different aspects of LN.[29]

NETs are increased in LN biopsies, and impairment of NET degradation is significantly associated with LN.[46] NETs are identified in kidney samples of diseased lupus-prone mice and patients with LN[28,52,53] (see **Fig. 1**). In addition, NETs containing mitochondrial DNA were also detected in LN renal biopsy specimens.[61] The presence of NETs in glomeruli correlated with severity of proteinuria.[52] NETs can alter endothelial cell-cell contacts and induce vascular leakage and transendothelial albumin passage through elastase-mediated proteolysis of the intercellular junction protein vascular endothelial cadherin.[52] Further, in a murine model of glomerulonephritis (GN), histones released by neutrophils during NET formation can cause direct cytotoxicity to glomerular endothelial cells, podocytes, and parietal epithelial cells in a dose-dependent manner.[62] In addition, tissue factor (TF)–bearing and IL-17A–bearing NETs are present in the glomerular and tubulointerstitial compartment of proliferative LN biopsy specimens, suggesting their involvement in the thromboinflammatory and fibrotic potential in LN.[53] NETs containing high mobility group box-1 (HMGB1) show immunogenic properties.[35] The expression of HMGB1 in NETs is higher in patients with LN, which correlates with clinical and histopathologic features of active nephritis, suggesting a possible link of NETs-derived HMGB1 in LN.[63] One barrier to better understand the role of NETs in LN is that the presence of neutrophils and their potential damage may occur at preclinical stages before overt proteinuria and the need to perform a kidney biopsy. Analysis of urine samples, including transcriptomic and proteomic assessments, may allow the identification of neutrophil and NET biomarkers that could help predict prognosis in LN.

Neutrophils and NETs in Cardiovascular Disease in Systemic Lupus Erythematosus

SLE associates with a significant risk of cardiovascular disease (CVD), which is not fully explained by traditional Framingham risk factors.[64] Patients with LN show significantly increased risk of myocardial infarction and CVD mortality than patients with SLE without LN,[65] suggesting that some of the immune and metabolic factors that are implicated in LN may also contribute to the CVD in SLE. Both LDGs and NETs have been associated with endothelial damage as well as with induction of abnormal endothelial differentiation, with potential implications in the development of premature atherosclerosis in SLE.[66] The levels of LDGs were independently associated with noncalcified coronary plaque burden (NCB).[67] Further, an LDG gene signature obtained by RNA sequencing independently associated with the presence of high vascular inflammation, as measured by fluorodeoxyglucose PET computed tomography scans and with high NCB in SLE.[67] The involvement of LDGs in SLE CVD is further confirmed by a recent study that showed that CD16⁻ LDGs are increased in patients with SLE with subclinical cardiovascular disease.[68] Another study revealed that CD10⁺ LDGs, but not CD10⁻ LDGs, impair murine aortic endothelium-dependent vasorelaxation.[29] Thus, CD10⁺ LDGs could be used as biomarkers for cardiovascular risk in SLE in the future, if longitudinal assessments confirm this association.

NETs play a proatherogenic and a prothrombotic role in several disorders[69–72] (see **Fig. 1**). Activated endothelial cells can promote neutrophil recruitment to plaques and NET formation, which in turn amplifies and propagates local inflammatory process that lead to endothelial injury by eliciting endothelial cell activation and increased expression of adhesion molecules.[73] NETs can induce TF expression and accelerate clotting.[73] Lupus LDG-derived NETs contain higher levels of matrix metalloproteinase (MMP) 9, which activates endothelial MMP-2 and subsequently leads to endothelial cell death and vascular dysfunction.[74] In addition, NETs can promote nuclear translocation of junctional β-catenin and induced endothelial-to-mesenchymal transition in cultured endothelial cells, which may contribute endothelial dysfunction.[52]

The dyslipidemia in SLE is characterized by increased levels of oxidized and dysfunctional high-density lipoprotein (HDL) with impaired cholesterol efflux capacity and in association with atherosclerosis.[64] Increased levels of lupus LDGs are associated with impaired HDL cholesterol efflux,[67] which may be in part caused by the ability of LDGs to synthesize higher amounts of NETs. NETs show the ability to oxidize HDL in a region-specific proatherogenic manner, which impairs the cholesterol efflux capacity of HDL,[75] suggesting that NETs contribute to CVD through promoting dyslipidemia. Consistent with these findings, the levels of NETs were shown to be associated with CVD in patients with SLE.[76] In fact, accumulating evidence suggest that NETs promote thrombosis through a variety of mechanisms. NETs can recruit red blood cells, promoted fibrin deposition, and induced a red thrombus.[77] NETs can also provide a scaffold for the binding of a variety of coagulation components, including platelets, factor XII (FXII), von Willebrand factor, and TF.[53,77,78] The prothrombotic role of NETs is further supported by the findings that inhibiting NET formation or disruption of NETs protects animals from thrombosis.[70,77] Because thrombosis contributes to a substantial morbidity and mortality in patients with SLE,[79] blocking NET formation may provide additional benefit in preventing thrombotic events in SLE.

Neutrophils and NETs in Cutaneous Manifestations of Systemic Lupus Erythematosus

Cutaneous lupus erythematosus (CLE) can present as a manifestation within the clinical spectrum of SLE or can present in isolation without systemic features. Of note, NETs have been identified in the skin of patients with different subtypes of lupus skin disease[28,53,80] (see **Fig. 1**). NETs are more prominent in CLE with features of tissue damage and scarring, suggesting a pathogenic role.[80] In 1 report, acute, discoid, and panniculitis subtypes of lupus skin involvement showed significantly higher levels of NETs than the subacute subtype.[80] TF-containing and IL-17A–containing NETs, which were detected in skin lesions of patients with active discoid lupus, promoted thrombin generation and the fibrotic potential of cultured skin fibroblasts.[53] In addition, lupus murine models with skin manifestations show evidence of enhanced NET formation, implicating netting neutrophils in skin damage in SLE.[81]

Neutrophils and NETs in Diffuse Alveolar Hemorrhage in Systemic Lupus Erythematosus

Diffuse alveolar hemorrhage (DAH) is a rare but life-threatening pulmonary manifestation of SLE.[82] Interstitial infiltration of neutrophils is common in pulmonary capillaritis.[83] NETs have been identified in lungs in the pristane model of DAH (see **Fig. 1**), where lung injury was attenuated through disruption of NETs by DNases, suggesting a pathogenic role of NETs in DAH.[84] The involvement of NETs in lung disorder has also been shown in multiple lung diseases, including cystic fibrosis, neutrophilic asthma, and transfusion-related acute lung injury (TRALI). In patients with TRALI, a similar pulmonary injury to DAH in several aspects, the levels of circulating NETs were significantly increased.[85] In addition, NETs were detected in the lungs of mice with TRALI, and treatment with DNases significantly reduced disease severity and improved survival.[85,86] In vitro, NETs can induce proinflammatory cytokine production by human airway epithelial cells and can also cause cytotoxicity in these cells.[87,88] Further, NETs can break epithelial integrity by downregulating the expression of occludin and claudin-1.[87] These findings suggest a pathogenic role of NETs in lung manifestations in SLE, highlighting a therapeutic potential of targeting NETs in SLE DAH. Furthermore, LDGs have perturbed biomechanical properties that limit their migration through the microvasculature, with implications for lung complications.[34]

Neutrophils and NETs in Neuropsychiatric Lupus

Neurologic and psychiatric manifestations are serious but among the least understood complications of SLE. Although few studies have implicated neutrophils in neuropsychiatric SLE (NPSLE), neutrophil-associated molecules, including lipocalin-2 (LCN2), MMP-9, and IL-8, were found increased in patients with SLE with NPSLE compared with patients with SLE without NPSLE.[74,89–94] LCN2 is upregulated in the cerebrospinal fluid of patients with NPSLE, and LCN2 deficiency attenuates depression-like behavior and impaired spatial and recognition memory in lupus-prone mice.[89] Assessing whether neutrophils or NETs are involved in NPSLE is an understudied area that deserves further attention.

Neutrophil-Related Biomarkers in Systemic Lupus Erythematosus

Several neutrophil-related parameters have been proposed as biomarkers in SLE. For instance, LDG-to-lymphocyte ratio is a marker of immune dysregulation in SLE.[21] A blood neutrophil signature has been proposed as a biomarker for stratifying LN risk and for monitoring treatment response.[59] A recent study reported that 25% of patients with SLE showed high neutrophil gene expression, which associated with fever, serositis, leukopenia, and glucocorticoid use.[95] Further, combined IFN-I and neutrophil gene scores were significantly associated with high disease activity, which showed better performance than anti–double-stranded DNA and anti-C1q autoantibody and complement levels for predicting SLE activity.[95] Thus, simultaneous assessment of IFN-I and neutrophil gene scores may stratify patients with SLE at risk of high disease activity.

Further, circulating levels of NETs measured by MPO-DNA complexes may help predict and assess disease activity and organ damage, such as nephritis or CVD in

SLE.[76] Further, using circulating levels of NETs for disease stratification in SLE may represent a new diagnostic direction; however, standardization of the methodologies to quantify NETs, as well as standardization of the definition of what constitutes high levels of NETs, is needed to translate these approaches into clinical practice.

Neutrophil-Related Therapy in Systemic Lupus Erythematosus

Given the increased recognition of neutrophils and NETs in the pathogenesis of SLE, therapeutic modulation of neutrophil function or NET formation has received extensive recent attention (**Fig. 2**). For example, antimalarials, first-line treatment of SLE, can decrease NET formation in vitro and in vivo.[75,96] Cyclosporine A, a calcineurin inhibitor commonly used to treat SLE, can inhibit IL-8–induced NET formation.[97] In addition, a recent clinical trial reported that a combination therapy with rituximab (RTX) and belimumab achieved clinically significant responses in patients with SLE with severe, refractory disease, which associated with specific reductions in antinuclear antibodies and decreases in NET formation.[98] Metformin, which may reduce subsequent disease flares in patients with SLE with low disease activity,[99] was shown to inhibit NET formation in vitro and in vivo.[100] Further, treatment of lupus-prone mice with tofacitinib, a Janus kinase inhibitor, can significantly ameliorate disease severity and organ damage, partially through blocking NET formation.[101]

Because PADs, in particular PAD4 and PAD2, play an important role in NET formation, extensive efforts have been made to assess the relevance of inhibition of these enzymes in the treatment of SLE. Using preclinical models, PAD inhibitors have been effective at reducing NET formation and disease severity as well as kidney damage in several murine models of lupus.[69,81] The protective effect of PAD inhibition in

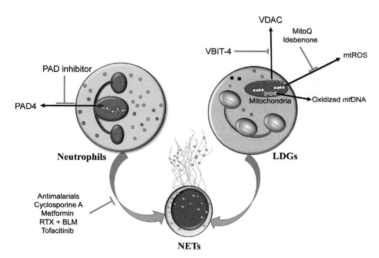

Fig. 2. Blocking NET formation as potential therapeutic targets in SLE. Lupus neutrophils, and particularly LDGs, are primed to form NETs. NET formation in LDGs depends on generation of mitochondrial ROS (mtROS). Compounds, including antimalarials, cyclosporine A, metformin, rituximab (RTX), and belimumab (BLM), and Jak inhibitors such as tofacitinib may exert their beneficial immunomodulatory effect in SLE, partially through blocking NET formation. PAD inhibitors are effective at reducing NET formation and may have protective effect in SLE. Idebenone and MitoQ, which target mtROS, can block NET formation in SLE LDGs. VBIT-4, a voltage-dependent anion channel (VDAC) oligomerization inhibitor, can inhibit mtROS in immune cells, thus suppressing NET formation in SLE LDGs.

amelioration of kidney injury was further confirmed in an anti–glomerular basement membrane nephritis model.[62] NETs promote the development of atherosclerosis,[72,102] and inhibition of NET formation by PAD4 inhibitors protects mice from atherosclerosis[70] and ameliorates vascular damage in murine models of lupus.[69,81] Therefore, PAD inhibition may also provide additional benefit in preventing vasculopathy and premature atherosclerosis in SLE, and future studies will be required to assess safety and efficacy. Of interest, controversies also exist regarding the role PADs in SLE. PAD4 deficiency protects mice from kidney damage in a model of TLR7-induced lupus,[103,104] but had little effect on lupus autoimmunity in the MRL.Fas[lpr] lupus model[105] and even exacerbated disease severity in a pristane-induced lupus model.[106] These discrepancies may be caused by the differences in the experimental models that cannot explain in full the complicated and heterogeneous clinical entities in SLE, indicating a clear need for additional preclinical and clinical studies to determine whether PAD inhibition is a viable therapeutic strategy in SLE.

Modulating mitochondrial dysfunction in LDGs represents a novel therapeutic target in SLE. Idebenone, a coenzyme Q10 synthetic quinone analogue that improves mitochondrial physiology, inhibited spontaneous NET formation in lupus LDGs by blocking mitochondrial ROS (mtROS) production.[107] Treatment of lupus-prone mice with idebenone reduced renal inflammation, attenuated systemic immune dysregulation, and improved mitochondrial metabolism.[107] Similarly, targeting mtROS with MitoQ, a mitochondrial antioxidant, significantly improved renal disease and immune dysregulation in murine lupus, in association with inhibition of NET formation.[108] A recent study showed that mitochondria stress can lead to release of mtDNA into the cytosol through pores formed by the voltage-dependent anion channel (VDAC) oligomers in the mitochondrial outer membrane and subsequent activation of the STING pathway.[109] Of interest, VBIT-4, a VDAC oligomerization inhibitor, decreased mtDNA release, IFN signaling, NET formation, and disease severity in a murine model of lupus.[109] In vitro, VBIT-4 inhibited mtROS in immune cells, and thus suppressed NET formation in SLE LDGs.[109] Taken together, these findings further confirm mitochondrial dysfunction in the pathogenesis of SLE, suggesting that correcting this dysregulation may represent a novel therapeutic direction in modulation of aberrant neutrophil responses and the treatment of SLE.

Because unique biomechanical properties of lupus LDGs enable their retention in the microvasculature, with potential pathogenic implications in lung and kidney damage and in development of small vessel vasculopathy,[34] development of therapeutics that modulate neutrophil biomechanical properties may represent a new direction to correct the neutrophil dysregulation in SLE.

SUMMARY

Neutrophil dysfunction, in particular aberrant neutrophil subsets and an imbalance between NET formation and degradation, are implicated in SLE pathogenesis. The mechanisms include bidirectional interactions of LDGs/NETs with different components of the innate and adaptive immune arms, modification and externalization of autoantigens, and direct induction of organ and vascular damage. Although correcting neutrophil dysfunction may provide additional efficacy to the current therapeutic strategies, continued efforts are needed to determine how to translate these findings into clinical practice. In addition, further prospective studies will help to understand whether neutrophil-associated biomarkers can provide clinicians with a precision-medicine approach to complex clinical problems, thus improving the clinical decision-making process. Because SLE is a heterogeneous disease with wide range of clinical and laboratory abnormalities, it remains unclear the extent to which NETs may contribute to certain aspects of SLE pathogenesis. In addition, it remains to be determined at which disease stage LDGs and NETs are main contributors to disease pathogenesis. Further investigation on other mechanisms that lead to neutrophil dysregulation in SLE are also needed to provide better molecular candidates for therapeutic targeting.

DISCLOSURE

The authors have nothing to disclose.

REFERENCES

1. Tsokos GC. Autoimmunity and organ damage in systemic lupus erythematosus. Nat Immunol 2020;21(6):605–14.
2. Crow MK, Olferiev M, Kirou KA. Type I interferons in autoimmune disease. Annu Rev Pathol 2019;14:369–93.
3. Liu Y, Kaplan MJ. Neutrophils in the pathogenesis of rheumatic diseases: fueling the fire. Clin Rev Allergy Immunol 2020;60(1):1–16.
4. Mutua V, Gershwin LJ. a review of neutrophil extracellular traps (NETs) in disease: potential anti-NETs therapeutics. Clin Rev Allergy Immunol 2020. https://doi.org/10.1007/s12016-020-08804-7.
5. Mantovani A, Cassatella MA, Costantini C, et al. Neutrophils in the activation and regulation of innate and adaptive immunity. Nat Rev Immunol 2011;11(8):519–31.
6. van Gisbergen KP, Sanchez-Hernandez M, Geijtenbeek TB, et al. Neutrophils mediate immune modulation of dendritic cells through glycosylation-dependent interactions between Mac-1 and DC-SIGN. J Exp Med 2005;201(8):1281–92.
7. Pelletier M, Maggi L, Micheletti A, et al. Evidence for a cross-talk between human neutrophils and Th17 cells. Blood 2010;115(2):335–43.
8. Puga I, Cols M, Barra CM, et al. B cell-helper neutrophils stimulate the diversification and production of immunoglobulin in the marginal zone of the spleen. Nat Immunol 2011;13(2):170–80.
9. Brandt L, Hedberg H. Impaired phagocytosis by peripheral blood granulocytes in systemic lupus erythematosus. Scand J Haematol 1969;6(5):348–53.
10. Donnelly S, Roake W, Brown S, et al. Impaired recognition of apoptotic neutrophils by the C1q/calreticulin and CD91 pathway in systemic lupus erythematosus. Arthritis Rheum 2006;54(5):1543–56.
11. Lood C, Blanco LP, Purmalek MM, et al. Neutrophil extracellular traps enriched in oxidized mitochondrial DNA are interferogenic and contribute to lupus-like disease. Nat Med 2016;22(2):146–53.
12. Hom G, Graham RR, Modrek B, et al. Association of systemic lupus erythematosus with C8orf13-BLK and ITGAM-ITGAX. N Engl J Med 2008;358(9):900–9.
13. Zhou Y, Wu J, Kucik DF, et al. Multiple lupus-associated ITGAM variants alter Mac-1 functions on neutrophils. Arthritis Rheum 2013;65(11):2907–16.
14. Olsson LM, Johansson AC, Gullstrand B, et al. A single nucleotide polymorphism in the NCF1 gene leading to reduced oxidative burst is associated with systemic lupus erythematosus. Ann Rheum Dis 2017;76(9):1607–13.
15. Jacob CO, Eisenstein M, Dinauer MC, et al. Lupus-associated causal mutation in neutrophil cytosolic factor 2 (NCF2) brings unique insights to the structure and function of NADPH oxidase. Proc Natl Acad Sci U S A 2012;109(2):E59–67.

16. Crow MK, Ronnblom L. Type I interferons in host defence and inflammatory diseases. Lupus Sci Med 2019;6(1):e000336.

17. Psarras A, Emery P, Vital EM. Type I interferon-mediated autoimmune diseases: pathogenesis, diagnosis and targeted therapy. Rheumatology (Oxford) 2017; 56(10):1662–75.

18. Ronnblom L, Leonard D. Interferon pathway in SLE: one key to unlocking the mystery of the disease. Lupus Sci Med 2019;6(1):e000270.

19. Lindau D, Mussard J, Rabsteyn A, et al. TLR9 independent interferon alpha production by neutrophils on NETosis in response to circulating chromatin, a key lupus autoantigen. Ann Rheum Dis 2014;73(12):2199–207.

20. Palanichamy A, Bauer JW, Yalavarthi S, et al. Neutrophil-mediated IFN activation in the bone marrow alters B cell development in human and murine systemic lupus erythematosus. J Immunol 2014;192(3):906–18.

21. Rahman S, Sagar D, Hanna RN, et al. Low-density granulocytes activate T cells and demonstrate a non-suppressive role in systemic lupus erythematosus. Ann Rheum Dis 2019;78(7):957–66.

22. van der Linden M, van den Hoogen LL, Westerlaken GHA, et al. Neutrophil extracellular trap release is associated with antinuclear antibodies in systemic lupus erythematosus and anti-phospholipid syndrome. Rheumatology (Oxford) 2018;57(7):1228–34.

23. Midgley A, Beresford MW. Increased expression of low density granulocytes in juvenile-onset systemic lupus erythematosus patients correlates with disease activity. Lupus 2016;25(4):407–11.

24. Denny MF, Yalavarthi S, Zhao W, et al. A distinct subset of proinflammatory neutrophils isolated from patients with systemic lupus erythematosus induces vascular damage and synthesizes type I IFNs. J Immunol 2010;184(6):3284–97.

25. Carmona-Rivera C, Kaplan MJ. Low-density granulocytes: a distinct class of neutrophils in systemic autoimmunity. Semin Immunopathol 2013;35(4):455–63.

26. Sagiv JY, Michaeli J, Assi S, et al. Phenotypic diversity and plasticity in circulating neutrophil subpopulations in cancer. Cell Rep 2015;10(4):562–73.

27. Wu H, Zhen Y, Ma Z, et al. Arginase-1-dependent promotion of TH17 differentiation and disease progression by MDSCs in systemic lupus erythematosus. Sci Transl Med 2016;8(331):331ra340.

28. Villanueva E, Yalavarthi S, Berthier CC, et al. Netting neutrophils induce endothelial damage, infiltrate tissues, and expose immunostimulatory molecules in systemic lupus erythematosus. J Immunol 2011;187(1):538–52.

29. Mistry P, Nakabo S, O'Neil L, et al. Transcriptomic, epigenetic, and functional analyses implicate neutrophil diversity in the pathogenesis of systemic lupus erythematosus. Proc Natl Acad Sci U S A 2019;116(50):25222–8.

30. Grayson PC, Carmona-Rivera C, Xu L, et al. Neutrophil-related gene expression and low-density granulocytes associated with disease activity and response to treatment in antineutrophil cytoplasmic antibody-associated vasculitis. Arthritis Rheum 2015;67(7):1922–32.

31. Liu Y, Xia C, Chen J, et al. Elevated circulating pro-inflammatory low-density granulocytes in adult-onset Still's disease. Rheumatology (Oxford) 2020;60(1): 297–303.

32. Seto N, Torres-Ruiz JJ, Carmona-Rivera C, et al. Neutrophil dysregulation is pathogenic in idiopathic inflammatory myopathies. JCI Insight 2020;5(3): e134189.

33. Coit P, Yalavarthi S, Ognenovski M, et al. Epigenome profiling reveals significant DNA demethylation of interferon signature genes in lupus neutrophils. J Autoimmun 2015;58:59–66.

34. Bashant KR, Aponte AM, Randazzo D, et al. Proteomic, biomechanical and functional analyses define neutrophil heterogeneity in systemic lupus erythematosus. Ann Rheum Dis 2020;80(2):209–18.

35. Garcia-Romo GS, Caielli S, Vega B, et al. Netting neutrophils are major inducers of type I IFN production in pediatric systemic lupus erythematosus. Sci Transl Med 2011;3(73):73ra20.

36. Lande R, Ganguly D, Facchinetti V, et al. Neutrophils activate plasmacytoid dendritic cells by releasing self-DNA-peptide complexes in systemic lupus erythematosus. Sci Transl Med 2011;3(73):73ra19.

37. Brinkmann V, Reichard U, Goosmann C, et al. Neutrophil extracellular traps kill bacteria. Science 2004;303(5663):1532–5.

38. Boeltz S, Amini P, Anders HJ, et al. To NET or not to NET:current opinions and state of the science regarding the formation of neutrophil extracellular traps. Cell Death Differ 2019;26(3):395–408.

39. Apel F, Zychlinsky A, Kenny EF. The role of neutrophil extracellular traps in rheumatic diseases. Nat Rev Rheumatol 2018;14(8):467–75.

40. Li P, Li M, Lindberg MR, et al. PAD4 is essential for antibacterial innate immunity mediated by neutrophil extracellular traps. J Exp Med 2010;207(9):1853–62.

41. Odqvist L, Jevnikar Z, Riise R, et al. Genetic variations in A20 DUB domain provide a genetic link to citrullination and neutrophil extracellular traps in systemic lupus erythematosus. Ann Rheum Dis 2019;78(10):1363–70.

42. Chang HH, Dwivedi N, Nicholas AP, et al. The W620 polymorphism in PTPN22 disrupts its interaction with peptidylarginine deiminase type 4 and enhances citrullination and NETosis. Arthritis Rheumatol 2015;67(9):2323–34.

43. Li D, Matta B, Song S, et al. IRF5 genetic risk variants drive myeloid-specific IRF5 hyperactivation and presymptomatic SLE. JCI Insight 2020;5(2):e124020.

44. Goel RR, Nakabo S, Dizon BLP, et al. Lupus-like autoimmunity and increased interferon response in patients with STAT3-deficient hyper-IgE syndrome. J Allergy Clin Immunol 2020;147(2):746–9.e9.

45. Blazkova J, Gupta S, Liu Y, et al. Multicenter systems analysis of human blood reveals immature neutrophils in males and during pregnancy. J Immunol 2017; 198(6):2479–88.

46. Hakkim A, Furnrohr BG, Amann K, et al. Impairment of neutrophil extracellular trap degradation is associated with lupus nephritis. Proc Natl Acad Sci U S A 2010;107(21):9813–8.

47. Kahlenberg JM, Carmona-Rivera C, Smith CK, et al. Neutrophil extracellular trap-associated protein activation of the NLRP3 inflammasome is enhanced in lupus macrophages. J Immunol 2013;190(3):1217–26.

48. Gehrke N, Mertens C, Zillinger T, et al. Oxidative damage of DNA confers resistance to cytosolic nuclease TREX1 degradation and potentiates STING-dependent immune sensing. Immunity 2013;39(3):482–95.

49. Carmona-Rivera C, Bicker KL, Thompson PR, et al. Response to comment on "synovial fibroblast-neutrophil interactions promote pathogenic adaptive immunity in rheumatoid arthritis". Sci Immunol 2018;3(21):eaar3701.

50. Tillack K, Breiden P, Martin R, et al. T lymphocyte priming by neutrophil extracellular traps links innate and adaptive immune responses. J Immunol 2012;188(7): 3150–9.

51. Gestermann N, Di Domizio J, Lande R, et al. Netting neutrophils activate autoreactive B cells in lupus. J Immunol 2018;200(10):3364–71.
52. Pieterse E, Rother N, Garsen M, et al. Neutrophil extracellular traps drive endothelial-to-mesenchymal transition. Arterioscler Thromb Vasc Biol 2017; 37(7):1371–9.
53. Frangou E, Chrysanthopoulou A, Mitsios A, et al. REDD1/autophagy pathway promotes thromboinflammation and fibrosis in human systemic lupus erythematosus (SLE) through NETs decorated with tissue factor (TF) and interleukin-17A (IL-17A). Ann Rheum Dis 2019;78(2):238–48.
54. Sollberger G, Choidas A, Burn GL, et al. Gasdermin D plays a vital role in the generation of neutrophil extracellular traps. Sci Immunol 2018;3(26):eaar6689.
55. Chen KW, Monteleone M, Boucher D, et al. Noncanonical inflammasome signaling elicits gasdermin D-dependent neutrophil extracellular traps. Sci Immunol 2018;3(26):eaar6676.
56. Wang X, Blanco LP, Carmona-Rivera C, et al. Effects of gasdermin D in modulating murine lupus and its associated organ damage. Arthritis Rheumatol 2020; 72(12):2118–29.
57. Nishi H, Mayadas TN. Neutrophils in lupus nephritis. Curr Opin Rheumatol 2019; 31(2):193–200.
58. Banchereau R, Hong S, Cantarel B, et al. Personalized immunomonitoring uncovers molecular networks that stratify lupus patients. Cell 2016;165(3):551–65.
59. Jourde-Chiche N, Whalen E, Gondouin B, et al. Modular transcriptional repertoire analyses identify a blood neutrophil signature as a candidate biomarker for lupus nephritis. Rheumatology (Oxford) 2017;56(3):477–87.
60. Russell DA, Markiewicz M, Oates JC. Lupus serum induces inflammatory interaction with neutrophils in human glomerular endothelial cells. Lupus Sci Med 2020;7(1):e000418.
61. Wang H, Li T, Chen S, et al. Neutrophil extracellular trap mitochondrial DNA and its autoantibody in systemic lupus erythematosus and a proof-of-concept trial of metformin. Arthritis Rheumatol 2015;67(12):3190–200.
62. Kumar SV, Kulkarni OP, Mulay SR, et al. Neutrophil extracellular trap-related extracellular histones cause vascular necrosis in severe GN. J Am Soc Nephrol 2015;26(10):2399–413.
63. Whittall-Garcia LP, Torres-Ruiz J, Zentella-Dehesa A, et al. Neutrophil extracellular traps are a source of extracellular HMGB1 in lupus nephritis: associations with clinical and histopathological features. Lupus 2019;28(13):1549–57.
64. Liu Y, Kaplan MJ. Cardiovascular disease in systemic lupus erythematosus: an update. Curr Opin Rheumatol 2018;30(5):441–8.
65. Hermansen ML, Lindhardsen J, Torp-Pedersen C, et al. The risk of cardiovascular morbidity and cardiovascular mortality in systemic lupus erythematosus and lupus nephritis: a Danish nationwide population-based cohort study. Rheumatology (Oxford) 2017;56(5):709–15.
66. Rajagopalan S, Somers EC, Brook RD, et al. Endothelial cell apoptosis in systemic lupus erythematosus: a common pathway for abnormal vascular function and thrombosis propensity. Blood 2004;103(10):3677–83.
67. Carlucci PM, Purmalek MM, Dey AK, et al. Neutrophil subsets and their gene signature associate with vascular inflammation and coronary atherosclerosis in lupus. JCI Insight 2018;3(8):e99276.
68. Lopez P, Rodriguez-Carrio J, Martinez-Zapico A, et al. Low-density granulocytes and monocytes as biomarkers of cardiovascular risk in systemic lupus erythematosus. Rheumatology (Oxford) 2020;59(7):1752–64.

69. Knight JS, Zhao W, Luo W, et al. Peptidylarginine deiminase inhibition is immunomodulatory and vasculoprotective in murine lupus. J Clin Invest 2013;123(7): 2981–93.

70. Knight JS, Luo W, O'Dell AA, et al. Peptidylarginine deiminase inhibition reduces vascular damage and modulates innate immune responses in murine models of atherosclerosis. Circ Res 2014;114(6):947–56.

71. Doring Y, Soehnlein O, Weber C. Neutrophil extracellular traps in atherosclerosis and atherothrombosis. Circ Res 2017;120(4):736–43.

72. Liu Y, Carmona-Rivera C, Moore E, et al. Myeloid-specific deletion of peptidylarginine deiminase 4 mitigates atherosclerosis. Front Immunol 2018;9:1680.

73. Folco EJ, Mawson TL, Vromman A, et al. Neutrophil extracellular traps induce endothelial cell activation and tissue factor production through interleukin-1alpha and cathepsin G. Arterioscler Thromb Vasc Biol 2018;38(8):1901–12.

74. Carmona-Rivera C, Zhao W, Yalavarthi S, et al. Neutrophil extracellular traps induce endothelial dysfunction in systemic lupus erythematosus through the activation of matrix metalloproteinase-2. Ann Rheum Dis 2015;74(7):1417–24.

75. Smith CK, Vivekanandan-Giri A, Tang C, et al. Neutrophil extracellular trap-derived enzymes oxidize high-density lipoprotein: an additional proatherogenic mechanism in systemic lupus erythematosus. Arthritis Rheumatol 2014;66(9): 2532–44.

76. Moore S, Juo HH, Nielsen CT, et al. Role of neutrophil extracellular traps regarding patients at risk of increased disease activity and cardiovascular co-morbidity in systemic lupus erythematosus. J Rheumatol 2020;47(11):1652–60.

77. Fuchs TA, Brill A, Duerschmied D, et al. Extracellular DNA traps promote thrombosis. Proc Natl Acad Sci U S A 2010;107(36):15880–5.

78. von Bruhl ML, Stark K, Steinhart A, et al. Monocytes, neutrophils, and platelets cooperate to initiate and propagate venous thrombosis in mice in vivo. J Exp Med 2012;209(4):819–35.

79. Ramirez GA, Efthymiou M, Isenberg DA, et al. Under crossfire: thromboembolic risk in systemic lupus erythematosus. Rheumatology (Oxford) 2019;58(6): 940–52.

80. Safi R, Al-Hage J, Abbas O, et al. Investigating the presence of neutrophil extracellular traps in cutaneous lesions of different subtypes of lupus erythematosus. Exp Dermatol 2019;28(11):1348–52.

81. Knight JS, Subramanian V, O'Dell AA, et al. Peptidylarginine deiminase inhibition disrupts NET formation and protects against kidney, skin and vascular disease in lupus-prone MRL/lpr mice. Ann Rheum Dis 2015;74(12):2199–206.

82. Xu T, Zhang G, Lin H, et al. Clinical characteristics and risk factors of diffuse alveolar hemorrhage in systemic lupus erythematosus: a systematic review and meta-analysis based on observational studies. Clin Rev Allergy Immunol 2020;59(3):295–303.

83. Colby TV, Fukuoka J, Ewaskow SP, et al. Pathologic approach to pulmonary hemorrhage. Ann Diagn Pathol 2001;5(5):309–19.

84. Jarrot PA, Tellier E, Plantureux L, et al. Neutrophil extracellular traps are associated with the pathogenesis of diffuse alveolar hemorrhage in murine lupus. J Autoimmun 2019;100:120–30.

85. Thomas GM, Carbo C, Curtis BR, et al. Extracellular DNA traps are associated with the pathogenesis of TRALI in humans and mice. Blood 2012;119(26): 6335–43.

86. Caudrillier A, Kessenbrock K, Gilliss BM, et al. Platelets induce neutrophil extracellular traps in transfusion-related acute lung injury. J Clin Invest 2012;122(7): 2661–71.

87. Pham DL, Ban GY, Kim SH, et al. Neutrophil autophagy and extracellular DNA traps contribute to airway inflammation in severe asthma. Clin Exp Allergy 2017;47(1):57–70.

88. Lachowicz-Scroggins ME, Dunican EM, Charbit AR, et al. Extracellular DNA, neutrophil extracellular traps, and inflammasome activation in severe asthma. Am J Respir Crit Care Med 2019;199(9):1076–85.

89. Mike EV, Makinde HM, Gulinello M, et al. Lipocalin-2 is a pathogenic determinant and biomarker of neuropsychiatric lupus. J Autoimmun 2019;96:59–73.

90. Trysberg E, Blennow K, Zachrisson O, et al. Intrathecal levels of matrix metalloproteinases in systemic lupus erythematosus with central nervous system engagement. Arthritis Res Ther 2004;6(6):R551–6.

91. Ainiala H, Hietaharju A, Dastidar P, et al. Increased serum matrix metalloproteinase 9 levels in systemic lupus erythematosus patients with neuropsychiatric manifestations and brain magnetic resonance imaging abnormalities. Arthritis Rheum 2004;50(3):858–65.

92. Trysberg E, Carlsten H, Tarkowski A. Intrathecal cytokines in systemic lupus erythematosus with central nervous system involvement. Lupus 2000;9(7): 498–503.

93. Li H, Feng D, Cai Y, et al. Hepatocytes and neutrophils cooperatively suppress bacterial infection by differentially regulating lipocalin-2 and neutrophil extracellular traps. Hepatology 2018;68(4):1604–20.

94. Trysberg E, Nylen K, Rosengren LE, et al. Neuronal and astrocytic damage in systemic lupus erythematosus patients with central nervous system involvement. Arthritis Rheum 2003;48(10):2881–7.

95. Chasset F, Ribi C, Trendelenburg M, et al. Identification of highly active systemic lupus erythematosus by combined type I interferon and neutrophil gene scores vs classical serologic markers. Rheumatology (Oxford) 2020;59(11):3468–78.

96. Zhang S, Zhang Q, Wang F, et al. Hydroxychloroquine inhibiting neutrophil extracellular trap formation alleviates hepatic ischemia/reperfusion injury by blocking TLR9 in mice. Clin Immunol 2020;216:108461.

97. Gupta AK, Giaglis S, Hasler P, et al. Efficient neutrophil extracellular trap induction requires mobilization of both intracellular and extracellular calcium pools and is modulated by cyclosporine A. PLoS One 2014;9(5):e97088.

98. Kraaij T, Kamerling SWA, de Rooij ENM, et al. The NET-effect of combining rituximab with belimumab in severe systemic lupus erythematosus. J Autoimmun 2018;91:45–54.

99. Sun F, Geng S, Wang H, et al. Effects of metformin on disease flares in patients with systemic lupus erythematosus: post hoc analyses from two randomised trials. Lupus Sci Med 2020;7(1):e000429.

100. Menegazzo L, Scattolini V, Cappellari R, et al. The antidiabetic drug metformin blunts NETosis in vitro and reduces circulating NETosis biomarkers in vivo. Acta Diabetol 2018;55(6):593–601.

101. Furumoto Y, Smith CK, Blanco L, et al. Tofacitinib ameliorates murine lupus and its associated vascular dysfunction. Arthritis Rheumatol 2017;69(1):148–60.

102. Warnatsch A, Ioannou M, Wang Q, et al. Inflammation. Neutrophil extracellular traps license macrophages for cytokine production in atherosclerosis. Science 2015;349(6245):316–20.

103. Liu Y, Lightfoot YL, Seto N, et al. Peptidylarginine deiminases 2 and 4 modulate innate and adaptive immune responses in TLR-7-dependent lupus. JCI Insight 2018;3(23):e124729.
104. Hanata N, Shoda H, Hatano H, et al. Peptidylarginine deiminase 4 promotes the renal infiltration of neutrophils and exacerbates the TLR7 agonist-induced lupus mice. Front Immunol 2020;11:1095.
105. Gordon RA, Herter JM, Rosetti F, et al. Lupus and proliferative nephritis are PAD4 independent in murine models. JCI Insight 2017;2(10):e92926.
106. Kienhofer D, Hahn J, Stoof J, et al. Experimental lupus is aggravated in mouse strains with impaired induction of neutrophil extracellular traps. JCI Insight 2017; 2(10):e92920.
107. Blanco LP, Pedersen HL, Wang X, et al. Improved mitochondrial metabolism and reduced inflammation following attenuation of murine lupus with coenzyme Q10 analog idebenone. Arthritis Rheumatol 2020;72(3):454–64.
108. Fortner KA, Blanco LP, Buskiewicz I, et al. Targeting mitochondrial oxidative stress with MitoQ reduces NET formation and kidney disease in lupus-prone MRL-lpr mice. Lupus Sci Med 2020;7(1):e000387.
109. Kim J, Gupta R, Blanco LP, et al. VDAC oligomers form mitochondrial pores to release mtDNA fragments and promote lupus-like disease. Science 2019; 366(6472):1531–6.

The Power of Systems Biology

Insights on Lupus Nephritis from the Accelerating Medicines Partnership

Andrea Fava, MD[a,*], Soumya Raychaudhuri, MD, PhD[b,c,d,e], Deepak A. Rao, MD, PhD[b,*]

KEYWORDS

- Lupus nephritis • SLE • Accelerating medicines partnership • AMP • scRNA-seq
- Proteomics • Transcriptomics • Biomarker

KEY POINTS

- The Accelerating Medicines Partnership (AMP) SLE network developed a set of protocols for multiomic analyses of renal tissue, urine, and blood to study lupus nephritis.
- Single-cell transcriptomic studies from the AMP cataloged the kidney-infiltrating immune cell populations and the parenchymal cell signatures that characterize lupus nephritis kidney biopsies, and the immune cells that accumulate in urine.
- Proteomic studies of urine from patients with lupus nephritis identified protein biomarkers highly enriched in disease, which provided insights into pathogenesis and advanced progress toward liquid biopsies.
- Mass cytometry analyses of blood cells highlighted specific CD4[+] T-cell and B-cell phenotypes expanded in lupus nephritis.

INTRODUCTION

Lupus nephritis (LN) affects 50% to 70% of patients with systemic lupus erythematosus (SLE), especially those of non-European ancestry. Up to 20% of patients with LN

[a] Division of Rheumatology, Johns Hopkins University, 1830 East Monument Street, Suite 7500, Baltimore, MD 21205, USA; [b] Division of Rheumatology, Inflammation, Immunity, Department of Medicine, Brigham and Women's Hospital, Harvard Medical School, Boston, MA, USA; [c] Center for Data Sciences, Brigham and Women's Hospital, Building for Transformative Medicine, 60 Fenwood Road, Boston, MA 02115, USA; [d] Program in Medical and Population Genetics, Broad Institute of MIT and Harvard, Cambridge, MA, USA; [e] Centre for Genetics and Genomics Versus Arthritis, Centre for Musculoskeletal Research, Manchester Academic Health Science Centre, The University of Manchester, Oxford Road, Manchester, UK
* Corresponding authors.
E-mail addresses: afava1@jh.edu (A.F.); darao@bwh.harvard.edu (D.A.R.)
Twitter: @andreafava (A.F.); @soumya_boston (S.R.); @Deepakarao (D.A.R.)

Rheum Dis Clin N Am 47 (2021) 335–350
https://doi.org/10.1016/j.rdc.2021.04.003
0889-857X/21/© 2021 Elsevier Inc. All rights reserved.
rheumatic.theclinics.com

develop end-stage kidney disease, and up to 40% of those with International Society of Nephrology/Renal Pathology Society class III, IV, or V nephritis progress to renal impairment.[1–4] Despite optimal treatment, the response rate is only 30% to 40%.[5,6] These findings support the heterogeneity of SLE and LN in terms of histologic, clinical, and immunologic features and suggest that distinct pathogenic mechanisms may drive disease in distinct patient subgroups, who converge in the LN diagnosis. Deep molecular dissection of LN may reveal novel disease mechanisms or unique patient subgroups to help understand this heterogeneity, leading to novel therapeutic strategies and more efficient treatment selection.[7]

The Accelerating Medicines Partnership (AMP) is a collaborative initiative led by the National Institutes of Health bringing together academia, government, nonprofit, and pharmaceutical industry partners to pursue moonshot projects to accelerate discovery, development, and validation of new disease treatments. There are currently five AMP projects evaluating a range of diseases: (1) Alzheimer disease, (2) type 2 diabetes, (3) Parkinson disease, (4) schizophrenia, and (5) autoimmunity. The AMP project on autoimmunity has focused on two rheumatic diseases, SLE and rheumatoid arthritis (RA), forming the joint AMP RA/SLE Network. To achieve the ambitious goal of new target discovery and validation in SLE, the AMP SLE Network took the approach of systems biology to dissect the complex immune and parenchymal responses in patients with LN, using multiple omics technologies (multiomics) including single-cell RNA-sequencing (scRNA-seq) of renal tissue, urine sediment, skin, and peripheral blood; longitudinal urine proteomics; peripheral blood mass cytometry; and genotyping. Between 2014 and 2020, the AMP SLE Network enrolled more than 300 patients with class III, IV, or V LN who underwent a clinically indicated kidney biopsy from 15 clinical sites in the United States.

The AMP SLE effort developed in three phases (**Fig. 1**). Multiple experimental protocols and pipelines were envisioned, tested, and optimized in phase 0. In phase 1, the candidate pipelines were applied to small cohorts of patients (n = 20–40) to assess feasibility, detect pitfalls, and generate preliminary data. Phase 1 was central to identify sources of biologic variability to optimize patient selection, develop computational tools, and make initial discoveries. Phase 2 entails the generation of large-scale (n >150 patients) multiomic data and its dissemination as a public resource. Here, we review the results from the analyses of phase 1 data, which have already produced several important discoveries impacting the understanding of LN, and the anticipated directions of the ongoing phase 2 analyses.

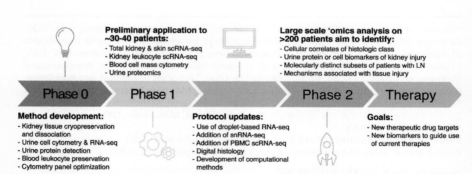

Fig. 1. The AMP in SLE project timeline. The AMP developed in three major operational phases. PBMC, peripheral blood mononuclear cells; snRNA-seq, single nucleus sequencing.

SINGLE-CELL ANALYSIS OF KIDNEY IN LUPUS NEPHRITIS

A central goal of the AMP SLE Network has been to generate a detailed catalog of the cell types and cell states present in kidneys affected by LN using single-cell transcriptomics. To achieve this, the network developed standardized protocols to collect and store kidney biopsy tissue for research and to generate scRNA-seq data from cells obtained from LN kidney tissue. Three aspects of the kidney scRNA-seq experience merit particular emphasis: (1) methods to develop a biorepository of kidney tissue samples containing viable cells; (2) flexible, multipronged approaches to generate single-cell omics datasets; and (3) catalogs of cell types that accumulate in LN kidneys. We discuss of these features in the following paragraphs.

Generation of a Biorepository of Tissue Samples with Viable Cells

Collection, transport, and storage of tissue samples is a major challenge for studies using high-dimensional analyses of patient samples. The AMP SLE Network established institutional review board protocols at participating sites to allow for collection of a specimen of kidney biopsy designated for research, separate from the tissue used for diagnostic pathology. This was typically collected as an independent biopsy core obtained specifically for research; in some cases, a portion of a biopsy core obtained for diagnostic evaluation was allocated for research after sufficient diagnostic material was obtained.

One major innovation from the AMP SLE Network experience was the development of protocols to preserve and store kidney biopsy tissue after collection. Kidney biopsy samples had to be collected at multiple sites across the country, yet only a few sites had the equipment and facilities needed to dissociate kidney tissue into single cells and generate scRNA-seq data. Furthermore, given the high sensitivity of single-cell transcriptomics to variation because of technical effects in sample processing, the network prioritized running samples through a uniform tissue processing pipeline at a single site to minimize experimental noise in the data.[8] Multiple shipping and storage strategies were evaluated, including shipping fresh tissue overnight on wet ice or dissociating kidney tissue and freezing cells at each site, yet the strategy with most advantages was perhaps the simplest: cryopreserving the intact kidney tissue biopsy at each site for short- or long-term storage.[9,10] Head-to-head comparisons of different storage and processing conditions demonstrated that kidney tissue can be cryopreserved in a dimethyl sulfoxide–containing cryoprotectant solution, similar to the manner in which peripheral blood mononuclear cells (PBMC) are cryopreserved.[9,10] Cryopreserved kidney tissue is stored for prolonged periods and shipped on dry ice. After thawing, tissue is dissociated as is done for freshly collected tissue, yielding viable cells for cytometry or transcriptomic analyses. The viability of different cell types varies with cryopreservation; most leukocytes and stromal cells surviving freeze/thaw well, whereas epithelial cells may be more susceptible to injury in the process.[9,10] This strategy, which has also recently been used for synovium, skin, and gut biopsies,[11–13] allows for the collection of a large biorepository of tissue samples containing viable cells. In phase 2, the AMP SLE Network has used this approach to amass a collection of greater than 200 kidney biopsies, which were stored through the recruitment phase so that they could be processed in a uniform manner after all samples were collected. The ability to run all samples in a short time period, with a defined set of reagents from the same lot, is likely to minimize technical variation that can accrue over time with subtle changes in reagents, technical details, personnel, and equipment. Generation of this type of biorepository also allows the potential to use new technologies that emerge in the future.

Parallel Pipelines to Ask Distinct Questions

scRNA-seq transcriptomics applied to patient samples, such as kidney biopsies, can generate rich datasets for discovery without requiring prespecified hypotheses. However, critical decisions must be made in the experimental design to generate datasets appropriate to evaluate key questions of the study. For example, to understand the cellular characteristics of global inflammatory responses induced in LN kidneys, it is of interest to gather a broad look at the transcriptomic signatures of all cells in the kidney. This is achieved by subjecting the total single-cell suspension of cells obtained from kidney tissue to scRNA-seq. However, it is also of major interest to analyze in detail the infiltrating leukocytes, which represent approximately 5% of total cells in kidney yet are key inducers of tissue injury. Analyzing sufficient numbers of leukocytes requires an effort to enrich these cells so they are not swamped out by the much larger numbers of tubular epithelial cells.

To balance these priorities, the AMP SLE Network ran two parallel pipelines in phase 1. One pipeline generated single-cell transcriptomes of total kidney cells, which was heavily represented by epithelial cells. This analysis revealed a clear interferon signature among tubular epithelial cells in LN and also highlighted a fibrosis-associated signature in tubular epithelium.[14] An interferon signature was also detected in keratinocytes from nonlesional, non-sun-exposed skin in patients with LN in a parallel study.[15] A separate pipeline specifically isolated CD45[+] leukocytes by flow cytometric cell sorting, providing a high-resolution view of the infiltrating leukocytes in the kidney.[10] These two pipelines were required to generate datasets to evaluate two distinct but complementary questions.

As new methods have emerged, additional options have become available to help analyze kidney biopsy samples. For one, the rapid maturation of droplet-based single-cell analyses has dramatically increased the number of cells that are analyzed by scRNA-seq.[16,17] After additional pipeline development following phase 1, the AMP SLE Network adopted droplet-based scRNA-seq via the 10X Genomics platform for analysis of samples in phase 2. In addition, single-nucleus sequencing (snRNA-seq) opened the possibility to more efficiently capture and analyze cells that are difficult to extract from intact tissues.[18] In kidney, this seems particularly useful for podocytes, which are challenging to isolate from kidney as intact, viable cells through mechanical dissociation and enzymatic digestion.[19] snRNA-seq offers a different approach, in which intact nuclei are collected even from tissues that do not easily yield intact cells.[18,20] This method facilitates study of cells that are underrepresented in scRNA-seq data and can avoid technical artifacts induced by enzymatic tissue digestion.[21] However, direct comparisons of scRNA-seq and snRNA-seq demonstrated that snRNA-seq is less effective at capturing and analyzing leukocytes.[20,21] In phase 2, again two parallel analyses are being used, using 10X Genomics platforms, with parallel snRNA-seq and scRNA-seq run on the same tissue samples. Given the rapid development of new technologies, including chromatin profiling in individual cells with single-cell ATAC-seq[22,23] and spatially resolved transcriptomics and proteomics,[24–26] the menu of options for single-cell analysis is likely to continue to expand.

Catalog of Immune Cells that Accumulate in Lupus Nephritis

The flagship achievement of the AMP SLE Network thus far has been the description of single-cell transcriptomic catalogs of parenchymal cells and leukocytes from within LN kidneys generated in phase 1. Analyses of the CD45[+] leukocytes revealed multiple clusters of different immune cell subsets, with some surprising patterns (**Fig. 2A**). The single largest cluster of immune cells was comprised of natural killer (NK) cells,

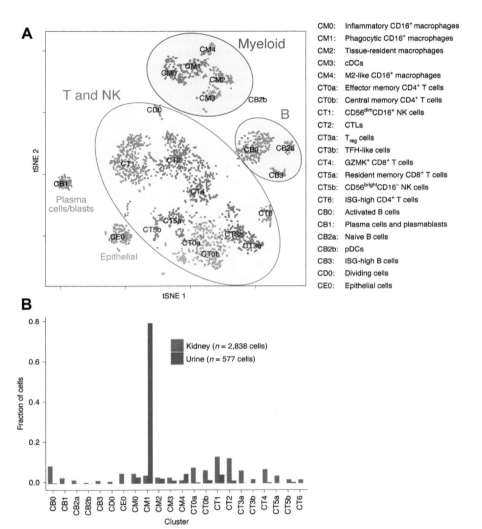

CM0:	Inflammatory CD16+ macrophages
CM1:	Phagocytic CD16+ macrophages
CM2:	Tissue-resident macrophages
CM3:	cDCs
CM4:	M2-like CD16+ macrophages
CT0a:	Effector memory CD4+ T cells
CT0b:	Central memory CD4+ T cells
CT1:	CD56dimCD16+ NK cells
CT2:	CTLs
CT3a:	Treg cells
CT3b:	TFH-like cells
CT4:	GZMK+ CD8+ T cells
CT5a:	Resident memory CD8+ T cells
CT5b:	CD56brightCD16− NK cells
CT6:	ISG-high CD4+ T cells
CB0:	Activated B cells
CB1:	Plasma cells and plasmablasts
CB2a:	Naïve B cells
CB2b:	pDCs
CB3:	ISG-high B cells
CD0:	Dividing cells
CE0:	Epithelial cells

Fig. 2. Summary of kidney-infiltrating immune cells and urine cells in LN by scRNA-seq. (*A*) tSNE plot displaying the 22 cell clusters identified in kidney biopsies from 24 patients with LN and 10 healthy donors; their identities are specified on the right. (*B*) The relative frequency of each cluster in urine and in kidney. NK, natural killer cell; tSNE; t-distributed stochastic neighbor embedding. (*Adapted from* Arazi A, Rao DA, Berthier CC, et al. The immune cell landscape in kidneys of patients with lupus nephritis. *Nat Immunol.* 2019;20(7):902-914; with permission.)

followed next by a substantial cluster of cytotoxic CD8 T cells with transcriptomic features that largely overlapped with the NK cells.[10] These cell populations suggest a significant cytotoxic cell component to LN, although the locations, cellular targets, and downstream effects of these cytotoxic leukocytes remain to be determined. Clustering approaches also highlighted a second, distinct population of CD8 T cells with little resemblance to cytotoxic CD8 cells; this second cluster was characterized by high expression of granzyme K but little granzyme B.[10] This granzyme K+ CD8 population also appears in scRNA-seq datasets of other inflamed tissues, including in RA synovium[11] and in immune-infiltrated tumors,[27] yet the functions of these cells are not yet understood. T-cell clusters also included a T-follicular helper (Tfh)-like population that may contain Tfh cells and T-peripheral helper (Tph) cells, both of which help stimulate B-cell activation and antibody production in SLE.[10,28] B-cell clusters in LN included a population of plasmablasts/plasma cells, and a range of activated B cells including some with features of CD11c+ Tbet+ age-associated B cells.[10,29] Myeloid cell clusters included subsets of patrolling monocytes, tissue resident macrophages, and a dendritic cell population.[10]

These observations provide an initial view of the immune cells that infiltrate LN kidneys, yet many steps remain to use these observations to improve care of patients with LN. Although a landmark effort, the phase 1 analysis provided in total 2736 leukocytes obtained from 24 patient samples; no correlations between cellular phenotypes and either histologic or clinical features were identified, possibly because of the low numbers of cells and patients. Major questions of clinical relevance remain, such as (1) which cell types are associated with different glomerulonephritis classes or with the presence of interstitial infiltrates, (2) are there cellular phenotypes that are associated with better prognosis or a good clinical response to treatment, and (3) can cellular phenotypes be used to identify patients with immunologically distinct disease that should be treated differently? Phase 2 analyses of kidney biopsies from more than 150 patients will offer more power to begin to inform these questions. Phase 1 results also raise mechanistic questions that can be asked in subsequent studies, including (1) which signals draw specific cell types into the kidney, (2) where are specific cell populations located and with what cell types do they interact, and (3) which cell types are most responsible for damage to tubules or damage to glomeruli?

URINE AS A SURROGATE TISSUE

In parallel to analyses of kidney cells, the AMP SLE Network has studied urine from patients with LN in the hope of finding features in the urine that convey the upstream pathology in the kidney. Urinary biomarkers may revolutionize the diagnosis and management of LN by enabling noninvasive determination of nephritis type or activity, tracking response to treatment longitudinally, and description of intrarenal biology, thus guiding treatment selection. Urine biomarkers may in fact enhance information obtained from kidney biopsies not only by providing information about active biologic pathways in real time, but also encompassing the totality of kidneys, not just the sampled tissue at time of biopsy. Such features have the potential to obviate a kidney biopsy.

Two major types of assays have been run on urine by the AMP SLE Network: cytometric and transcriptomic analyses of immune cells from urine, and broad analyses of proteins in the urine. We discuss each of these analyses in the following sections.

Analysis of Cells in Urine

It has been well appreciated that immune cells accumulate in the urine in multiple conditions of kidney inflammation, including in LN and in renal allograft rejection.[10,30–33] Despite the harsh conditions in urine, these cells are pelleted from urine and collected for cytometric and transcriptomic analyses. Cytometry studies have at times been complicated by the autofluorescence caused by proteins abundant in urine; however, careful selection of fluorophores allows for clear identification of immune cell subsets from urine samples, including monocytes, CD4 T cells, and CD8 T cells.[9] Compared with kidney tissue, the relative frequencies of T cells and monocytes are skewed in urine, with monocytes representing by far the most abundant mononuclear leukocyte in urine (**Fig. 2**B).[10,34,35] Although B cells are rare in urine from patients with LN, T cells are collected in sufficient numbers for detailed analyses. Prior work has highlighted an increased number of T cells in the urine of patients with LN,[36,37] in particular CXCR3[+] T cells,[36] and follow-up work in larger cohorts of patient with SLE indicated that urinary CD4[+] T cells are a robust marker of proliferative nephritis that improves with treatment.[30] In addition to cytometry, high-quality RNA-seq transcriptomes are generated from sorted bulk T-cell and monocyte populations and from leukocytes sorted as single cells from urine of patients with LN.[9,10] Single-cell transcriptomes of urine leukocytes in LN correspond to cell populations from within LN kidney tissue (see **Fig. 2**B)[10]; these analyses suggested enrichment of a specific population of phagocytic patrolling monocytes in LN urine.[10] Although single-cell transcriptomes have been reported thus far from only a small number of patients in AMP SLE Network, the promising preliminary work suggests that it may be possible to detect and quantify components of intrarenal immune response by studying in detail the cells that accumulate in urine, a possibility that will be explored in phase 2.

Proteomic Analyses of Urine

Urine collects the by-products of intrarenal biologic processes, such as inflammation, tubular damage, or tissue remodeling. Because these molecules can be quantified, urine proteomics provides a powerful opportunity to discover new mechanisms of disease and to develop noninvasive biomarkers.

Several urinary biomarkers have shown promise in LN, but none are currently used in clinical practice, because most lack the sensitivity and specificity to detect active renal inflammation or do not provide benefit over measuring other available biomarkers, such as proteinuria.[38,39] Unbiased proteomic screenings carry a high potential for discovery, but these have been limited to the evaluation of proteins or peptides sufficiently abundant to be detectable by mass spectrometry.[40] In the phase 0, the AMP SLE Network explored different approaches, such as mass spectrometry, peptidome analysis by capillary electrophoresis/mass spectrometry, and a sensitive large proteomic array to longitudinally quantify 1000 urinary proteins in patients with biopsy-proven LN. Compared with the mass spectrometry–based assays, proteomic arrays provided the most biologically interpretable data and undetectable evidence of batch effect. Urine samples were collected at or near the time of biopsy to study their association with real-time histologic features and renal single-cell transcriptomics, and then prospectively after 3, 6, and 12 months.

The approach to high-dimensional data is data-driven (agnostic) or hypothesis-driven. In an agnostic approach, the AMP SLE Network explored the biologic patterns emerging from an unbiased analysis of urine proteomics in LN.[41] Although the initial expectation was to detect clusters of patients characterized by distinct biologic processes (ie, B, T, or myeloid cell activation, tissue remodeling, ischemia), it became evident that patients stratified over a gradient characterized by interferon-γ-inducible chemokines (**Fig. 3**A, B). Higher gradient values identified patients with proliferative LN. Renal single-cell transcriptomics confirmed that interferon-γ was one of the most expressed cytokines in the kidney. Integrating the urine proteomics with single-cell transcriptomics of kidney biopsies revealed that the urinary chemokines defining the gradient were predominantly produced by infiltrating CD8[+] T cells, along with NK and myeloid cells (**Fig. 3**C). The urine chemokine gradient significantly correlated with the number of kidney-infiltrating CD8[+] cells (**Fig. 3**D). These promising preliminary findings suggest that urine proteomics can capture and quantify the complex biology of the kidney in LN. These results also indicate that urine studies may enhance

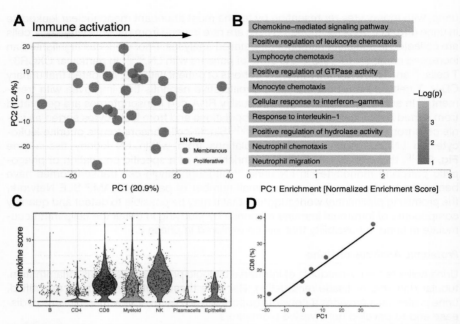

Fig. 3. Integration of urine proteomics and kidney single-cell transcriptomics identified an interferon-γ response gradient in LN. (*A*) PCA of the first two PCs of the urine proteome (% variance explained is indicated). Patients with higher PC1 value almost exclusively have proliferative LN (class III, IV, or mixed). (*B*) Top 10 enriched pathways detected by PC1 using Gene Ontology Biological Process, indicating the biologic significance of PC1. (*C*) Chemokine response scores (GO:0070098) in LN single-cell transcriptional profiles identified kidney-infiltrating myeloid, CD8$^+$, and NK cells as the main producers of the chemokines in response to interferon-γ detected in the urine by PC1. (*D*) Urine PC1 values correlated with the frequency of kidney-infiltrating CD8$^+$ T cells. PCA, principal component analysis. (*Adapted from* Fava A, Buyon J, Mohan C, et al. Integrated urine proteomics and renal single-cell genomics identify an IFN-γ response gradient in lupus nephritis. *JCI Insight.* 2020;5(12); with permission).

the information obtained by kidney histology. Analyses from hypothesis-driven approaches to identify novel urinary biomarkers and potentially treatable targets and additional studies on peptidome-based classifiers are underway. Larger scale longitudinal proteomic studies in the AMP phase 2 (n ~ 200), bolstered by their integration with matching omics, will provide a discovery springboard to develop novel biomarkers and better understand LN pathogenesis.

PERIPHERAL BLOOD CELL ANALYSES

To be able to assess alterations in circulating immune cells in LN, the AMP SLE Network pursued high-dimensional cytometry of blood samples from the same cohorts of patients with LN. Immune cells from blood were collected by two methods to enable detailed analyses of different cell types. PBMC were isolated by density centrifugation of anticoagulated whole blood, as is routinely done. In addition, a separate sample of blood was subjected to hypotonic red blood cell lysis, and the total leukocytes, including neutrophils, were cryopreserved to enable evaluation of granulocytes, which are lost during density centrifugation to isolate PBMC.

Neutrophils typically do not survive freeze/thaw well, therefore a method was developed to stabilize the neutrophils with light fixation immediately after thawing the cells. This novel approach allowed for detailed phenotyping of PBMC and neutrophils by mass cytometry. Both PBMC and total leukocytes were analyzed with greater than 35 marker mass cytometry panels, with panels emphasizing T-cell and B-cell markers used on PBMC, and panels emphasizing granulocyte makers used on total leukocytes. In both cases, samples from patients with SLE were run in with samples from patients with RA and control subjects in barcoded batches of 20 samples each.

Thus far, the CD4 and B-cell phenotypes have been explored in the most depth in this cohort. Dimensional reduction and clustering analyses of CD4$^+$ T cells revealed a marked expansion of PD-1^{hi} ICOS$^+$ CXCR5$^-$ Tph cells, a B-cell-helper T-cell subset enriched in inflamed tissues,[42] as the most prominently expanded CD4$^+$ T-cell population in the circulation of patients with LN.[28] Expansion of Tph cells exceeded that of PD-1^{hi} CXCR5$^+$ Tfh cells and was positively associated with clinical disease activity measured by systemic lupus erythematosus disease activity index (SLEDAI) in this cohort. Similar analysis of the B cells highlighted an expansion of CD11c$^+$ CD21$^-$ CXCR5$^-$ B cells in patients with LN. Both expansion of Tph cells and CD11c$^+$ B cells was greater in patients with SLE than in the patients with RA studied in phase 1 of the AMP.[28] The frequencies of Tph cells and CD11c$^+$ B cells were strongly positively correlated in patients with SLE and RA.[28] These observations highlight the dramatic changes in circulating T-cell and B-cell phenotypes evident in patients with LN. Correlating circulating immune cell phenotypes with intrarenal phenotypes will be of substantial interest as larger cohorts are analyzed. In addition, exploring phenotypes of other immune cell types, such as NK cells, or neutrophils captured in total leukocyte preparations[43] may add additional dimensions to the understanding of immune dysregulation in LN.

COMPUTATIONAL DEVELOPMENTS
Novel Computational Approaches

The recent explosion in the ability to systematically measure thousands of features at the single-cell level has brought new analytical challenges. Because the crude comprehension of high-dimensional data far exceeds the capability of the human brain,[44] computational tools to accurately resolve multilayered information are necessary to generate results for biologic interpretation.

Identification of expanded cell populations across groups
Case-control single-cells studies have the potential to reveal expanded pathogenic cell populations in immune-mediated diseases. A typical starting approach for analysis of high-dimensional single-cell data, including scRNA-seq or mass cytometry data, is to aggregate individual cells into populations using Louvain clustering or other clustering methods, and then to evaluate whether the frequencies of specific cell clusters are altered in disease samples compared with control subjects. However, direct comparison of the frequency of each cell cluster in disease and control using univariate approaches, such as a Student t test or a nonparametric Mann-Whitney test, poses several challenges. This approach is markedly underpowered because it relies on reducing single-cell data to potentially inaccurate per-sample subset frequencies. Furthermore, technologies, such as scRNA-seq and mass cytometry may be sensitive to unwanted sources of variation, such as processing batch, sample quality, or donor-specific features. To overcome these challenges, a method to measure mixed-effects association of single cells was developed.[45] Mixed-effects association of single cells takes full advantage of single-cell measurements by using a "reverse association"

framework to test whether case-control status influences the membership of a given cell in a population (ie, each single cell was treated as a single event). In addition, the use of a mixed-effects logistic regression model allowed to account for covariance in single-cell data induced by technical and biologic factors that could confound association signals, without inflated association tests. The application of mixed-effects association of single cells enabled the discovery of expanded cell populations in several conditions including SLE,[43] RA,[11] and COVID-19.[46]

Harmonization of single-cell omics datasets and mitigation of batch effect

Unbiased single-cell transcriptional profiling provides precise information as to the transcriptional identity of each single cell. As such, knowledge derived from distinct experiments could be combined to generate comprehensive catalogs to define the cellular basis of health and disease as aspired by the Human Cell Atlas project.[47] This effort requires the ability to integrate multiple datasets across studies, donors, and technological platforms. Harmony[48] was developed to tackle this challenge. Harmony is a fast and scalable algorithm that enables robust integration of multiple scRNA-seq datasets.[48] In addition, the implementation of Harmony in the AMP and other project pipelines allowed to minimize batch effect from technical and biologic confounders.[11,49] In a step further, Symphony[50] was developed to efficiently map single-cell transcriptional profiles to a reference dataset.

These analytical methods have been instrumental in extracting insights from the AMP datasets and provide critical tools to investigators across the scientific community to analyze and integrate single-cell studies, potentially paving the path to get closer to the ground truth of cell biology. To promote the goal of accelerating discovery and development of new treatments, the AMP RA/SLE Network provides open access to the data generated so as to provide a worldwide resource and foster all possible contributions. The scRNA-seq data from phase 1 are accessed and easily browsed at https://immunogenomics.io/ampsle/ and https://singlecell.broadinstitute.org/single_cell/study/SCP279/amp-phase-1. A World Wide Web portal to allow access and use of the phase 2 data is being developed.

ANTICIPATING THE POTENTIAL OF PHASE 2

Although the results from the preliminary phases of AMP SLE effort have provided novel insights into LN pathology, the major advance in phase 2 is that multiomics studies are being pursued on a much larger group of patients, including a core cohort of greater than 150 patients with kidney, urine, and blood samples collected at or near the time of kidney biopsy (**Fig. 4**, **Table 1**). These comprehensive biologic data from multiple omics modalities will be matched to detailed longitudinal clinical information, providing unprecedented power to associate cellular or molecular features with clinical disease phenotypes. The potential discoveries that may emerge from this dataset will likely far outstrip what one can imagine here, yet we highlight two promising directions where this dataset may be particularly valuable.

Identifying Clinical and Demographic Correlates of Cellular Pathology, and Vice Versa

The AMP SLE Network has collected detailed demographic and longitudinal clinical features for patients enrolled in the study. The patients enrolled by the AMP SLE Network well represent the demographics of LN in the United States, including 83% female, 44% Black/African American, 29% White, 17% Asian, and 28% Hispanic/Latinx patients, with a mean age of 35.6 years.[51] This is of particular importance because even though Blacks and African-Americans make up almost 50%

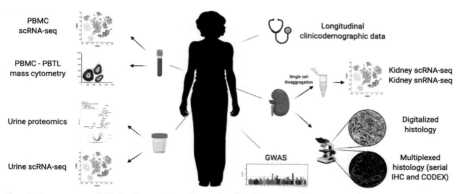

Fig. 4. Summary of AMP phase 2 studies. The final phase of the LN AMP involves the generation of multiomics as detailed in **Table 1**. CODEX, CO-Detection by indexing; GWAS, genome-wide association study; IHC, immunohistochemistry; PBTL, peripheral blood total leukocytes.

of LN cases in the United States,[52] their representation in clinical trials is less than 15% and declining,[53] highlighting the critical need to include this group in LN studies.

The integration of multiomic studies in phase 2 AMP with granular clinicodemographic information is critical to define the clinical correlates of novel patient subsets that may be revealed by molecular studies. Conversely, the AMP SLE studies enable investigators to explore the differences at the molecular level in groups with distinct clinicodemographic features (ie, membranous LN and proliferative LN, or treatment responders and nonresponders). Although ambitious, we find it likely that the phase 2 data will enable sequences such as this: (1) correlating scRNA-seq cell clusters with renal metrics highlights a specific kidney-infiltrating immune cell associated

Table 1
AMP phase 2 studies

	Visit (mo)			
	0	3	6	12
Renal scRNA-seq	x			
Renal snRNA-seq	s			
Urine scRNA-seq	x	s		s
PBMC scRNA-seq	x	s		s
PBMC mass cytometry	x	s		s
PBTL mass cytometry	x			
Urine proteomics	x	x	x	x
Multiplexed histology	x			
Digital histology	x			
GWAS	x			
Clinical parameters	x	x	x	x

A core set of at least 160 samples from unique patients has been collected at or near the time of kidney biopsy (visit Month 0). Visits with available study data for all the patients ("x") or a subset ("s") are shown.
Abbreviations: GWAS, genome-wide association study; PBTL, peripheral blood total leukocytes.

with poor prognosis; (2) receptor-ligand expression patterns predict associated cell networks; (3) multiplexed histology pinpoints the localization of the infiltrating cell population; (4) quantification of the specific cell type in blood or urine is found to correlate with intrarenal levels and prognosis, providing a surrogate biomarker; and (5) differential expression analyses identify unique features of the cell population that are leveraged to develop a new biologic therapy to target this cell population in patients in whom the cell type is expanded.

Looking Across Diseases for Tissue Agnostic Disease Mechanisms

Defining characteristic cellular and molecular abnormalities in high resolution across many patients will allow for a detailed and nuanced description of the range of immunologic phenotypes in SLE, which will help in comparison with other autoimmune disease. Relatives of patients with SLE have higher risk of developing other autoimmune diseases,[54] suggesting that common core mechanisms may drive distinct autoimmune and inflammatory diseases. The parallel study of LN kidney and RA synovium in the AMP phase 1 provided further support for this idea, revealing striking similarities among the immune cell types infiltrating these distinct tissues.[10,11,46] For example, discrete regulatory T-cell clusters, distinct from other effector T-cell population, were present in both tissues. CXCL13-associated Tph or Tfh cell clusters appeared in both tissues. In addition, distinct populations of CD8 T cells, distinguished in part by reciprocal expression of granzyme B and granzyme K, were present in both tissues. However, cross-disease comparisons also suggest differentially active pathways, such as a much more prominent interferon signature in cells from LN compared with RA synovium and a more pronounced representation of cytotoxic lymphocytes in LN kidneys, which may have important therapeutic implications.[10,11] Studies from AMP RA/SLE phase 2 should have enough power to define differences in the transcriptional profiles within similar tissue-infiltrating cell populations as compared between SLE and RA. Importantly, initial analyses integrating LN and RA studies with scRNA-seq data obtained from colon in inflammatory bowel disease, lung in interstitial lung disease, and bronchoalveolar lavage in COVID-19 infection revealed a shared and expanded macrophage phenotype driven by tumor necrosis factor and interferon-γ.[46] The success of baricitinib as an RA and also a COVID-19 medication suggests further the important role of interferon-γ.[55,56] A broader comparison across tissues from multiple autoimmune diseases, tumors, and infections may provide a roadmap and a rationale for repurposing medications in clinically dissimilar diseases and to envision the development of "tissue agnostic"[57] treatments based on molecular mechanisms rather than clinical syndromes.

SUMMARY

The AMP efforts have demonstrated the power of collaboration of a richly diverse network. The AMP SLE Network united expertise in clinical, basic, and data science across several specialties. Importantly, the partnership among multiple academic research groups with the National Institutes of Health, industry, and nonprofit partners allowed an efficient use of funding and resources. The discovery framework developed by the AMP is in itself a powerful resource that can be applied to further advancements in SLE and other conditions. The results from the initial AMP phases led to a novel understanding of the molecular environment in LN and the nomination of new candidate biomarkers and therapeutic targets. Future directions will involve the study of additional tissues and diseases to better understand what is SLE specific and what is not and novel technologies, such as epigenomics and spatially resolved omics. The phase 2 of AMP SLE effort will generate an unprecedented, publicly available resource for discovery that will lead closer to the ground truth of LN and will likely stimulate new therapeutic strategies to treat LN.

CLINICS CARE POINTS

- Ongoing multiomics studies in the AMP network may molecularly redefine LN classification and suggest new management strategies to be tested in clinical trials.
- Proteinuria is an imperfect LN indicator. Novel urine-based biomarkers derived from phase 2 of AMP network effort may contribute to the development of a liquid biopsy to noninvasively infer intrarenal activity or class.
- Future deep molecular phenotyping in clinically dissimilar diseases may provide the rationale for repurposing medications and for developing "tissue agnostic" treatments based on molecular mechanisms rather than clinical syndromes.

ACKNOWLEDGMENTS

A. Fava is supported by the Accelerated Medicines Partnership (AMP) NIH UH2 AR067679, the Hopkins Lupus Cohort NIH R01 AR069572, the Cupid Foundation, and the Jerome L Greene Foundation. D.A. Rao is supported by the AMP NIH UH2 AR06768, Lupus Research Alliance, Burroughs Wellcome Fund Career Award for Medical Sciences, and NIH NIAMS K08 AR072791.

DISCLOSURE

Dr D.A. Rao reports personal fees from Pfizer, Janssen, Merck, Bristol-Myers Squibb, and Scipher Medicine; and grants from Janssen and Bristol-Myers Squibb outside the submitted work. Dr S. Raychaudhuri reports personal fees from Gilead, Mestag, Biogen, and Merck; and grants from Biogen and Bristol-Myers Squibb.

REFERENCES

1. Contreras G, Pardo V, Cely C, et al. Factors associated with poor outcomes in patients with lupus nephritis. Lupus 2005;14(11):890–5.
2. Costenbader KH, Desai A, Alarcón GS, et al. Trends in the incidence, demographics, and outcomes of end-stage renal disease due to lupus nephritis in the US from 1995 to 2006. Arthritis Rheum 2011;63(6):1681–8.
3. Davidson A. What is damaging the kidney in lupus nephritis? Nat Rev Rheumatol 2016;12(3):143–53.
4. Petri M, Barr E, Magder LS. Risk of renal failure within ten or twenty years of SLE diagnosis. J Rheumatol 2020. https://doi.org/10.3899/jrheum.191094.
5. Teng YKO, Arriens C, Polyakova S, et al. OP0277 aurora phase 3 study demonstrates voclosporin statistical superiority over standard of care in lupus nephritis (LN). Ann Rheum Dis 2020;79(Suppl 1):172–3.
6. Furie R, Rovin BH, Houssiau F, et al. Two-year, randomized, controlled trial of belimumab in lupus nephritis. N Engl J Med 2020;383(12):1117–28.
7. Rosen A. Moments of wonder. Am J Med 2018;131(7):852–3.
8. Rao DA, Arazi A, Wofsy D, et al. Design and application of single-cell RNA sequencing to study kidney immune cells in lupus nephritis. Nat Rev Nephrol 2020;16(4):238–50.

9. Rao DA, Berthier CC, Arazi A, et al. A protocol for single-cell transcriptomics from cryopreserved renal tissue and urine for the Accelerating Medicine Partnership (AMP) RA/SLE network. bioRxiv 2018;53(9):275859.

10. Arazi A, Rao DA, Berthier CC, et al. The immune cell landscape in kidneys of patients with lupus nephritis. Nat Immunol 2019;20(7):902–14.

11. Zhang F, Wei K, Slowikowski K, et al. Defining inflammatory cell states in rheumatoid arthritis joint synovial tissues by integrating single-cell transcriptomics and mass cytometry. Nat Immunol 2019;20(7):928–42.

12. Mirizio E, Tabib T, Wang X, et al. Single-cell transcriptome conservation in a comparative analysis of fresh and cryopreserved human skin tissue: pilot in localized scleroderma. Arthritis Res Ther 2020;22(1):1–10.

13. Konnikova L, Boschetti G, Rahman A, et al. High-dimensional immune phenotyping and transcriptional analyses reveal robust recovery of viable human immune and epithelial cells from frozen gastrointestinal tissue. Mucosal Immunol 2018; 11(6):1684–93.

14. Der E, Suryawanshi H, Morozov P, et al. Tubular cell and keratinocyte single-cell transcriptomics applied to lupus nephritis reveal type I IFN and fibrosis relevant pathways. Nat Immunol 2019;20(7):915–27.

15. Der E, Ranabothu S, Suryawanshi H, et al. Single cell RNA sequencing to dissect the molecular heterogeneity in lupus nephritis. JCI Insight 2017;2(9):1–12.

16. Macosko EZ, Basu A, Satija R, et al. Highly parallel genome-wide expression profiling of individual cells using nanoliter droplets. Cell 2015;161(5):1202–14.

17. Klein AM, Mazutis L, Akartuna I, et al. Droplet barcoding for single-cell transcriptomics applied to embryonic stem cells. Cell 2015;161(5):1187–201.

18. Krishnaswami SR, Grindberg RV, Novotny M, et al. Using single nuclei for RNA-seq to capture the transcriptome of postmortem neurons. Nat Protoc 2016;11(3): 499–524.

19. Wu H, Kirita Y, Donnelly EL, et al. Advantages of single-nucleus over single-cell RNA sequencing of adult kidney: rare cell types and novel cell states revealed in fibrosis. J Am Soc Nephrol 2019;30(1):23–32.

20. Slyper M, Porter CBM, Ashenberg O, et al. A single-cell and single-nucleus RNA-Seq toolbox for fresh and frozen human tumors. Nat Med 2020;26(5):792–802.

21. Denisenko E, Guo BB, Jones M, et al. Systematic assessment of tissue dissociation and storage biases in single-cell and single-nucleus RNA-seq workflows. Genome Biol 2020;21(1):130.

22. Buenrostro JD, Wu B, Litzenburger UM, et al. Single-cell chromatin accessibility reveals principles of regulatory variation. Nature 2015;523(7561):486–90.

23. Cusanovich DA, Daza R, Adey A, et al. Multiplex single-cell profiling of chromatin accessibility by combinatorial cellular indexing. Science 2015;348(6237):910–4.

24. Chen KH, Boettiger AN, Moffitt JR, et al. Spatially resolved, highly multiplexed RNA profiling in single cells. Science 2015;348(6233):1360–3.

25. Rodriques SG, Stickels RR, Goeva A, et al. Slide-seq: a scalable technology for measuring genome-wide expression at high spatial resolution. Science 2019; 363(6434):1463–7.

26. Goltsev Y, Samusik N, Kennedy-Darling J, et al. Deep profiling of mouse splenic architecture with CODEX multiplexed imaging. Cell 2018;174(4):968–81.e15.

27. Zhang L, Yu X, Zheng L, et al. Lineage tracking reveals dynamic relationships of T cells in colorectal cancer. Nature 2018;564(7735):268–72.

28. Bocharnikov AV, Keegan J, Wacleche VS, et al. PD-1hiCXCR5– T peripheral helper cells promote B cell responses in lupus via MAF and IL-21. JCI Insight 2019; 4(20):e130062.

29. Wang S, Wang J, Kumar V, et al. IL-21 drives expansion and plasma cell differentiation of autoreactive CD11chiT-bet+ B cells in SLE. Nat Commun 2018;9(1):1758.

30. Enghard P, Rieder C, Kopetschke K, et al. Urinary CD4 T cells identify SLE patients with proliferative lupus nephritis and can be used to monitor treatment response. Ann Rheum Dis 2014;73(1):277–83. https://doi.org/10.1136/annrheumdis-2012-202784.

31. Goerlich N, Brand HA, Langhans V, et al. Kidney transplant monitoring by urinary flow cytometry: biomarker combination of T cells, renal tubular epithelial cells, and podocalyxin-positive cells detects rejection. Sci Rep 2020;10(1):796.

32. Suthanthiran M, Schwartz JE, Ding R, et al. Urinary-cell mRNA profile and acute cellular rejection in kidney allografts. N Engl J Med 2013;369(1):20–31.

33. Anglicheau D, Suthanthiran M. Noninvasive prediction of organ graft rejection and outcome using gene expression patterns. Transplantation 2008;86(2):192–9.

34. Kopetschke K, Klocke J, Grießbach A-S, et al. The cellular signature of urinary immune cells in Lupus nephritis: new insights into potential biomarkers. Arthritis Res Ther 2015;17:94.

35. Bertolo M, Baumgart S, Durek P, et al. Deep phenotyping of urinary leukocytes by mass cytometry reveals a leukocyte signature for early and non-invasive prediction of response to treatment in active lupus nephritis. Front Immunol 2020;11:1–12.

36. Enghard P, Humrich JY, Rudolph B, et al. CXCR3+CD4+ T cells are enriched in inflamed kidneys and urine and provide a new biomarker for acute nephritis flares in systemic lupus erythematosus patients. Arthritis Rheum 2009;60(1):199–206.

37. Dolff S, Abdulahad WH, van Dijk MCRF, et al. Urinary T cells in active lupus nephritis show an effector memory phenotype. Ann Rheum Dis 2010;69(11):2034–41.

38. Birmingham DJ, Merchant M, Waikar SS, et al. Biomarkers of lupus nephritis histology and flare: deciphering the relevant amidst the noise. Nephrol Dial Transpl 2017;32(1):i71–9.

39. Soliman S, Mohan C. Lupus nephritis biomarkers. Clin Immunol 2017;185:10–20.

40. Pejchinovski M, Siwy J, Mullen W, et al. Urine peptidomic biomarkers for diagnosis of patients with systematic lupus erythematosus. Lupus 2018;27(1):6–16.

41. Fava A, Buyon J, Mohan C, et al. Integrated urine proteomics and renal single-cell genomics identify an IFN-γ response gradient in lupus nephritis. JCI Insight 2020;5(12):e138345.

42. Rao DA. T cells that help B cells in chronically inflamed tissues. Front Immunol 2018;9:1924.

43. Grieshaber-Bouyer R, Keegan J, Nigrovic P, et al. Mass cytometry reveals activation heterogeneity of circulating neutrophils in systemic lupus erythematosus. Arthritis Rheumatol 2020;72(suppl) [Abstract].

44. Tyukin I, Gorban AN, Calvo C, et al. High-dimensional brain: a tool for encoding and rapid learning of memories by single neurons. Bull Math Biol 2019;81(11):4856–88.

45. Fonseka CY, Rao DA, Teslovich NC, et al. Mixed-effects association of single cells identifies an expanded effector CD4 + T cell subset in rheumatoid arthritis. Sci Transl Med 2018;10(463):eaaq0305.

46. Zhang F, Mears JR, Shakib L, et al. IFN-γ and TNF-α drive a CXCL10+ CCL2+ macrophage phenotype expanded in severe COVID-19 and other diseases with tissue inflammation. bioRxiv 2020. https://doi.org/10.1101/2020.08.05.238360.

47. Regev A, Teichmann SA, Lander ES, et al. The human cell atlas. Elife 2017;6: e27041.
48. Korsunsky I, Millard N, Fan J, et al. Fast, sensitive and accurate integration of single-cell data with Harmony. Nat Methods 2019;16(12):1289–96.
49. Carvelli J, Demaria O, Vély F, et al. Association of COVID-19 inflammation with activation of the C5a–C5aR1 axis. Nature 2020;588(7836):146–50.
50. Kang JB, Nathan A, Millard N, et al. Efficient and precise single-cell reference atlas mapping with symphony 1. bioRxiv 2020;617–25.
51. Fava A, Li J, Carlucci P, et al. Lupus nephritis and renal outcomes in African-Americans: the accelerating medicines partnership cohort experience. Arthritis Rheumatol 2020;72(suppl):496–7.
52. Feldman CH, Hiraki LT, Liu J, et al. Epidemiology and sociodemographics of systemic lupus erythematosus and lupus nephritis among US adults with Medicaid coverage, 2000–2004. Arthritis & Rheumatism 2013;65:753–63, https://doi-org.ezp-prod1.hul.harvard.edu/10.1002/art.37795.
53. Falasinnu T, Chaichian Y, Bass MB, et al. The Representation of Gender and Race/Ethnic Groups in Randomized Clinical Trials of Individuals with Systemic Lupus Erythematosus. Curr Rheumatol Rep 2018;20. https://doi-org.ezp-prod1.hul.harvard.edu/10.1007/s11926-018-0728-2.
54. Ulff-Møller CJ, Simonsen J, Kyvik KO, et al. Family history of systemic lupus erythematosus and risk of autoimmune disease: nationwide cohort study in Denmark 1977-2013. Rheumatology (Oxford) 2017;56(6):957–64.
55. Genovese MC, Kremer J, Zamani O, et al. Baricitinib in patients with refractory rheumatoid arthritis. N Engl J Med 2016;374(13):1243–52.
56. Kalil AC, Patterson TF, Mehta AK, et al. Baricitinib plus remdesivir for hospitalized adults with Covid-19. N Engl J Med 2020. https://doi.org/10.1056/NEJMoa2031994. NEJMoa2031994.
57. Garber K. In a major shift, cancer drugs go "tissue-agnostic". Science 2017;356(6343):1111–2.

Patient-Reported Outcomes in Lupus

Narender Annapureddy, MD[a], Meenakshi Jolly, MD[b],*

KEYWORDS

- Patient-reported outcome (PRO) • Quality of life (QOL)
- Systemic lupus erythematosus (SLE)

KEY POINTS

- Patient-reported outcomes, a core outcome measure for systemic lupus erythematosus (SLE), is important for patient care, education, and research.
- Currently, legacy generic tool, such as the 36-Item Short Form Health Survey, is used primarily for research in SLE.
- Research is needed urgently to evaluate responsiveness and minimally important differences of PRO tools currently available for SLE.

INTRODUCTION

Mortality in systemic lupus erythematosus (SLE) has improved over the past few decades; however, patients continue to have significant morbidity and poor health outcomes. SLE and medications used for treatment contribute toward morbidity and have an impact on patient quality of life (QOL).

The Outcomes Measures in Rheumatology Clinical Trials (OMERACT) IV identified 4 core outcomes in SLE: disease activity, damage, medication side effects, and health-related QOL (HRQOL). Disease activity is the primary outcome in SLE clinical trials, but it does not capture patient perspectives. Patient-reported outcomes (PROs) capture unique information not assessed by disease activity or damage.[1] Physician–patient discordance in evaluations of lupus activity indicate the differences in priorities and relative importance placed by each in their evaluations of the disease status. Patient with SLE have worse QOL than the general population as well other more common chronic diseases.[2] Capturing PROs (eg, QOL) is important to include patient evaluations and preferences in developing management plans and for their understanding

[a] Department of Medicine, Vanderbilt University, 1160 21st Avenue, Suite T3113 MCN, Nashville, TN 37232, USA; [b] Department of Medicine, Rush University, 1611 West Harrison Street, Suite 510, Chicago, IL 60615, USA
* Corresponding author.
E-mail address: Meenakshi_Jolly@Rush.edu

Rheum Dis Clin N Am 47 (2021) 351–378
https://doi.org/10.1016/j.rdc.2021.04.004
0889-857X/21/© 2021 Elsevier Inc. All rights reserved.

of the disease. Furthermore, because PROs predict mortality in SLE, they also may be used to triage resources to those at greater risk.[3]

PRO tools may be utilized to systematically evaluate the impact of SLE on patients' daily lives (eg, QOL), a symptom (eg, fatigue), and disease severity (disease activity or damage) (**Table 1**). For a long time, only generic PROs were used in SLE research, but recently both generic PROs and disease-specific PROs have begun to be used for research and sometimes with patient care. Generic PRO tools have the advantage of ease of use in clinics, and, because they can be applied to varied diseases, they allow for comparisons. Also, because generic PROs (eg, 36-Item Short Form Health Survey-36) are legacy tools, a large body of published literature exists compared with the disease-specific PROs for SLE. Generic PRO tools however, may lack disease-specific concepts deemed relevant and important by SLE patients, thus making such evaluations incomplete when used independently. Examples of such SLE-relevant concepts include body image, cognition, medications, flares, burden, sleep, procreation, and intimacy, among others. Disease-specific PRO tools capture SLE-relevant concepts, thus providing a comprehensive evaluation, but do not allow comparisons across diseases. This article describes some of the PRO tools utilized in SLE (see **Table 1**) for patient care and/or research. Details on the commonly used generic and disease-specific PRO tools in SLE are included (**Tables 2** and **3**).

Table 1
Patient-reported outcomes used in lupus

Impact on Daily Life			
Generic		**Disease Specific**	
QOL	MOS Short Form-36	QOL	LupusPRO
	EQ-5D		LIT
	PROMIS		SLEQOL
	MDHAQ		L-QOL
	CHAQ		LupusQOL
Symptoms	FACIT-Fatigue		SIQ
	Anxiety (Beck Anxiety Inventory and Positive and Negative Affect Schedule)		LEQOL
	Depression (Center for Epidemiologic Studies Depression Scale and PHQ-9)		SMILEY
	Pain (Brief Pain Inventory)	Symptoms	SSC, SSD
	Cognition (Multiple Sclerosis Neuropsychological Questionnaire)		
	Stress (Perceived Stress Scale)	Medication	SSQ
	Sleep (Insomnia Severity Index)	Other concepts	BILS
			LSQ
			SLE-FAMILY questionnaire
			SLENQ
			SLICC-FI
Disease Severity			
Disease activity	SLAQ	Damage	BILD
	SIMPLE		LDIQ
	LFA-REAL PRO		

Table 2
Description and psychometric properties of commonly used generic patient-reported outcomes in systemic lupus erythematosus

Description	Medical Outcomes Study 36-Item Short Form Survey	EQ-5D	Patient-Reported Outcomes Measurement Information System	Multidimensional Health Assessment Questionnaire	Childhood Health Assessment Questionnaire	Functional Assessment of Chronic Illness Therapy–Fatigue Scale
Age group (adult/pediatrics)	Adult	Adult	Adult/pediatric	Adult	Pediatric	Adult
Item generation from patients	No	No	No	No	No	Expert and patients
Number items	36	6	29 in PROMIS-29	Variable by new patient or return and iteration (>100 + 3 VAS)	30	13
Domains	8: physical function, role physical, bodily pain, vitality, general health, social function, mental health, role emotional	5: mobility, self-care, usual activities, pain/discomfort, anxiety/depression	7 PROMIS-29: depression, anxiety, physical function, pain interference, fatigue, sleep disturbance, ability to participate in social roles and	Function, pain, joints, patient global, review of systems, fatigue among others	8: dressing and grooming, arising, eating, walking, hygiene, reach, grip, activities	1: fatigue
Scores	0–100	0–100 (VAS)	T score metric, 50 = average general population, SD = 10	0–10 for RAPID3	0–10	0–52

(continued on next page)

Table 2
(continued)

Description	Medical Outcomes Study 36-Item Short Form Survey	EQ-5D	Patient-Reported Outcomes Measurement Information System	Multidimensional Health Assessment Questionnaire	Childhood Health Assessment Questionnaire	Functional Assessment of Chronic Illness Therapy–Fatigue Scale
Recall	4 wk	Same day	Physical function does not have recall period. "Lately" for social roles and activity. 1 wk for PROMIS-CAT	1 wk for function. pain, fatigue, current far patient global, last month far ROS	1 wk	1 wk
Ease of reading	Fairly easy-FRE 74.6, FK 7.L	Standard ease-FRE 66.6, FK 6.7	Not available	Not available	Not available	Target was sixth-grade level. Details not available
Reliability						
Internal consistency (Cronbach α)	>0.7 (except for SF and MH)	Not available	PROMIS SF >0.7	0.88	0.96	>0.85
Test Retest Reliability	>0.7 (except for RE)	<0.3 (anxiety/depression)	PROMIS-10, PROMIS CAT >0.8	0.65–0.81 (not specific to SLE)	0.79	0.95 (not specific to SLE)
Validity						
Content	Yes	Not available	Yes	Yes	Yes (but not for SLE)	Yes
Convergent (rho)	Yes (with EQ-5D, LupusPRO, LIT, LupusQOL)	Yes (with Short Form-36, LupusQOL, LupusPRO)	Yes (with Short Form-36, LupusQOL, PedsQOL-GC, CHQ, CHAQ, LIT)	Yes (LupusPRO)	Yes (with CHQ PROMIS, SMILEY, LIT)	Yes (with vitality domains of Short Form-36 and LupusPRO and SLEQOL)

Discriminant	Good	Good	Poor based in SFI	Good	Good for disease activity	Poor
Criterion (rho)	None to weak with SLEDAI (<0.15) and BILAG	Moderate (042) with SLAM, weak (0.23) with SLEDAI	RAPID3 correlated with SLAQ (r= 0.60), none with PhGA,, SLEDAI or SDI	None for SLEDAI, weak for SDI, moderate with SLAQ and BILD	Weak with SLEDAI (−0.21) and SDI (−0.20)	None–modest with SDI (none to −0.35), weak with BILAG (none to −0.41)
Structural	Yes, for general population Factor loadings for 13 items were 0.38–0.89	Not available for SLE	Two-factor loadings for FN Cross-loadings for 1 a, e and f	Yes. Fatigue loads on physical and mental health	Not available	4 factors loadings (Factor1 = PF, RP, BP, RE. Factor2 = GH, VT, MH)
Floor-ceiling effect (>15%)	Not available for SLE	Floor, and ceiling effects + (non-SLE)	Floor effects + in SLE	Ceiling effects +	Ceiling effects +	Floor +, ceiling effects +
Responsiveness (anchor)	Yes PhGA, SLEDAI, SFI)	Yes (global assessment of patient well-being and)	Not responsive in SLE	Yes (reported changes)	Yes (self-reported Improvement but not)	Yes (patient global rating of disease)
Minimally Important Differences	3–7	Not available	Not available for SLE	Approximately 2 points	Not available	1.9–11.3 (improvement) −4.4 to −15.6 (worsening)
Cross-cultural validation	Not available (for SLE)	Yes (not in SLE)	Not available (for SLE)	Not available (for SLE)	Yes (Chinese version tested in SLE)	Yes

Table 3
Description and psychometric properties of commonly used generic patient-reported outcomes in systemic lupus erythematosus

Description	Lupus Patient Reported Outcome	Lupus Impact Tracker	Lupus Quality of Life	Systemic Lupus Erythematosus –Specific Quality of Life	Systemic Lupus Erythematosus Quality of Life Questionnaire	Simple Measure of Impact of Lupus Erythematosus on Youngsters
Age group (adult/pediatrics)	Adult	Adult and pediatrics	Adult	Adult	Adult	Pediatric
Item generation from patients	Yes	Yes	Yes	No	Yes	No Modified later
Number items	49 (V1.8)	10	34	40	25	26
Domains	14: HRQOL (lupus symptoms, cognition, lupus medications, procreation, physical health, pain, sleep, vitality, emotional health, body image) Non-HRQOL (desires-goals, social support, coping, satisfaction with care)	Unidimensional: impact	8: physical health, emotional health, body image, pain planning, fatigue, intimate relationships, burden to others	6: physical functioning, activities, symptoms, treatment, mood, self-image	Unidimensional: impact	4: effect on self, limitations, social, burden of life
Scores	0–100	0–100	0–100	40–280	0–100	0–100

Recall	4 wk (HRQOL), 3 month (non-HRQOL)	4 wk	4 wk	1 wk	4 wk	1 mo (except first 2 items, which refer to current SLE status and QOL)
Ease of reading	Fairly easy—FRE score 78.9, FK 5.5	Fairly easy—FRE score 73.8, FK 6.6	Fairly difficult—FRE score 59.6, FK 11.8 (LupusQOL-US)	Fairly easy—FRE score 70.2, FK 6	Not available	Fifth grade
Reliability						
Internal consistency (Cronbach α)	0.7 (except procreation: 0.68, coping: 0.69)	>0.9	≥0.85	0.95	0.93	0.9
Test Retest Reliability	>0.7	>0.9	≥0.7	0.83 (0.52–0.80 for subsections)	0.92	0.6–0.9
Validity						
Content	Yes	Yes	Yes	Yes	Yes	Yes
Convergent (rho)	Yes (Short Form-36, EQ-5D, LupusQOL, Facit-Fatigue, depression, sleep, pain, cognition, body image on relevant domains)	Yes (SF-12, Short Form-36, EQ-5D, LupusQOL, and PHQ-9, in children with CHAQ, PROMIS)	Yes (Short Form-36, SF-6D, EQ-5D, LIT)	Poor with Short Form-36	Yes (Nottingham Health Profile, Health Assessment Questionnaire, ratings of general health)	Yes for Child-SMILEY, Parent-SMILEY, CHAQ-DI, Global QOL, PedsQOL, PedsQL-GC
Discriminant	Yes (patient, physician global, SFI, DORIS remission)	Yes (SELENA-SLEDAI, SLAQ, SFI, SRI, patient-reported health status)	Yes (BILAG, SLEDAI, SLAQ, and SDI)	Yes (low disease activity state, SLEDAI-2K, flare, Damage)	Yes (perceived disease activity QOL)	Yes (PhGA and SDI)
Criterion	Weak correlated with PhGA (r= -0.34), SELENA-SLEDAI (r= -0.32) and BILAG (-0.21 to -0.23)	Weak PhGA (0.31), SLEDAI (0.26) SFI and SDI strong (SLAQ [0.76])	Moderate with SLAQ (≥0.50), none to weak with SLEDAI (-0.09 to -0.26)	None to weak (SLEDAI [0.02], SLAM [0.018] and SDI [0.05])	None (SLEDAI-2K [0.29])	None (PhGA,, SLEDAI, or SDI)

(continued on next page)

Table 3
(continued)

Description	Lupus Patient Reported Outcome	Lupus Impact Tracker	Lupus Quality of Life	Systemic Lupus Erythematosus –Specific Quality of Life	Systemic Lupus Erythematosus Quality of Life Questionnaire	Simple Measure of Impact of Lupus Erythematosus on Youngsters
Structural	Yes	Yes-unidimensional	Yes (2–8 factor models noted in other languages)	8 Factors structure noted	Yes-unidimensional	Not available
Floor-ceiling effect (>15%)	Ceiling effects +	None	Floor +, ceiling +	Floor effects+	Floor effects (10.9%)	Not available
Responsiveness	Yes (patient-reported change in health, PhGA and SLEDAI): 2.0–3.8 (improvement), −2.7 to −3.5 (worsening)	Yes (patient-reported change in health, PhGA, SLEDAI, SLAQ, SFI T2T and SRI): −4.2 (improvement), 2.3 (worsening)	Yes (patient-reported change in health): 5.6–10.4 (improvement), −2.5 to −7.7 (deterioration)	Yes (patient global QOL)	Not available	Yes (global HRQOL, SLE status, SLEDAI and SDI, r range 0.3–0.4)
MID	Not available	2–4	3.5–7.3 (improvement), −2.4 to 8.7 (deterioration)	25	Not available	Not available
Cross-cultural validation	Yes	Yes	Yes	Yes	Yes—Turkish	Yes

PATIENT-REPORTED OUTCOMES TO EVALUATE IMPACT OF SYSTEMIC LUPUS ERYTHEMATOSUS ON PATIENT LIFE
Generic Patient-Reported Outcome Instruments

Most generic PRO tools used in SLE measure impact on patients' daily lives (QOL). Various generic PRO measures have been used and validated in SLE (see **Table 1**) (eg, Short Form-36). Generic PROs can be used to evaluate symptoms (eg, fatigue) in SLE.

The **Medical Outcomes Study (MOS) Short Form-36** is the most widely used PRO in SLE. It was not derived from patient feedback. It has 36 questions that assess HRQOL and 8 domains: physical functioning (PF), role-physical (RP), bodily pain (BP), general health (GH), vitality (VT), social functioning (SF), role-emotional (RE), and mental health (MH).[4] Summary scores are physical component summary (PCS) and mental component summary (MCS). Shorter versions, the 8-Item Short Form Health Survey and the 12-Item Short Form Health Survey, are available. The 6-dimensional health state short form (Short Form six-dimension) index, calculated from Short Form-36,[5,6] may be used in cost-effectiveness evaluations. Recall period is 4 weeks (1 week for acute version). SLE patients completed Short Form-36 in less than 7 minutes.[7] Short Form-36 scores range from 0 to 100 (higher = better health). Flesch Reading Ease (FRE) score is 74.6 (fairly easy) and Flesch Kincaid (FK) grade is 7.1.[8] Another reported literacy level of eighth grade.[9]

Psychometric properties are shown in **Table 2**. Short Form-36 has good internal consistency reliability (ICR), with Cronbach α coefficient greater than 0.7. ICR for SF (0.27) and MH (0.46) domains, however, is poor.[10] Test-retest (TRT) reliability is good (r $\geq$0.7) across most domains except RE.[11,12] Structural validity with items loading on 4 different factors is reported.[11] Short Form-36 has good convergent validity with the EuroQoL EQ-5D, Lupus Patient Reported Outcome (LupusPRO), Lupus Impact Tracker (LIT), and LupusQOL (r= 0.48–0.83).[6,13–17] Short Form-36 domains, PCS and MCS, could not differentiate among SLE patients by disease activity and damage.[6] Short Form-36 has weak to moderate correlation with disease activity and SDI for criterion validity (see **Table 2**).[11,18–20] Floor effects ($\geq$15%) exist for RE (25%) and RP (42.8%), whereas ceiling effects ($\geq$15%) are seen for BP (16.2%), RE (53.4%), RP (36.2%), and SF (23.7%).[16]

In a longitudinal study, only PF domain scores declined over 8 years, which was not attributable to changes in SLE but to fibromyalgia.[21] Baba and colleagues[22] did not find changes in Short Form-36 with worsening in Systemic Lupus Erythematosus Disease Activity Index (SLEDAI) of greater than or equal to 3.[14] Changes in Short Form-36 domains, PCS and MCS, using anchors of Safety of Estrogens in Systemic Lupus Erythematosus National Assessment (SELENA)-SLEDAI, SELENA Flare Index (SFI), British Isles Lupus Assessment Group (BILAG), and SLE responder Index (SRI), are available from BLISS-52 trial data. Mean change in Short Form-36 domains exceeded 5 with attainment of SRI.[23] Short Form-36 is responsive to worsening and improvement in patient-reported global rating of change (GRC)[24] but not to worsening in BILAG. Using a distribution-based approach, standardized response means (SRMs) were 0.32 to 0.58 for improvement and −0.14 to −0.72 for worsening in health. SRMs were larger for worsened health status than for improved.[25] In a recent study, PCS was responsive to change in patient global assessment (PaGA) (effect size [ES] 0.15) but not to changes in Physician Global Assessment (PhGA) or SELENA-SLEDAI.[26]

Using anchors of patient-reported change in GRC, minimally important differences (MIDs) for deterioration ranged from −2.0 (GH) to −11.1 (RP) and for improvement ranged from 2.8 (GH) to 10.9 (BP and VT).[24] MIDs were greater than 5 for deterioration: BP {−6.7}, MH {−5.1}, RE {−10.4}, and RP {−11.1}; and for improvement: BP {10.9}, MH {7.5}, VT {10.9}, RE {10.2}, RP {10.8}, and SF {9.6}. Using the distribution-based approach (SD = 0.5), MID was greater than or equal to 10 for 7/8 domains: PF (13.4), RP (13.8), BP (11.6), MH (10.3), VT (10.0), GH (9.3), RE (19.7), and SF (14.9).[24] In a second study, MIDs were 1.9 to 11.3 for improvement and −4.4 to −15.6 for worsening using a 7-point Likert score.[25] MID estimates noted in this study were significantly different for the domains than those noted in the study by McElhone and colleagues.[24] For example, MIDs for worsening using 2 different patient-reported health status anchors for Devilliers and colleagues[25] and McElhone and colleagues[24] studies were −12.8 and −6.7, respectively for BP domain and −2.0 and −7.8, respectively for the GH domain. MIDs for improvement also were significantly different in the 2 studies: MIDs for MH domain were 3.7 and 7.5, respectively; whereas for VT domain were 2 and 10.9, respectively. The differences could be partly from use of 2 different scales as anchors or number of observations in each study. Short Form-36 has been translated and validated among SLE patients in many languages.[11,12,27,28]

The **European Quality of Life Five Dimension (EQ-5D)** is a short 6-item questionnaire with 5 dimensions (mobility, self-care, usual activities, pain/discomfort, and anxiety/depression) and includes a EuroQol EQ visual analog scale (VAS) score. The dimensions were selected based on review of existing health status tools.[29,30] Versions for response options (5 levels or 3 levels [EQ-5D-3L]) and youth are available. Same-day recall is used, and it takes less than 2 minutes to complete. For EQ-5D-3L, higher level is equal to greater problems. Five-digit descriptive score represents level of impairment endorsed for each dimension. The EQ-5D VAS score is obtained from the 0 to 100 VAS health rating scale (worst to best imaginable health) for quality of adjusted life years analysis. Single summary index (EQ-5D index) is obtained using weights according to the preferences of the general population of a country or region. The scores range from −0.11 to 1 (1 = perfect health, 0 = death, and <0 = health worse than death). FRE and FK grade scores are 66.6 (standard ease) and 6.7,[8] whereas another study reported eighth-grade literacy level.[9]

ICR in SLE is not reported. TRT reliability for anxiety/depression is poor (<0.30)[31] whereas content validity in SLE is not known. Convergent validity of EQ-5D dimensions, VAS, and EQ-5D index in SLE is good with Short Form-36 domains PCS and MCS, SF-6D domains,[6] most LupusQOL domains, and all LupusPRO domains.[31-33] As with all PRO tools, EQ-5D index and EQ-5D VAS correlations with SLEDAI and SDI (r= −0.22 and 0.20) and (r= −0.21 and −0.20), respectively, are weak.[6] Other reported correlations, however, between EQ-5D and SLEDAI and SDI were −0.59 and −0.51, respectively, from China,[34] supporting construct validity. The EQ-5D index can discriminate between patients based on disease activity, but discrimination by damage is conflicting.[6,31] Its structural validity in SLE is not known. No floor effects were observed, but ceiling effects were observed in SLE for EQ-5D index (34%), and EQ-5D dimensions (22.8%–47.9%), especially self-care and pain/discomfort.[34]

The EQ-5D index is responsive to self-reported improvement in health status (ES 0.35) but not to deterioration or to changes in disease activity.[6] In the clinical trials with belimumab and rituximab, there were no changes in EQ-5D (belimumab study), whereas in the rituximab group, there were improvements in EQ-5D at 6 months but not significant at month 12.[35] MIDs for EQ-5D in SLE are not available. Translations are available but validated only among Chinese SLE patients.[34]

The **Patient-Reported Outcomes Measurement Information System (PROMIS)** was developed to assess health status across various chronic illness for clinical research among adults and children.[36,37] Static short forms (SFs) with 4 to 20 items also are available. Anywhere from 4 to 14 PROMIS SFs have been used in SLE.[38,39] The PROMIS-29 health profile is composed of 4 items from 7 domains (depression, anxiety, physical function, pain interference, fatigue, sleep disturbance, and ability to participate in social roles and activities) and a pain intensity item. Physical function has no recall period, whereas "lately" is used for ability to participate in social roles and satisfaction with social roles and activities.[38] All PROMIS computer adaptive tests (CATs) have a recall of 1 week. A score of 50 represents the average of the general US population (SD= 10).[40] For all PROMIS scales, higher scores denote more of the construct being evaluated. During development, targeted reading level mentioned was less than ninth grade or less than 12 years of education.[41] Readability metrics, however, are not published. Some challenges were reported by SLE patients and readability may be a concern among vulnerable populations[42]; 28% participants commented on challenges completing the survey or provided suggestions for improvement, which included confusion and variation in recall period.[38] Mean CAT items administered was 72.8, and it took greater than 11 minutes to complete.[7]

The PROMIS SF has acceptable ICR across domains (>0.7) among adults and children with SLE.[7,43] TRT reliability of the PROMIS-10 global physical health and global mental health component scores were greater than 0.8[44] and was greater than 0.7 for PROMIS CAT.[7] Focus group interviews among English-speaking Asian SLE patients confirmed the content validity and identified gaps in it.[45] In support of convergent validity, PROMIS SFs have moderate to strong correlation with corresponding domains of Short Form-36,[46] whereas PROMIS CAT has good correlation with Short Form-36 and LupusQOL–US version in adults with SLE.[7] Similarly, among children with SLE, moderate to strong correlations for PROMIS SFs are noted with HRQOL tools (PEDSQL-GC, Child Health Questionnaire [CHQ], and Childhood Health Assessment Questionnaire [CHAQ]) and LIT.[43,47] Among adults with SLE, there were no to weak correlations of PROMIS SFs with SELENA-SLEDAI and SDI.[7,46] There were moderate correlations, however, between PROMIS SFs and patient-reported measures of disease activity (Systemic Lupus Activity Questionnaire [SLAQ] and damage Brief Index of Lupus Damage [BILD]).[46] In children, PROMIS SFs weekly correlated with disease activity (SLEDAI, BILAG, and PhGA) or damage (SDI).[43] Structural validity shows fatigue and sleep disturbance to load equally on physical and mental health factors (non-SLE).

PROMIS-10 showed better responsiveness to patient-reported changes in health status compared with Short Form-36.[26] ESs were small to moderate for global physical and global mental health for deterioration and small for improvement in health status. PROMIS-10, however, did not show responsiveness to PhGA or SELENA-SLEDAI.[26] In a recent study by Katz and colleagues,[39] PROMIS was responsive to changes using patient-reported changes in HRQOL (HAQ, Short Form-36 PF, and VT) or patient assessment of disease activity (for fatigue and pain interference) as anchors. SRMs were small to moderate. Among children with SLE, there were signals for responsiveness using anchors of physician-assessed improvement in health status (anger) and SLE (anger, anxiety, mobility, and pain), SLEDAI (anger and mobility), and BILAG (mobility, upper extremity, and pain).[43] MIDs for PROMIS SFs have been published by Katz and colleagues.[39] MID estimate for all PROMIS scales using anchor and distribution methods was approximately 2 points. Ceiling effects (>15%) exist for physical health (physical function, 20.3%); mental health (psychosocial illness impact, 21.7%); social health (ability to participate in social roles and activities, 24.8%); satisfaction, discretionary social activities (20%); satisfaction, social roles (24.1%); and social isolation (27.5%) in the CLUES cohort.[46] In another study, ceiling effects were as follows: physical function (28.3%), satisfaction with social roles (21.8%), pain interference (23.9%), anxiety (44.6%), and depression (56.7%).[48] PROMIS item banks for CAT are available in English and Spanish. SFs are available in some other languages.[46,49] Validation studies of translated versions in varied languages are not yet available for SLE.

The **Multidimensional Health Assessment Questionnaire (MDHAQ)** originally was developed in rheumatoid arthritis patients. It subsequently has been used in various other rheumatic conditions, including SLE.[50] It includes evaluation of function (0–10), visual numeric scale (VNS) pain (0–10), VNS PaGA (0–10), VNS fatigue (0–10), and other components. Number of items vary based on the iteration, new patient or return patient. Items are greater than 100 along with 3 VNS. Initial versions included helplessness and ability to cope with stress items. Latter versions include adherence with medications and widespread pain index items. Rheumatology Assessment of Patient Index Data 3 (RAPID3) is a composite score of pain, PaGA and function. Recall period for function, pain and fatigue is 1 week, "at this time" for PaGA, and 1-month for review of systems. It is completed in 7 minutes to 10 minutes. RAPID3 scores range from 0 to 10 (higher = worse health). Data on readability of MDHAQ are not available.

ICR for the 10 FN items in SLE was 0.88.[51] TRT reliability of earlier versions is noted to be 0.65 to 0.81 among varied rheumatological disease patients. Structural validity of function items shows loadings on 2 factors, with significant cross-loadings for items 1(a), 1(e), and 1(f).[51] RAPID3 has convergent validity with LupusPRO (composite HRQOL [r= −0.68] and physical health domain [r= −0.86]).[51] RAPID3 (but not function, pain, and PaGA) can discriminate among SLE patients with flare and without flare (SFI).[51] MDHAQ can distinguish between SLE patients with few and many noninflammatory symptoms and with fibromyalgia.[52] RAPID3 and PaGA correlate with SLAQ (r= 0.60 and 0.59), but not with PhGA, SLEDAI-2K, SELENA-SLEDAI, or SDI.[52] Significant floor effects for the 10 function items were noted. Floor effects were greater than 50% for 8/10 function items in SLE.[51]

RAPID3 does not respond to changes in PhGA, SELENA-SLEDAI, or SFI[51] SLE-specific MIDs are not available. Decline in RAPID3 score of 3.6 is significant in rheumatoid arthritis.[53] Data on cross-cultural validation studies for varied languages are not available in SLE.

The **Childhood Health Assessment Questionnaire (CHAQ)**, a 30-item PRO (or parent-reported) questionnaire, evaluates a child's ability to perform functions in 8 areas (dressing and grooming, arising, eating, walking, hygiene, reach, grip, and activities). The Stanford Health Assessment Questionnaire was modified by adding questions specific for children of all ages for each functional area.[54] It is targeted for children 1 year to 19 years of age. It may be completed by children greater than or equal to 8 years and by the parent for children less than 8 years. Parent global assessment VAS and pain include "previous week" recall period. It takes 10 minutes to complete. Parent global assessment VAS and parent global assessment of the child's pain ranges from 0 to 10 (higher = worse health). CHAQ disability index (DI), ranges from 0 to 3 (higher = greater disability).

Less than 5% missing data on CHAQ suggests excellent feasibility and ease with understanding. Information is not available on ease of readability. ICR for the 8 CHAQ function domains in SLE was 0.96.[55] TRT reliability in juvenile rheumatoid arthritis patients was 0.79.[54] Face validity was established through expert feedback.[54] Convergent validity with CHQ physical score (r= −0.61), parent global VAS (r= 0.53), and PROMIS mobility (r= -0.60) is established.[55,56] CHAQ also correlates with 2 disease-specific PROs: Parent–Simple Measure of Impact of Lupus Erythematosus on Youngsters (SMILEY) scores (r= 0.50). and the LIT (r= 0.74).[47,57] CHAQ-DI can discriminate between patients using the Paediatric Rheumatology International Trials Organisation (PRINTO)/American College of Rheumatology (ACR) responder definition for improvement.[55] CHAQ has moderate correlation with Systemic Lupus Activity

Measure (SLAM) (r= 0.42) but weak with SLEDAI (r= 0.23). In another study, child-CHAQ scores correlated with SLEDAI (r= 0.40) and SDI (r= 0.52).[58] CHAQ has floor effects in non-SLE patients.[59] CHAQ-DI has been reported to have 50% ceiling effect in patients with childhood arthritis and juvenile dermatomyositis.[56] Structural validity in SLE is not known.

Using modified PRINTO/ACR improvement definition for responder among juvenile SLE patients, significant changes in CHAQ were noted among responders, in all areas. SRMs were large for the parents' global assessment of patients' overall well-being and pain VAS (SRMs >0.90) but moderate for other areas (0.59 for eating and 0.78 for activities), and CHAQ-DI (0.74).[55] SLE-specific MIDs are not available. CHAQ is validated for use in other cultures and languages, including Spanish, Portuguese, Italian, Dutch, Swedish, and Norwegian.[60]

Generic Patient-Reported Outcome Tools for Symptom Evaluation

The **Functional Assessment of Chronic Illness Therapy–Fatigue Scale (FACIT-Fatigue)** is a 13-item questionnaire that assesses self-reported fatigue and its effect. It was developed based on expert and patient feedback. One week is standard recall but for validation study by Lai and colleagues[61] it was 4 weeks. It takes 2 minutes to 3 minutes to complete. Scores range from 0 to 52 (higher = less fatigue). Targeted reading level was less than or equal to sixth grade, but specifics are not available.

It has excellent ICR (Cronbach α >0.85).[10,61] TRT reliability in SLE is not available. Most items have good content validity, but concerns were raised by the SLE participants in a qualitative study regarding 4/13 items.[62] These centered around wording, relevance, relatability, clarity on response options, and suggestions around recall period. Convergent validity with Short Form-36 vitality, PCS and MCS (r= .5), LupusPRO vitality (r= −0.86), and SLE-specific QOL (SLEQOL) (r= 0.64) is good.[10,63] It can differentiate between groups defined by BILAG general and musculoskeletal domain grades.[61]

There was no to weak correlation with other physician-assessed outcomes, such as SLEDAI (r <0.15) and BILAG.[64] Structural validity of unidimensionality in the general population is present but factor loadings range from 0.38 to 0.89.[65] Floor and ceiling effects estimates in SLE are not available.

It is responsive to changes in the PaGA with ES range of 0.5 to 0.8. Mean change in FACIT-Fatigue in patients with SLE in response to improvement (SLEDAI decline ≥7) and worsening (SLEDAI increase ≥8) was +/-2.[23] Mean changes in response to SFI flare were 1.9 (improvement) and −1.3 (worsening), whereas 3.9 for achieving SLE responder Index 4 response.[23] MIDs using anchor and distribution based approach range from 3 to 7.[61,66,67] The tool is available in multiple languages but cross-cultural validation in SLE is not available.

Several other PRO tools are used in SLE patient care and research to evaluate varied symptoms, traits, and states, such as anxiety, depression, pain, stress, and sleep, among others (see **Table 1**). Some have been evaluated for reliability and validity in SLE.[68]

Disease-Specific Patient-Reported Outcome Tools

Several PRO tools are available for use in SLE specifically (see **Table 1**). Detailed features of commonly used tools are summarized in **Table 3**.

The **Lupus Patient-Reported Outcome tool (LupusPRO)** was developed in the United States using Food and Drug Administration (FDA) guidelines for development of PROs, from SLE patients (male and female) of varied race and ethnicity.[13] It utilizes gender neutral language and evaluates both HRQOL and non-HRQOL. Version 1.8 has

49 items: HRQOL domains (lupus symptoms, cognition, lupus medications, procreation, physical health, pain, sleep, vitality, emotional health, and body image), and non-HRQOL domains (desires/goals, social support, coping, and satisfaction with care).[10] LupusPRO version 1.7 had 43 items (pain, vitality, and sleep domains combined for parsimony). Recall for HRQOL domains is 4 weeks, whereas it is 3 months for the non-HRQOL domains. It takes 7 minutes to 8 minutes to complete. Scores range from 0 to 100 (higher = better QOL). FRE score is 78.9 (fairly easy) and FK grade is 5.5.[10]

ICR is greater than 0.7 except for procreation (0.68) and coping (0.69) domains.[10] In other studies, ICR for these domains is noted to be greater than 0.7.[13,27] TRT reliability is greater than 0.7.[13,27,69] Because it was developed from patients and underwent clinometric analysis, it has good face and content validity. Structural validity is well established. It has convergent validity against corresponding domains of MOS Short Form-36, EQ-5D, LupusQOL, FACIT-Fatigue, depression (Physician Health Questionnaire [PHQ]-9 and Center for Epidemiologic Studies Depression Scale), sleep (Insomnia Severity Index), pain (Brief Pain Inventory), cognition (Multiple Sclerosis Neuropsychological Questionnaire), and body image (Body Image Quality of Life Inventory and Situational Inventory of Body Image Dysphoria [SIBID]). Lupus symptom domain correlates with PhGA (-0.35), SELENA-SLEDAI (r= -0.36), total BILAG (-0.43), Cutaneous Lupus Disease Area and Severity Index (r= -0.38).[10,13,70] It discriminates between SLE patients based on change in health status (patient-reported, PhGA, Lupus Foundation of American [LFA] flare, and Definition of Remission in SLE (DORIS) remission status).[10,13,71] Total HRQOL scores correlate with PhGA (r= -0.34), SELENA-SLEDAI (r= -0.32), and BILAG (-0.21 to -0.23).[10,13] Ceiling effects in excess of 15%, especially with procreation, cognition, and some of the non-HRQOL domains, are noted.

There is evidence of responsiveness to changes in patient-reported health status and in PhGA, SELENA-SLEDAI, SFI flare, and LFA flare status.[72,73] Mean changes in LupusPRO-HRQOL scores in response to change in patient-reported health status were -3.5 for worsening and 2.3 for improvement. Mean changes in LupusPRO-HRQOL in response to PhGA and SLEDAI worsening in were -3.2 and -2.7, respectively, whereas for improvement were 2.03 and 3.8, respectively.[73] In response to an intervention, changes in body-image domain were noted.[74] MID data are not available. The tool is available and has undergone cross cultural validation studies in multiple languages.

The **Lupus Impact Tracker (LIT)** is a unidimensional, 10-question, PRO tool to assess and monitor the impact of SLE.[17] Psychometric, analytical, and focus group approaches were used to select items from LupusPRO. It is validated among adults and children with SLE.[47] Recall is 4 weeks. Scores range from 0 to 100 (higher =''' greater impact). FRE is 73.8 (fairly easy), and FK grade is 6.6. Scoring is easy and quick. The tool takes less than or equal to 3 minutes to complete and was noted by patients and physicians to not be disruptive or burdensome.[14] Feasibility was similarly good among children with SLE and adult SLE patients in European countries.[47,75]

Among adults and children with SLE, ICR is 0.91 and TRT reliability is 0.98.[14,47,76] Face and content validity are well established (LupusPRO developed from patients, and LIT included focus group interviews in its derivation).[17] Approximately 80% of patients and 70% of rheumatologists reported that the LIT helped them discuss the impact of SLE on a patient's life. Similarly, approximately 75% of patients and 50% of rheumatologists reported LIT improved communication between them.[14] Similar findings were noted from 5 European countries.[75] Structural validity confirmed its unidimensionality. LIT has good convergent validity against SF-12, Short Form-36,

EQ-5D, LupusQOL, and PHQ-9 (r= −0.55 to −0.83) among adults.[14,75,77] It has convergent validity with CHAQ-DI (r= 0.74) and PROMIS SFs (r ranges from 0.45 to 0.81, except for PROMIS SF depression with r= 0.35 [*P* = .05]) among children with SLE.[47] It can discriminate among patients based on patient-reported health status, disease activity (PhGA, SELENA-SLEDAI, and SLAQ), Flare (SFI), treat-to-target categories, patient-reported health status (global evaluation, Short Form-36, EQ-5D, and patient acceptable symptom state).[14,75–78] LIT scores correlate with activity (PhGA [0.31], SLEDAI [0.26], SLAQ [0.76]), flare (SFI), and damage[14,47,75,77] and do not exhibit floor or ceiling effects.[79]

It is responsive to change in the patient-reported health ratings, PhGA, SLEDAI, SLAQ, SFI, treat-to-target, and SRI.[14,77,79–81] Mean change was −4.2 (improvement) and 2.3 (worsening) in patient-reported health status.[80] Mean decline was −7.9 (SRM −0.68; ES −0.36) among SRI4 responders compared with −2.9 (SRM −0.19; ES −0.12) among SRI4 nonresponders (*P* = .02).[79] A mean change of 2 to 4 represents a significant clinical change in LIT.[80] It has been translated and validated in Australia, France, Germany, Italy, Spain, and Sweden. It has undergone analysis for differential item functioning (DIF) across 5 languages and cultures, and showed DIF at lower level of moderate magnitude for 1/10 items.[75]

The **Lupus Quality of Life (LupusQOL)** was developed from feedback from women SLE patients (mostly white) in the United Kingdom. It has 34 items that evaluate HRQOL across 8 domains—physical health, emotional health, body image, pain, planning, fatigue, intimate relationships, and burden to others.[82] Recall is 4 weeks and takes less than 10 minutes to complete.[82] Scores range from 0 to 100 (higher = better QOL). Feedback from patients was good as were completion rates.[28] Readability data are not available for LupusQOL. FRE and FK grade are 59.6 (fairly difficult) and 11.8 (LupusQOL-US).

ICR of LupusQOL domains is greater than or equal to 0.85 and TRT reliability greater than or equal to 0.70.[82] Face and content validity are established. Structural validity has varied, with 2 to 8 factors.[28,83] Some items have problematic fit statistics (Questions 8, 16, 19, 26, and 29–31), and/or factor loadings.[28,33,84] Wording of a few questions may be confusing regarding the concept being evaluated.[33] LupusQOL has good convergent validity against Short Form-36, SF-6D, EQ-5D, and LIT,[14,33,83–85] and it can differentiate between patients based on patient-reported health, BILAG, SLEDAI, SLAQ, and SDI.[28,33,82] Good correlations (r ≥0.50) between LupusQOL and SLAQ are reported; however, correlation with SLEDAI was none to weak (r= −0.09 to −0.26).[15,28,84] Floor and ceiling effects are reported.[16,28,84,86]

It is responsive to changes in patient-reported GRC.[24] Mean change in domains ranged from −2.5 to −7.7 (deterioration) and from 5.6 to 10.4 (improvement in GRC).[24] It is responsive to changes in SLEDAI-2K among those who improve or flare but not among those who undergo remission, and the ES are small to moderate.[87] The number of patient visits with changes in disease activity, however, overall were small. Its responses to change in disease activity (BILAG) were less consistent in 6/8 domains to no changes.[24] MIDs for patient-reported health status deterioration ranged from −2.4 to −8.7 and for improvement from 3.5 to 7.3.[24] Distribution based MIDs are larger than anchor-based estimates. In another study, using patient-reported change in health, mean change ranged from 1.1 to 9.2 for minimal improvement and from −0.5 to −6.4 for minimal deterioration.[25] It has been translated and validated in multiple languages for use in SLE.

The **Systemic Lupus Erythematosus Quality of Life (SLEQOL)** was developed in Singapore.[88] It has 40 items across 6 subsections measuring HRQOL—physical functioning, activities, symptoms, treatment, mood, and self-image. Items were generated from health care provider experts. Recall is 1 week and takes less than 8 minutes to complete.[89] Scores range from 40 to 280 (higher = worse QOL).[88] The FRE is 70.2 (fairly easy) and FK grade is 6.0.

SLEQOL–Thai Version evaluated understandability and embarrassment. Patients reported some difficulty with few of the items (6, 11, 12, 25, 29, and 34). ICR for total score was 0.95. TRT reliability for summary score was 0.83 (range 0.52–0.80 for subsections).[88] Face validity is present. Content validity was tested in SLE patients during tool development.[88] The items of SLEQOL loaded into eight factors.[88] Convergent validity with the Short Form-36 rheumatology attitudes index and helplessness subscale was poor.[88] Strong correlations, however, with Short Form-36 PCS and MCS were reported in another study.[90] It can distinguish between patients based on low disease activity state, SLEDAI-2K, flare, and damage.[90] It correlated negligibly to poorly with SLEDAI (r= 0.02), SLAM (r= 0.018), and Systemic Lupus Erythematosus International Collaborating Clinics (SLICC)/ACR-SDI (0.05).[88] There are significant floor effects reported.[88]

In a smaller study, it was more sensitive but less specific to changes using patient-reported improvements in global QOL. Subsections 3 to 5 of SLEQOL were the best indicators of improvements in QOL.[88] In another study, SLEQOL scores were associated with deterioration in patient-reported global change in health status but not to improvement.[90] MID suggested is 25, using anchor of patient-reported change in global QOL.[88] It has been translated and validated in some languages. It has undergone evaluation of DIF between the Thai and the original version. Eight items showed moderate DIF.[89]

The **Simple Measure of the Impact of Lupus Erythematosus in Youngsters (SMILEY)** was developed for children with SLE. There are child and parent versions. It has 26 items, across 4 domains: effect on self, limitations, social, and burden of life. Items related to school are spread across all domains.[91] It was developed by experts and then modified based on qualitative feedback from children with SLE and their parents.[91] It includes pictorial response options. The first 2 items refer to "current" SLE status and QOL, whereas rest of the items use "previous month" for recall.[91] It is completed in less than or equal to 10 min.[91] Scores range from 0 to 100 (higher =''' better QOL). Reading level for SMILEY is fifth grade.[91]

ICRs for total Child-SMILEY and Parent-SMILEY were 0.9. There was moderate agreement between child and parent total and domain scores (r= 0.4–0.6). TRT reliability for total and domain scores for child and parent reports is 0.6 to 0.9.[91] Face validity was confirmed from SLE patients, parents, and experts. Moderate correlations were noted between Child-SMILEY, Parent-SMILEY, and corresponding domains of other tools (CHAQ-DI [r= 0.6 and r= 0.5, respectively], global QOL [r= 0.5 and r= 0.6, respectively], PedsQOL generic tool [0.4–0.6 and 0.5–0.6, respectively], and PedsQL-GC rheumatology [r= 0.4–0.6 and r= 0.4–0.6, respectively). SMILEY summary score correlated only weakly,[43] however, whereas some of the SMILEY subscales had mild to moderate correlation with the PROMIS SFs.[92] Total or domain scores of Child-SMILEY and Parent-SMILEY do not correlate with PhGA, SLEDAI, or SDI. Limitation domain of Child-SMILEY can differentiate by PhGA and SDI. Structural validity and floor or ceiling effects information is not available.

Correlation between changes in Child-SMILEY total scores and changes in global HRQOL, SLE status, SLEDAI, and SDI were present (r= range 0.3–0.4). Changes in Parent-SMILEY total scores correlated with changes in global HRQOL and SLE status but not with changes in PhGA and SLEDAI.[93] MID information is not available. It has been translated and adapted in 17 languages and validated in Portuguese.

The **Systemic Lupus Erythematosus Quality of Life Questionnaire (L-QOL)** initially was developed in the United Kingdom.[92] It has 25 items and provides unidimensional index of impact of SLE.[92] It was developed using the needs-based model from patients with SLE. It has face and content validity. It takes less than 3 minutes to complete.[94] Scores range from 0 to 100 (higher = worse health). TRT reliability and ICR are excellent, 0.92 and 0.93, respectively. Structural validity is good. Moderate correlations were seen with Nottingham Health Profile, perceived disease activity, perceived SLE severity, ratings of general health, QOL, and Health Assessment Questionnaire.[92,94] No correlation with SLEDAI-2K and 10.9% floor effects were noted in the Turkish validation study.[94] No data on reading ease, responsiveness, or MIDs are available.

Lupus Erythematosus Quality of Life (LEQOL) was developed in Spain to evaluate QOL in lupus erythematosus (SLE and cutaneous lupus erythematosus).[95] It was derived from literature review, and its content validity tested in lupus erythematosus patients and experts. It has 7 sociodemographic and 21 items that load on 5 factors: physical, appearance, emotions, cognition, and relationships. ICR was 0.92, and structural validity confirmed 5 factors.

The **SLE Impact Questionnaire (SIQ)** was developed from SLE patients and experts to evaluate patients' ability to make plans, work, and physical/social/emotional functioning.[96] It contains 50 items with a 7-day recall period. It takes 12 minutes to complete and had good feasibility and face and content validity.

Disease-Specific Patient-Reported Outcome Tools for Symptom Evaluation

The **SLE Symptom Checklist (SSC)** was developed in Netherlands.[97] It utilized literature review, experts, and SLE patients in its development. The tool assesses the number (0–38) and perceived burden of symptoms (0–152) on patients' lives in the past 4 weeks. ICR (0.89) and TRT reliability (>0.75) are good. Structural validity did not support the 2-factor model: disease and treatment-related symptoms. There was fair correlation with Short Form-36. Responsiveness to change in VAS was noted.

The **SLE Symptom Severity Diary (SSD)** was designed from literature review and SLE patient feedback to capture daily variability in SLE symptoms. It contains 17 items assessing energy/vitality, joint and muscle pain/stiffness/swelling, flulike symptoms, cognition, numbness/tingling, skin symptoms, and hair loss.[96] It utilizes 24-hour recall period (except for hair loss) and includes steroid status and dose. It takes 6 minutes to complete. It has good face and content validity.

Disease-Specific Patient-Reported Outcome Tools for Other Dimensions

The **SLE Steroid Questionnaire (SSQ)** evaluates general impact, benefits, side effects, and impacts with the use of oral steroids in SLE.[98] Its development was guided through literature review and patient and expert feedback. It has 50 items. One-week recall is used for benefits and side effects of steroids. General impact of steroids questions does not include a recall period. Feasibility and content validity are good.

The SLE Fatigue, Activity participation, Mental health, Isolation, Love and Intimacy, and You/Fulfilling Family Roles (SLE-FAMILY) questionnaire is a 6-domain measure to assess the impact of SLE on family role functioning.[99] It was developed through review of literature and patient feedback. Scores range from 1 to 7 (higher = worse family role functioning). It had good ICR (0.71) and TRT reliability (0.75). There was good correlation with family subscale of Sheehan Disability Scale, Short Form-36, SLAQ, and social support.

The **Body Image Lupus Scale (BILS)** is a 5-item, unidimensional tool, developed from SLE patients to screen for body image (BI) concerns.[100] Scores range from 0 to 100 (higher = better BI), with 4-week recall. It has excellent ICR (>0.90) and

TRT reliability (>0.90). It correlates with validated BI measures (SIBID and BIQLI), and with HRQOL. It is responsive to changes in health status.

The **Lupus Satisfaction Questionnaire (LSQ)** is a 39-item tool to evaluate patient satisfaction with treatment, treatment options, and medical care.[101] It was developed from SLE patients. Recall is 3 months, and it is completed in 5 minutes. It has face and content validity.

The **SLE Needs Questionnaire (SLENQ)** was developed in Australia to evaluate needs of SLE patients.[102] It is derived from literature review and patient and expert feedback. There are 97 items and 6 domains: physical needs, daily living issues, social support, psychological needs, interpersonal communications, health information, and access to services (lower score = more unmet need). Recall is 6 months. Time to complete is less than 30 minutes. ICR for all domains is greater than 0.75. It has good face and content validity. Convergent validity against Short Form-36 was noted (r= −0.31 to −0.60).

The **SLICC Frailty Index (SLICC-FI)** was developed from SLICC cohort data, to assess vulnerability to adverse outcomes among SLE patients.[103] It includes 14 PRO variables related to function, mobility, health attitude, and mental health. Correlation, as expected, is strong with Short Form-36 PCS, but weak with SDI and higher SLEDAI. Changes of greater than or equal to 0.3 are significant.

The **Patient Uncertainty Questionnaire-Rheumatology (PUQ-R)** was developed in the United Kingdom, from patients, for SLE and rheumatoid arthritis.[104] It has 49 items across 5 scales: symptoms and flares, medication, trust in doctor, self-management, and impact. ICR was greater than 0.70. There is convergent validity against other measures of treatment compliance, depression, anxiety, and physical and mental QOL.

PATIENT-REPORTED OUTCOME TOOLS TO EVALUATE DISEASE SEVERITY IN SYSTEMIC LUPUS ERYTHEMATOSUS
Disease Activity

The **Systemic Lupus Activity Questionnaire (SLAQ),** based on SLAM, was developed to track SLE disease activity and flares in epidemiologic studies remotely and as a screening tool to direct further evaluation.[105] It has 3 components: PaGA about presence and severity of lupus activity (over the past month), set of 24 specific symptoms of disease activity (items amenable to self-report from SLAM), and a numeric rating scale to rate disease activity (0–10). Symptoms and a numeric rating scale use a 3-month recall. Scores for symptoms range from 0 to 44. It takes 10 minutes to complete. ICR is 0.87.[106] Convergent validity against SF-12 global health rating, SF-12 PCS, and Short Form-36 PF is noted. It correlates with SLAM-nolab version (r= 0.62). Positive predictive value is 56% to 89% for detecting a clinically significant disease activity. SLAQ shows small to moderate degree of responsiveness to patient-reported change in disease status. SRMs were 0.66 (worsening) and −0.37 (improvement) to changes in PaGA of disease activity. SLAQ is translated and validated in German, Swedish, Italian, and Japanese languages.[107–110]

The **SIMple Disease Assessment for People with Lupus Erythematosus (SIMPLE) Index (SI)** is a composite outcome with PRO items and 2 laboratory values (complements C3-C4 and proteinuria, utilizing SELENA-SLEDAI definition).[111] PRO items include LupusPRO lupus-symptoms domain (3), LIT (10), change in the health status (1), current glucocorticoids use (1), and daily dose of current glucocorticoids (1). SI explains 55% of the variance in SELENA-SLEDAI. With the addition of double-stranded (ds)DNA (SI-3) and dsDNA and leukopenia (SI-4), the variance in SELENA-SLEDAI explained increased to 59% and 62%, respectively. Both SI and SI-4 correlate strongly with SELENA-SLEDAI (r= 0.74 and r= 0.79, respectively). In another study, SI correlated with SELENA-SLEDAI (r= 0.76). SI of greater than 27 predicts a clinical SLEDAI score of 1 to 6 (area under the curve 0.78 [0.73–0.84]; sensitivity 0.75; specificity 0.71), whereas greater than 36.8 predicts a clinical SLEDAI score of greater than or equal to 7 (area under the curve 0.87 [0.69–1.00]; sensitivity 0.88; specificity 0.85).[112]

The **LFA–Rapid Evaluation of Activity in Lupus (REAL)**[113] has a physician version (Clinician Reported Outcome [ClinRO]) and a patient version (PRO).[114] The latter was derived from SLE patients and includes 11 items to evaluate rashes, arthritis (pain/stiffness/swelling), muscle pain, fatigue, hair loss, and symptoms from inside the body. Anchored VAS (0–100 mm) is used for each manifestation (higher = greater activity).[115] Recall is 4 weeks. FRE is 71.5 (fairly easy) and FK grade is 7. Content validity is good. Although it was designed to improve concordance between patients'–physicians' evaluations of disease activity, correlations between LFA-REAL-PRO and LFA-REAL-ClinRO (r= 0.16) and other measures of disease activity completed by physicians (PhGA [r= 0.16] SLEDAI-2K [r= 0.12], and clinical SLEDAI [r= 0.14]) were poor.[115]

Damage

The **Lupus Damage Index Questionnaire (LDIQ)** assesses organ damage and was developed from the SDI.[116] It includes 56 items over 12 organ damage domains. It targets the eighth-grade level. Scores range from 0 to 22 and it takes less than 10 minutes to complete. It has good TRT reliability (0.85).[117] It has moderate correlation with SDI (r= 0.48), comorbidity index (r= 0.45), and Short Form-36 PCS (r= 0.43). ES and SRM for change greater than or equal to 1 in the SDI are 0.43 and 0.59, respectively. It has been validated in Spanish, French, and Japanese.[117,118]

The **Brief Index of Lupus Damage (BILD)** is an interviewer-administered PRO proxy for damage in SLE for use in population studies.[119] It is shorter than LDIQ and excludes rare and nonspecific SDI items. It has 26 items; scores range from 0 to 31. It takes 10 minutes to complete. A self-administered version is available. TRT reliability of self-administered version is 0.93. Acceptability was good, and correlation with SDI strong (r= 0.64). It discriminates between patients by health status (Short Form-36 PCS), employment, disability, and health care utilization. It has been validated in Italian and German.

DISCUSSION

There is an agreement that a patient's viewpoint needs to be included in their care and in research. OMERACT defined PRO as a core outcome in SLE in 1998.[120] Because information captured by PROs is unique and important, there is a need to prioritize their inclusion in SLE care and research. The authors have made progress in the development, adaptation, and validation of varied PRO tools for clinical care and research in SLE in the past decade. Further work urgently is indicated, however, for more effective and efficient integration of appropriate PROs in SLE.

Because development and validation of PRO tools are an iterative process, they require significant patient, personnel, time, and financial resources. The FDA document on guidance for industry on PROs states, "Early in medical product development, sponsors planning to use a PRO instrument in support of a labeling claim are encouraged to determine whether an adequate PRO instrument exists to assess and measure the concepts of interest. If it does not, a new PRO instrument can be developed. In some situations, the new instrument can be developed by modifying an existing instrument."[121] There is consensus on the unique advantages and disadvantages of using a generic versus a disease-specific PRO. Disease-specific PRO tools comprehensively evaluate relevant concepts as identified and prioritized by the patients the disease. Therefore, not only do they provide full breadth of relevant information but also they may be more sensitive to changes in the disease state than generic PRO tools. The choice of PRO tool to be used depends ultimately on the purpose for its use and its measurement properties.

Significant advances already have been made in qualitative work to identify relevant domains of interest for SLE. There are a fair number of generic and disease-specific PRO tools for use in SLE, and some of these are further along in evaluation of their measurement properties than others. Some were developed using the FDA guidelines. It is now time to shift focus and resources from developing new PRO tools for SLE to evaluations of responsiveness and MIDs of select PRO tools with documented feasibility, readability, validity (face, content, convergent, discriminant, structural, and cross-cultural) and reliability (ICR and TRT reliability) in clinical trials settings. Candidate PRO tools for accelerated studies include PROMIS, LupusPRO, LIT, and LupusQOL. Because Short Form-36 and LupusQOL already have been included in SLE clinical trials for several years, collated data would solidify their responsiveness and MIDs further. PROMIS and LIT have been validated among adults and children with SLE; they may have additional advantage in application.

Lastly, for application purposes, provision of readability statistics for existent PRO tools in SLE needs to be encouraged, because US norms recommend less than or equal to 8 years to 9 years of formal schooling for the general population and less than or equal to 5 years of formal schooling for vulnerable populations for surveys.

CLINICS CARE POINTS

- PROs are important to include in clinical care of patients in SLE, because they provide patients' viewpoints and unique information.
- Use of PRO tools allows for systematic measurement of PROs in SLE.
- In a routine clinical care setting, use of the 10-item LIT as a disease-specific PRO was found useful and less burdensome by patients (adults and children with SLE) and their rheumatologists. It is quick and easy to complete and score at point of care.

DISCLOSURE

M. Jolly receives a portion of proceeds from intellectual property use of LupusPRO LIT per Rush University intellectual property revenue distribution regulations. Rush University and University of Illinois at Chicago hold copyrights to the following intellectual property: LupusPRO, LIT, SIMPLE, and BILS.

REFERENCES

1. Jolly M, Utset TO. Can disease specific measures for systemic lupus erythematosus predict patients health related quality of life? Lupus 2004;13(12): 924–6.
2. Jolly M. How does quality of life of patients with systemic lupus erythematosus compare with that of other common chronic illnesses? J Rheumatol 2005;32(9): 1706–8.

3. Azizoddin DR, Jolly M, Arora S, et al. Patient-reported outcomes predict mortality in lupus. Arthritis Care Res 2019;71(8):1028–35.

4. Ware JE, Sherbourne CD. The MOS 36-item short-form health survey (SF-36). I. Conceptual framework and item selection. Med Care 1992;30(6):473–83.

5. Brazier J, Roberts J, Deverill M. The estimation of a preference-based measure of health from the SF-36. J Health Econ 2002;21(2):271–92.

6. Aggarwal R, Wilke CT, Pickard AS, et al. Psychometric properties of the EuroQol-5D and short form-6D in patients with systemic lupus erythematosus. J Rheumatol 2009;36(6):1209–16.

7. Kasturi S, Szymonifka J, Burket JC, et al. Validity and reliability of patient reported outcomes measurement information system computerized adaptive tests in systemic lupus erythematosus. J Rheumatol 2017;44(7):1024–31.

8. Paz SH, Liu H, Fongwa MN, et al. Readability estimates for commonly used health-related quality of life surveys. Qual Life Res 2009;18(7):889–900.

9. Adams J, Chapman J, Bradley S, et al. Literacy levels required to complete routinely used patient-reported outcome measures in rheumatology. Rheumatology (Oxford) 2013;52(3):460–4.

10. Azizoddin DR, Weinberg S, Gandhi N, et al. Validation of the LupusPRO version 1.8: an update to a disease-specific patient-reported outcome tool for systemic lupus erythematosus. Lupus 2018;27(5):728–37.

11. Thumboo J, Feng PH, Boey ML, et al. Validation of the Chinese SF-36 for quality of life assessment in patients with systemic lupus erythematosus. Lupus 2000; 9(9):708–12.

12. Baba S, Katsumata Y, Okamoto Y, et al. Reliability of the SF-36 in Japanese patients with systemic lupus erythematosus and its associations with disease activity and damage: a two-consecutive year prospective study. Lupus 2018;27(3): 407–16.

13. Jolly M, Pickard AS, Block JA, et al. Disease-specific patient reported outcome tools for systemic lupus erythematosus. Semin Arthritis Rheum 2012;42(1): 56–65.

14. Jolly M, Kosinski M, Garris CP, et al. Prospective validation of the lupus impact tracker: a patient-completed tool for clinical practice to evaluate the impact of systemic lupus erythematosus. Arthritis Rheum 2016;68(6):1422–31.

15. Jolly M, Pickard SA, Mikolaitis RA, et al. LupusQoL-US benchmarks for US patients with systemic lupus erythematosus. J Rheumatol 2010;37(9):1828–33.

16. Nantes SG, Strand V, Su J, et al. Comparison of the sensitivity to change of the 36-item short form health survey and the lupus quality of life measure using various definitions of minimum clinically important differences in patients with active systemic lupus erythematosus. Arthritis Care Res 2018;70(1):125–33.

17. Jolly M, Garris CP, Mikolaitis RA, et al. Development and validation of the lupus impact tracker: a patient-completed tool for clinical practice to assess and monitor the impact of systemic lupus erythematosus. Arthritis Care Res 2014; 66(10):1542–50.

18. Thumboo J, Fong KY, Ng TP, et al. Validation of the MOS SF-36 for quality of life assessment of patients with systemic lupus erythematosus in Singapore. J Rheumatol 1999;26(1):97–102.

19. Yilmaz-Oner S, Oner C, Dogukan FM, et al. Health-related quality of life assessed by LupusQoL questionnaire and SF-36 in Turkish patients with systemic lupus erythematosus. Clin Rheumatol 2016;35(3):617–22.

20. García-Carrasco M, Mendoza-Pinto C, Cardiel MH, et al. Health related quality of life in Mexican women with systemic lupus erythematosus: a descriptive study using SF-36 and LupusQoL(C). Lupus 2012;21(11):1219–24.

21. Kuriya B, Gladman DD, Ibañez D, et al. Quality of life over time in patients with systemic lupus erythematosus. Arthritis Rheum 2008;59(2):181–5.

22. Baba S, Katsumata Y, Okamoto Y, et al. Reliability of the SF-36 in Japanese patients with systemic lupus erythematosus and its associations with disease activity and damage: a two-consecutive year prospective study. Lupus 2018;27(3): 407–16. https://doi.org/10.1177/0961203317725586.

23. Jolly M, Annapureddy N, Arnaud L, et al. Changes in quality of life in relation to disease activity in systemic lupus erythematosus: post-hoc analysis of the BLISS-52 Trial. Lupus 2019;28(14):1628–39.

24. McElhone K, Abbott J, Sutton C, et al. Sensitivity to change and minimal important differences of the LupusQoL in patients with systemic lupus erythematosus. Arthritis Care Res 2016;68(10):1505–13.

25. Devilliers H, Amoura Z, Besancenot J-F, et al. Responsiveness of the 36-item short form health survey and the lupus quality of life questionnaire in SLE. Rheumatology (Oxford) 2015;54(5):940–9.

26. Kasturi S, Szymonifka J, Berman JR, et al. Responsiveness of the patient-reported outcomes measurement information system global health short form in outpatients with systemic lupus erythematosus. Arthritis Care Res 2020; 72(9):1282–8.

27. Jolly M, Toloza S, Block J, et al. Spanish LupusPRO: cross-cultural validation study for lupus. Lupus 2013;22(5):431–6.

28. Devilliers H, Amoura Z, Besancenot J-F, et al. LupusQoL-FR is valid to assess quality of life in patients with systemic lupus erythematosus. Rheumatology (Oxford) 2012;51(10):1906–15.

29. EuroQol Group. EuroQol–a new facility for the measurement of health-related quality of life. Health Policy 1990;16(3):199–208.

30. Izadi Z. Health-related quality of life measures in adult systemic lupus erythematosus. Arthritis Care Res 2020;72(Suppl 10):577–92.

31. Wang S, Hsieh E, Zhu L, et al. Comparative assessment of different health utility measures in systemic lupus erythematosus. Sci Rep 2015;5:13297.

32. Navarra SV, Tanangunan RMDV, Mikolaitis-Preuss RA, et al. Cross-cultural validation of a disease-specific patient-reported outcome measure for lupus in Philippines. Lupus 2013;22(3):262–7.

33. Jolly M, Pickard AS, Wilke C, et al. Lupus-specific health outcome measure for US patients: the LupusQoL-US version. Ann Rheum Dis 2010;69(1):29–33.

34. Wang S, Wu B, Zhu L, et al. Construct and criterion validity of the euro QoI-5D in patients with systemic lupus erythematosus. PLoS One 2014;9(6):e98883.

35. Parodis I, Benavides AHL, Zickert A, et al. The impact of belimumab and rituximab on health-related quality of life in patients with systemic lupus erythematosus. Arthritis Care Res 2019;71(6):811–21.

36. Bruce B, Fries JF. The arthritis, rheumatism and aging medical information system (ARAMIS): still young at 30 years. Clin Exp Rheumatol 2005;23(5 Suppl 39): S163–7.

37. Reeve BB, Burke LB, Chiang Y, et al. Enhancing measurement in health outcomes research supported by Agencies within the US Department of Health and Human Services. Qual Life Res 2007;16(Suppl 1):175–86.

38. Kasturi S, Burket JC, Berman JR, et al. Feasibility of patient-reported outcomes measurement information system (PROMIS®) computerized adaptive tests in systemic lupus erythematosus outpatients. Lupus 2018;27(10):1591–9.
39. Katz P, Pedro S, Alemao E, et al. Estimates of responsiveness, minimally important differences, and patient acceptable symptom state in five patient-reported outcomes measurement information system short forms in systemic lupus erythematosus. ACR Open Rheumatol 2019;2(1):53–60.
40. Rothrock NE, Hays RD, Spritzer K, et al. Relative to the General US population, chronic diseases are associated with poorer health-related quality of life as measured by the patient-reported outcomes measurement information system (PROMIS). J Clin Epidemiol 2010;63(11):1195–204.
41. DeWalt DA, Rothrock N, Yount S, et al, PROMIS Cooperative Group. Evaluation of item candidates: the PROMIS qualitative item review. Med Care 2007;45(5 Suppl 1):S12–21.
42. Paz SH, Jones L, Calderón JL, et al. Readability and comprehension of the geriatric depression scale and PROMIS® physical function items in older African Americans and Latinos. Patient 2017;10(1):117–31.
43. Jones JT, Carle AC, Wootton J, et al. Validation of patient-reported outcomes measurement information system short forms for use in childhood-onset systemic lupus erythematosus. Arthritis Care Res 2017;69(1):133–42.
44. Kasturi S, Szymonifka J, Burket JC, et al. Feasibility, validity, and reliability of the 10-item patient reported outcomes measurement information system global health short form in outpatients with systemic lupus erythematosus. J Rheumatol 2018;45(3):397–404.
45. Ow YLM, Thumboo J, Cella D, et al. Domains of health-related quality of life important and relevant to multiethnic English-speaking Asian systemic lupus erythematosus patients: a focus group study. Arthritis Care Res 2011;63(6):899–908.
46. Katz P, Yazdany J, Trupin L, et al. Psychometric evaluation of the national institutes of health patient-reported outcomes measurement information system in a multiracial, multiethnic systemic lupus erythematosus cohort. Arthritis Care Res 2019;71(12):1630–9.
47. Ganguli SK, Hui-Yuen JS, Jolly M, et al. Performance and psychometric properties of lupus impact tracker in assessing patient-reported outcomes in pediatric lupus: Report from a pilot study. Lupus 2020;29(13):1781–9.
48. Katz P, Pedro S, Michaud K. Performance of the patient-reported outcomes measurement information system 29-item profile in rheumatoid arthritis, osteoarthritis, fibromyalgia, and systemic lupus erythematosus. Arthritis Care Res 2017;69(9):1312–21.
49. Available translations. Available at: https://www.healthmeasures.net/explore-measurement-systems/promis/intro-to-promis/available-translations. Accessed January 7, 2021.
50. Pincus T, Maclean R, Yazici Y, et al. Quantitative measurement of patient status in the regular care of patients with rheumatic diseases over 25 years as a continuous quality improvement activity, rather than traditional research. Clin Exp Rheumatol 2007;25(6 Suppl 47):69–81.
51. Annapureddy N, Giangreco D, Devilliers H, et al. Psychometric properties of MDHAQ/RAPID3 in patients with systemic lupus erythematosus. Lupus 2018;27(6):982–90.
52. Askanase AD, Castrejón I, Pincus T. Quantitative data for care of patients with systemic lupus erythematosus in usual clinical settings: a patient

multidimensional health assessment questionnaire and physician estimate of noninflammatory symptoms. J Rheumatol 2011;38(7):1309–16.

53. Pincus T, Hines P, Bergman MJ, et al. Proposed severity and response criteria for routine assessment of patient index data (RAPID3): results for categories of disease activity and response criteria in abatacept clinical trials. J Rheumatol 2011;38(12):2565–71.

54. Singh G, Athreya BH, Fries JF, et al. Measurement of health status in children with juvenile rheumatoid arthritis. Arthritis Rheum 1994;37(12):1761–9.

55. Meiorin S, Pistorio A, Ravelli A, et al. Validation of the childhood health assessment questionnaire in active juvenile systemic lupus erythematosus. Arthritis Rheum 2008;59(8):1112–9.

56. Craig J, Feldman BM, Spiegel L, et al. Comparing the measurement properties and preferability of patient reported outcome measures in pediatric rheumatology: PROMIS versus CHAQ. J Rheumatol 2020. https://doi.org/10.3899/jrheum.200943.

57. Moorthy LN, Saad-Magalhães C, Sato JO, et al. Validation of the Portuguese simple measure of impact of lupus erythematosus in youngsters (SMILEY) in Brazil. Lupus 2013;22(2):190–7.

58. Moorthy LN, Harrison MJ, Peterson M, et al. Relationship of quality of life and physical function measures with disease activity in children with systemic lupus erythematosus. Lupus 2005;14(4):280–7.

59. Huber AM, Hicks JE, Lachenbruch PA, et al. Validation of the childhood health assessment questionnaire in the juvenile idiopathic myopathies. Juvenile dermatomyositis disease activity collaborative study group. J Rheumatol 2001; 28(5):1106–11.

60. Klepper SE. Measures of pediatric function: Child Health Assessment Questionnaire (C-HAQ), Juvenile Arthritis Functional Assessment Scale (JAFAS), Pediatric Outcomes Data Collection Instrument (PODCI), and Activities Scale for Kids (ASK). Arthritis Care Res 2011;63(Suppl 11):S371–82.

61. Lai J-S, Beaumont JL, Ogale S, et al. Validation of the functional assessment of chronic illness therapy-fatigue scale in patients with moderately to severely active systemic lupus erythematosus, participating in a clinical trial. J Rheumatol 2011;38(4):672–9.

62. Kosinski M, Gajria K, Fernandes AW, et al. Qualitative validation of the FACIT-fatigue scale in systemic lupus erythematosus. Lupus 2013;22(5):422–30.

63. Jiang H-Z, Lin Z-G, Li H-J, et al. The Chinese version of the SLEQOL is a reliable assessment of health-related quality of life in Han Chinese patients with systemic lupus erythematosus. Clin Rheumatol 2018;37(1):151–60.

64. Petri MA, Martin RS, Scheinberg MA, et al. Assessments of fatigue and disease activity in patients with systemic lupus erythematosus enrolled in the Phase 2 clinical trial with blisibimod. Lupus 2017;26(1):27–37.

65. Montan I, Löwe B, Cella D, et al. General population norms for the Functional Assessment of Chronic Illness Therapy (FACIT)-Fatigue Scale. Value Health 2018;21(11):1313–21.

66. Goligher EC, Pouchot J, Brant R, et al. Minimal clinically important difference for 7 measures of fatigue in patients with systemic lupus erythematosus. J Rheumatol 2008;35(4):635–42.

67. Pettersson S, Lundberg IE, Liang MH, et al. Determination of the minimal clinically important difference for seven measures of fatigue in Swedish patients with systemic lupus erythematosus. Scand J Rheumatol 2015;44(3):206–10.

68. Azizoddin DR, Gandhi N, Weinberg S, et al. Fatigue in systemic lupus: the role of disease activity and its correlates. Lupus 2019;28(2):163–73.

69. Bourré-Tessier J, Clarke AE, Mikolaitis-Preuss RA, et al. Cross-cultural validation of a disease-specific patient-reported outcome measure for systemic lupus erythematosus in Canada. J Rheumatol 2013;40(8):1327–33.

70. Jolly M, Kazmi N, Mikolaitis RA, et al. Validation of the Cutaneous Lupus Disease Area and Severity Index (CLASI) using physician- and patient-assessed health outcome measures. J Am Acad Dermatol 2013;68(4):618–23.

71. Mok CC, Ho LY, Tse SM, et al. Prevalence of remission and its effect on damage and quality of life in Chinese patients with systemic lupus erythematosus. Ann Rheum Dis 2017;76(8):1420–5.

72. Giangreco D, Devilliers H, Annapureddy N, et al. Lupuspro is responsive to changes in disease activity over time. ACR Meeting Abstracts. Available at: http://acrabstracts.org/abstract/lupuspro-is-responsive-to-changes-in-disease-activity-over-time/. Accessed March 30, 2016.

73. Mok CC, Block J, Jolly M. THU0264 Responsiveness of lupuspro v1.8 among chinese patients with lupus. Ann Rheum Dis 2017;76(Suppl 2):303–4.

74. Jolly M, Peters KF, Mikolaitis R, et al. Body image intervention to improve health outcomes in lupus: a pilot study. J Clin Rheumatol 2014;20(8):403–10.

75. Schneider M, Mosca M, Pego-Reigosa J-M, et al. Cross-cultural validation of lupus impact tracker in five European clinical practice settings. Rheumatology (Oxford) 2017;56(5):818–28.

76. Antony A, Kandane-Rathnayake RK, Ko T, et al. Validation of the lupus impact tracker in an Australian patient cohort. Lupus 2017;26(1):98–105.

77. Brandt JE, Drenkard C, Kan H, et al. External validation of the lupus impact tracker in a southeastern US longitudinal cohort with systemic lupus erythematosus. Arthritis Care Res 2017;69(6):842–8.

78. Rodriguez TRV, Figueroa IR, Perez VDC, et al. 245 Associations between patient acceptable symptom state and three domains of the disease in SLE: a cross-sectional study of 1,364 patients from the spanish society of rheumatology lupus registry. Lupus Sci Med 2019;6(Suppl 1). https://doi.org/10.1136/lupus-2019-lsm.245.

79. Devilliers H, Bonithon-Kopp C, Jolly M. The lupus impact tracker is responsive to changes in clinical activity measured by the systemic lupus erythematosus responder index. Lupus 2017;26(4):396–402.

80. Giangreco D, Devilliers H, Annapureddy N, et al. Lupus impact tracker is responsive to physician and patient assessed changes in systemic lupus erythematosus. Lupus 2015;24(14):1486–91.

81. Figueroa IR, Devilliers H, Reigosa JMP, et al. 72 Lupus impact tracker is responsive to changes in physician (T2T) and patient (SLAQ, EQ5D) relevant outcomes in a large spanish lupus registry cohort. Lupus Sci Med 2019;6(Suppl 1):A53–4.

82. McElhone K, Abbott J, Shelmerdine J, et al. Development and validation of a disease-specific health-related quality of life measure, the LupusQol, for adults with systemic lupus erythematosus. Arthritis Rheum 2007;57(6):972–9.

83. Wang S, Wu B, Leng L, et al. Validity of LupusQoL-China for the assessment of health related quality of life in Chinese patients with systemic lupus erythematosus. PLoS One 2013;8(5):e63795.

84. Meseguer-Henarejos A-B, Gascón-Cánovas J-J, López-Pina J-A. Components of quality of life in a sample of patients with lupus: a confirmatory factor analysis and Rasch modeling of the LupusQoL. Clin Rheumatol 2017;36(8):1789–95.

85. Meacock R, Harrison M, McElhone K, et al. Mapping the disease-specific Lu-pusQoL to the SF-6D. Qual Life Res 2015;24(7):1749–58.

86. Delis PC, Dowling J. An integrative review of the LupusQoL measure. J Nurs Meas 2020;28(2):E139–74.

87. Touma Z, Gladman DD, Ibañez D, et al. Is there an advantage over SF-36 with a quality of life measure that is specific to systemic lupus erythematosus? J Rheumatol 2011;38(9):1898–905.

88. Leong KP, Kong KO, Thong BYH, et al. Development and preliminary validation of a systemic lupus erythematosus-specific quality-of-life instrument (SLEQOL). Rheumatology 2005;44(10):1267–76.

89. Kasitanon N, Wangkaew S, Puntana S, et al. The reliability, validity and respon-siveness of the Thai version of Systemic Lupus Erythematosus Quality of Life (SLEQOL-TH) instrument. Lupus 2013;22(3):289–96.

90. Louthrenoo W, Kasitanon N, Morand E, et al. Comparison of performance of specific (SLEQOL) and generic (SF36) health-related quality of life question-naires and their associations with disease status of systemic lupus erythemato-sus: a longitudinal study. Arthritis Res Ther 2020;22(1):8.

91. Moorthy LN, Peterson MGE, Baratelli M, et al. Multicenter validation of a new quality of life measure in pediatric lupus. Arthritis Rheum 2007;57(7):1165–73.

92. Doward LC, McKenna SP, Whalley D, et al. The development of the L-QoL: a quality-of-life instrument specific to systemic lupus erythematosus. Ann Rheum Dis 2009;68(2):196–200.

93. Moorthy LN, Peterson MGE, Hassett AL, et al. Relationship between health-related quality of life and SLE activity and damage in children over time. Lupus 2009;18(7):622–9.

94. Duruöz MT, Unal C, Toprak CS, et al. The validity and reliability of Systemic Lupus Erythematosus Quality of Life Questionnaire (L-QoL) in a Turkish popula-tion. Lupus 2017;26(14):1528–33.

95. Castellano-Rioja E, Giménez-Espert MDC, Soto-Rubio A. Lupus Erythematosus Quality of Life Questionnaire (LEQoL): Development and Psychometric Proper-ties. Int J Environ Res Public Health 2020;17(22):8642.

96. Mathias SD, Berry P, De Vries J, et al. Patient experience in systemic lupus er-ythematosus: development of novel patient-reported symptom and patient-reported impact measures. J Patient Rep Outcomes 2018;2(1):11.

97. Grootscholten C, Ligtenberg G, Derksen RHWM, et al. Health-related quality of life in patients with systemic lupus erythematosus: development and validation of a lupus specific symptom checklist. Qual Life Res 2003;12(6):635–44.

98. Mathias SD, Berry P, De Vries J, et al. Development of the Systemic Lupus Ery-thematosus Steroid Questionnaire (SSQ): a novel patient-reported outcome tool to assess the impact of oral steroid treatment. Health Qual Life Outcomes 2017; 15(1):43.

99. Hassett AL, Li T, Radvanski DC, et al. Assessment of health-related family role functioning in systemic lupus erythematosus: Preliminary validation of a new measure. Arthritis Care Res 2012;64(9):1341–8.

100. Jolly M, Pickard AS, Sequeira W, et al. A brief assessment tool for body image in systemic lupus erythematosus. Body Image 2012;9(2):279–84.

101. Mathias SD, Berry P, Pascoe K, et al. Treatment satisfaction in systemic lupus erythematosus: development of a patient-reported outcome measure. J Clin Rheumatol 2017;23(2):94–101.

102. Moses N, Wiggers J, Nicholas C, et al. Development and psychometric analysis of the systemic lupus erythematosus needs questionnaire (SLENQ). Qual Life Res 2007;16(3):461–6.

103. Legge A, Kirkland S, Rockwood K, et al. Construction of a frailty index as a novel health measure in systemic lupus erythematosus. J Rheumatol 2020;47(1): 72–81.

104. Cleanthous S, Isenberg DA, Newman SP, et al. Patient Uncertainty Questionnaire-Rheumatology (PUQ-R): development and validation of a new patient-reported outcome instrument for systemic lupus erythematosus (SLE) and rheumatoid arthritis (RA) in a mixed methods study. Health Qual Life Outcomes 2016;14:33.

105. Karlson EW, Daltroy LH, Rivest C, et al. Validation of a Systemic Lupus Activity Questionnaire (SLAQ) for population studies. Lupus 2003;12(4):280–6.

106. Yazdany J, Yelin EH, Panopalis P, et al. Validation of the systemic lupus erythematosus activity questionnaire in a large observational cohort. Arthritis Rheum 2008;59(1):136–43.

107. Chehab G, Richter J, Sander O, et al. Validation and evaluation of the German version of the Systemic Lupus Activity Questionnaire (SLAQ). Clin Exp Rheumatol 2015;33(3):354–9.

108. Pettersson S, Svenungsson E, Gustafsson J, et al. A comparison of patients' and physicians' assessments of disease activity using the Swedish version of the systemic lupus activity questionnaire. Scand J Rheumatol 2017;46(6):474–83.

109. Tani C, Vagelli R, Stagnaro C, et al. Translation, cultural adaptation and validation of the Systemic Lupus Erythematosus Activity Questionnaire (SLAQ) in a cohort of Italian systemic lupus erythematosus patients. Lupus 2018;27(10): 1735–41.

110. Okamoto Y, Katsumata Y, Baba S, et al. Validation of the Japanese version of the Systemic Lupus Activity Questionnaire that includes physician-based assessments in a large observational cohort. Lupus 2016;25(5):486–95.

111. Gandhi N, Arora S, Sengupta M, et al. Validation of SIMPLE Index for lupus disease activity. J Clin Rheumatol 2018;24(6):313–8.

112. Validation of the SIMPLE Index for Disease Activity of Systemic Lupus Erythematosus in Chinese Patients. ACR Meeting Abstracts. Available at: https://acrabstracts.org/abstract/validation-of-the-simple-index-for-disease-activity-of-systemic-lupus-erythematosus-in-chinese-patients/. Accessed January 7, 2021.

113. Askanase A, Li X, Pong A, et al. Preliminary test of the LFA rapid evaluation of activity in lupus (LFA-REAL): an efficient outcome measure correlates with validated instruments. Lupus Sci Med 2015;2(1):e000075.

114. Askanase AD, Daly RP, Okado M, et al. Development and content validity of the Lupus Foundation of America rapid evaluation of activity in lupus (LFA-REAL™): a patient-reported outcome measure for lupus disease activity. Health Qual Life Outcomes 2019;17(1):99.

115. Ugarte-Gil MF, Gamboa-Cardenas RV, Reátegui-Sokolova C, et al. Evaluation of the LFA-REAL clinician-reported outcome (ClinRO) and patient-reported outcome (PRO): data from the Peruvian Almenara Lupus Cohort. Lupus Sci Med 2020;7(1):e000419.

116. Costenbader KH, Khamashta M, Ruiz-Garcia S, et al. Development and Initial Validation of the Self-Assessed Lupus Damage Index Questionnaire (LDIQ). Arthritis Care Res 2010;62(4):559–68.

117. Okamoto Y, Katsumata Y, Baba S, et al. Validation of the Japanese version of the Lupus Damage Index Questionnaire in a large observational cohort: A two-year

prospective study. Mod Rheumatol 2020;1–9. https://doi.org/10.1080/14397595.2020.1829341.

118. Pons-Estel BA, Sánchez-Guerrero J, Romero-Díaz J, et al. Validation of the Spanish, Portuguese and French Versions of the lupus damage index questionnaire: data from North and South America, Spain and Portugal. Lupus 2009; 18(12):1033–52.

119. Yazdany J, Trupin L, Gansky SA, et al. Brief index of lupus damage: a patient-reported measure of damage in systemic lupus erythematosus. Arthritis Care Res 2011;63(8):1170–7.

120. Strand V, Gladman D, Isenberg D, et al. Endpoints: consensus recommendations from OMERACT IV. Outcome measures in rheumatology. Lupus 2000; 9(5):322–7.

121. Patient-Reported Outcome Measures: Use in Medical Product Development to Support Labeling Claims | FDA. Available at: https://www.fda.gov/regulatory-information/search-fda-guidance-documents/patient-reported-outcome-measures-use-medical-product-development-support-labeling-claims. Accessed January 7, 2021.

T Cells in Systemic Lupus Erythematosus

Jacqueline L. Paredes, BA[a,1], Ruth Fernandez-Ruiz, MD, MSCI[a,b,1], Timothy B. Niewold, MD[a,*]

KEYWORDS

- Systemic lupus erythematosus • Lupus • T cells • Cytokines • Epigenetics
- Metabolism • T-cell subsets

KEY POINTS

- Predominance of pathogenic and dysfunctional T-cell subsets over regulatory T cells is central to systemic lupus erythematosus (SLE) pathogenesis.
- Abnormalities in metabolic pathways, such as oxidative stress, glycolysis, and lipid metabolism, contribute to the dysfunctional T-cell phenotypes in SLE.
- T-cell epigenetic and genetic alterations are associated with disease activity and clinical phenotypes.
- Although multiple drugs have failed to meet their primary outcomes in SLE, various promising therapeutic agents targeting T cell–related pathways are currently in different phases of development.

INTRODUCTION

T cells have a central role in systemic lupus erythematosus (SLE) pathogenesis. T-cell dysregulation affects peripheral tolerance and induces inappropriate activation of B cells.[1,2] Various T-cell subsets are implicated in disease pathogenesis. Via excessive production of proinflammatory cytokines and contact-dependent interactions, these subsets promote autoantibody production and lead to tissue damage through the recruitment of immune cells. In addition to traditional cytokine signals, several other factors influence T-cell dysregulation, including metabolic and epigenetic changes.[3,4] This article discusses the function of T cells in SLE, primarily focusing on the various roles of T-cell subsets, and how molecular, genetic, and epigenetic pathways affect T-cell dysregulation. It also addresses the development of T cell–targeted drugs and their role as potential SLE therapies.

[a] Colton Center for Autoimmunity, NYU Grossman School of Medicine, 550 1st Avenue, New York, NY 10016, USA; [b] Division of Rheumatology, NYU Grossman School of Medicine, 550 1st Avenue, New York, NY 10016, USA
[1] Authors contributed equally to this work.
* Corresponding author.
E-mail address: Timothy.Niewold@nyulangone.org

Rheum Dis Clin N Am 47 (2021) 379–393
https://doi.org/10.1016/j.rdc.2021.04.005
0889-857X/21/© 2021 Elsevier Inc. All rights reserved.

rheumatic.theclinics.com

OVERVIEW OF T CELLS AND T-HELPER SUBSETS, AND EVIDENCE OF T-CELL DYSFUNCTION IN SYSTEMIC LUPUS ERYTHEMATOSUS
CD 4⁺ T-helper Cells and Subsets

T-helper (Th) cells orchestrate the immune response against pathogens. These cells express cluster of differentiation (CD) 4 in their surface and are subdivided by cytokine expression profiles, which dictate their subtypes and function in host defense (**Fig. 1**).[5] The significant plasticity in differentiation and expression of signature cytokines between Th subsets contributes to maintaining the physiologic balance between proinflammatory and antiinflammatory states. Dysregulated Th responses, with disrupted cytokine homeostasis and predominance of pathogenic Th subsets, occur in many autoimmune and inflammatory diseases, including SLE.

T-helper 1 cells
Th1 cells, classically defined by their production of IL-2 and interferon (IFN)-γ, are involved in cell-mediated inflammatory responses and defense against intracellular pathogens. Effector Th1 cells express the transcription factor Tbet.[5] Th1 cytokines play central roles in the pathogenesis of SLE. IFN-γ promotes B-cell class switching and stimulates pathogenic autoantibody production, at least in part by induction of aberrant T-follicular helper (Tfh) cell activation and germinal center formation.[6] Levels of IFN-γ are increased in patients with SLE compared with controls and positively correlate with SLE disease activity index (SLEDAI) scores.[7,8]

T-helper 2 cells
Th2 cells play a major role in combating parasitic infections and contribute to atopic conditions. Th2 cells express the GATA3 transcription factor, and their cytokine profile includes IL-4, IL-5, and IL-13. IL-4 promotes B-cell differentiation into plasma cells and induces antibody class switching to immunoglobulin (Ig) G1 and IgE.[5] In lupus-prone mice, blocking IL-4 decreases anti–double-stranded DNA (anti-dsDNA) antibodies, whereas administration of IL-4 increases the levels of this autoantibody.[9] However, patients with SLE may have a decreased number of IL-4–producing

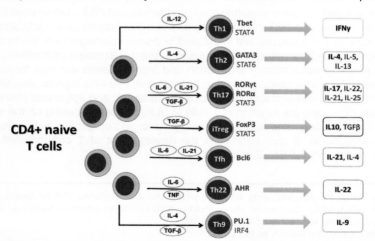

Fig. 1. Cluster of differentiation (CD) 4⁺ T-cell subsets relevant in SLE. Naïve CD4+ T cells differentiate into a specific subset (Th1, Th2, Th17, Treg, Tfh, Th22, or Th9) depending on the cytokine milieu. Activation of subset-specific transcription factors is necessary for CD4+ T cell differentiation and subsequent production of their signature cytokines. IFN, interferon; IL, interleukin; TGF, transforming growth factor; TNF, tumor necrosis factor.

T cells, with the increased IFN-γ/IL-4 CD4$^+$ T-cell ratio being positively correlated with SLEDAI scores.[10] IL-13 promotes the proliferation and differentiation of B cells, and induces the expression of major histocompatibility complex (MHC) class II, CD23, and IgE. In addition, IL-13 is a profibrotic cytokine and is a negative regulator of Th17 differentiation.[11] Previous studies have reported higher levels of circulating IL-13 in patients with SLE.[12,13] IL-5 has traditionally been described as a cytokine responsible for stimulating antibody production from activated B cells, and proliferation and differentiation of eosinophils from precursors to mature cells. Although the specific roles of IL-5 in SLE remain to be elucidated, IL-5 is overexpressed in keratinocytes from lesional skin and sera of patients with SLE compared with controls.[14,15]

T-helper 17 cells

Th17 cells are a major source of IL-17, a family of cytokines with potent inflammatory effects and major roles in host defense against extracellular bacteria and fungi. Th17 cells can also exacerbate tissue injury because of the proinflammatory roles of IL-17, including neutrophil recruitment, activation of the innate immune system, and enhancement of B-cell functions. The Th17 phenotype is regulated by the retinoic acid receptor-related orphan receptor (ROR)γt and RORα, which are induced by transforming growth factor (TGF) β and IL-6 in a STAT3-dependent manner.[5]

Several studies have shown a central role of Th17 cells and IL-17 in SLE pathogenesis. IL-17 and B cell–activating factor (BAFF) could have a synergistic effect at enhancing B-cell differentiation, proliferation, and antibody production.[16] Moreover, IL-17 levels correlate with SLEDAI scores, and baseline levels are higher in patients with persistently active nephritis despite therapy.[17,18] Similarly, levels of IL-23, which is required for Th17 maintenance, are increased in patients with SLE compared with controls, and high levels are associated with renal involvement.[19] In patients with active lupus nephritis, IL-23 levels were higher in those who did not respond to therapy compared with partial or complete responders.[18] In murine lupus, mice deficient in the IL-23 receptor have lower anti-dsDNA levels and less severe nephritis.[20]

T-helper 22 cells

Th22 cells predominantly produce IL-22, a member of the IL-10 family that is thought to play a role in protective immunity, limiting local intestinal and liver inflammation, as well as systemic inflammatory responses.[21] However, pathogenic roles of IL-22 have been reported in psoriasis and rheumatoid arthritis. The specific role of this cytokine in SLE remains controversial because of conflicting data and the potential for antiinflammatory or proinflammatory functions depending on the microenvironment.[22,23]

Previous studies have shown that patients with SLE have a greater proportion of Th22 cells compared with healthy controls. Similarly, a positive correlation between Th22 cells and IL-22 plasma concentration in patients with SLE, as well as between the percentage of Th22 cells and SLEDAI scores, has also been described.[17,22,24] In contrast, other studies have shown reduced levels of circulating IL-22 or IL-22-producing cells in active patients with SLE compared with patients with inactive SLE and healthy controls, as well as an inverse correlation between SLEDAI scores and IL-22 levels.[23,25–27] The conflicting results among different studies are possibly caused by timing of evaluation with respect to disease course, medication use, or clinical phenotype. For example, a study assessing patients with new-onset SLE found decreased plasma levels of IL-22 compared with patients with relapsing SLE, which increased after improved disease activity and treatment with hydroxychloroquine and systemic steroids.[23] Moreover, IL-22 levels are increased in patients with SLE with sole skin involvement and decreased in those with only lupus nephritis.[17] Patients with class III or class IV lupus nephritis were also shown to have significantly lower levels of urinary IL-22 messenger RNA (mRNA) than those with class V nephritis.[28]

T-helper 9 cells

Although originally classified as a Th2 cytokine, IL-9 is now thought to be mainly produced by a distinct subset identified as Th9 cells. IFN regulatory factor 4 (IRF4) is crucial for IL-9 production and Th9 development.[29] IL-9 acts in multiple cells as a growth factor, including mast cells and eosinophils. This cytokine also plays a central role in allergic airway disease, tumor immunity, and inflammatory bowel disease, although antiinflammatory functions have also been described.[29] In lupus-prone mice, IL-9 has been implicated in B-cell activation, proliferation, and heightened auto-antibody production, and improved nephritis outcomes when the mice were treated with IL-9 neutralizing antibodies.[30] However, only a few studies have assessed the role of Th9 and IL-9 in patients with SLE, suggesting increased circulating levels of this cytokine compared with healthy controls. Whether IL-9 and Th9 frequency are associated with SLE-specific characteristics is less clear.[31]

Regulatory T cells

Regulatory T cells (Tregs) are crucial in maintaining self-tolerance and immune homeostasis. These cells are characterized by expression of the IL-2 receptor alpha chain (CD25) and the nuclear transcription factor FoxP3. Tregs also express cytotoxic T lymphocyte–associated protein 4 (CTLA4), and the transcription factors neuropilin-1 and Helios.[32] These cells suppress activation and expansion of autoreactive lymphocytes, and thus are crucial in maintaining peripheral tolerance to self-antigens. Tregs have been further subdivided according to their developmental origin into thymic Tregs and peripherally induced Tregs.[32] No protein markers have been identified to date to accurately distinguish between these two populations of Tregs, although there are important epigenetic differences.[33]

Although both quantitative and qualitative differences in Tregs have been described in SLE, studies to date have shown contradictory results.[34,35] The selection of phenotypic markers to characterize the Treg population, the protocols used for isolation and stimulation of these cells, as well as the SLEDAI thresholds to differentiate between active and inactive SLE have potentially played a role in these discrepancies.[36] It is also possible that the number and function of Tregs are not uniformly affected in all patients with SLE or that other mechanisms, such as an acquired resistance of effector T cells to suppression by Tregs, may be involved.[37]

T-follicular helper cells

Tfhs localize in germinal centers and extrafollicular foci, providing B cells with key survival, differentiation, and maturation signals. The transcription factor BCL6 is required for Tfh development.[38] In the normal immune response, the main role of Tfh cells is to assist B cells during the response to T cell–dependent antigens, by releasing cytokines such as IL-21 and IL-4. SLE-specific autoantibodies such as anti-dsDNA acquire high antigen affinity through somatic hypermutation, indicating Tfh involvement in generating autoreactive B-cell clones in both murine and human SLE.[39] In lupus nephritis, Tfhs aggregate in renal tissue with B cells, similar to what is observed in germinal centers.[40] Contact-dependent molecules such as CD40L and inducible T cell co-stimulator (ICOS) from Tfhs also enhance activation of B cells in murine models of autoimmunity.[41] Therefore, cognate T-cell–B-cell interactions are crucial in the development and maintenance of self-reactive B cells and their differentiation into autoantibody-producing plasma cells.

Cluster of Differentiation 8 T Cells

CD8 T cells recognize peptide antigens presented by MHC class I molecules, and their main effector function consists of the release of perforin and granzymes.[42] These cells participate in infection control, antitumoral response, and autoimmunity. Circulating CD8 T cells from patients with SLE show functional defects, including impaired cytolytic function with decreased production of granzyme and perforin.[43] An exhausted phenotype in circulating CD8 T cells from patients with SLE has been associated with lower disease flare rates.[44] These qualitative abnormalities in CD8 T cells may contribute to the pathogenesis of autoimmunity in SLE and likely relate to the predisposition of patients with SLE to infections, which can be further exacerbated by the use of immunosuppressive drugs.[45]

In mice with lupus-like nephritis, most kidney-infiltrating T cells have reduced proliferative capacity, cytokine production, and increased expression of inhibitory receptors, including programmed cell death protein 1.[46] In contrast, recent single-cell transcriptomics data from human lupus nephritis indicate that kidney-infiltrating CD8 T cells express low levels of canonical exhaustion markers, whereas circulating CD8 T cells do show an exhausted phenotype in patients with SLE.[47] These contrasting study findings suggest potential discrepancies in human versus murine lupus data. Moreover, the differences in exhausted markers between the circulating and affected organ CD8 T cells in SLE show some of the complexities in understanding the disease pathogenesis.

Double-Negative T Cells

Mature double-negative T (DNT) cells express the $\alpha\beta$ T-cell receptor but lack the CD4 and CD8 coreceptors and natural killer cell markers.[48] Although these cells represent a small proportion of circulating lymphocytes in healthy individuals and are considered quiescent, patients with SLE and mice with lupus-like disease show expansion of the DNT cell population. DNT cells are proinflammatory in SLE and can infiltrate the kidneys, producing significant amounts of IL-17 and IFN-γ.[49] In lupus-prone mice, these cells also increase in parallel with worsening disease.[50]

DNT cells are thought to originate from activated self-reactive CD8 T cells after downregulation of CD8 expression on the cell surface in patients with SLE.[51] However, the exact mechanisms and specific factors by which these CD8 T cells escape activation-induced cell death and acquire the DNT-cell phenotype are not completely understood. It is possible that self-antigens from apoptotic cells can activate self-reactive CD8 T cells and give rise to DNT cells via downregulation of CD8.[48] This cell population has a proinflammatory phenotype, with enhanced tissue migration ability, IL-17 production, and promotion of autoantibody production and renal immune complex deposition.[48,49] Improved understanding of the origins, heterogeneity, plasticity, and function of DNT cells may reveal potential therapeutic targets in SLE.

$\gamma\delta$T Cells

$\gamma\delta$T cells represent a minor population of circulating lymphocytes. In contrast with conventional $\alpha\beta$ T cells, $\gamma\delta$T cells do not recognize antigens presented by MHC molecules. Instead, $\gamma\delta$T cells directly recognize a large variety of nonpeptide molecules such as transfer RNA synthetases and glycosides.[52] $\gamma\delta$T cells have pleiotropic roles and are potent effectors against pathogens, because these cells can identify specific antigens from biochemical pathways commonly used by bacteria, fungi, and parasites.[53] These cells are also involved in B-cell class switching (in germinal centers or extrafollicular aggregates) and enhancement of plasma cell survival.[54]

Previous studies have reported higher numbers of circulating γδT cells in general in patients with SLE compared with healthy controls.[55] However, on evaluation of γδT-cell subsets and when patients are stratified according to timing of SLE onset and disease activity, the differences between patients with SLE and controls become more complex. For example, a specific subset of γδT cells with regulatory functions (ie, CD27$^+$CD25^{high}FoxP3$^+$ Vδ1 T-cell population) is decreased in the blood of patients with SLE. In new-onset patients with SLE, a significantly lower proportion of circulating γδT cells was found compared with healthy controls. Moreover, absolute γδT-cell counts were found to be decreased in patients with active SLE. The counts increased to overall normal levels after SLE treatment. There were also greater counts of the γδ1 subtype in patients with SLE compared with healthy individuals.[56] In contrast, in target tissues such as the skin, there is a greater proportion of γδT cells, particularly in those with active disease.[57] Several in vitro and murine lupus models have also shown a potential pathogenic role of γδ T cells in SLE by multiple mechanisms.[52]

T-CELL METABOLISM IN SYSTEMIC LUPUS ERYTHEMATOSUS

Several studies have shown the impact of metabolic control on T-cell differentiation, signaling, and pathogenicity. Nutrient availability directly affects the function of immune cells. Abnormalities in oxidative stress, glycolysis, lipid metabolism, and mitochondrial dysfunction are thought to contribute to dysregulated T-cell responses in SLE, and may explain the aberrant phenotypes in patients and murine lupus models.[58] Specifically, glycolysis-derived oxidative phosphorylation is characteristic of T cells from patients and mice with lupus. A predominance of glycolysis and glutaminolysis is also known to promote the generation of Th17 cells, whereas fatty acid and pyruvate oxidation can favor Treg and memory T-cell differentiation.[4]

In SLE, T cells are prone to hyperactivation caused by T cell receptor (TCR) rewiring, in which the CD3ζ chain is replaced by FcεRIγ and couples with the spleen tyrosine kinase instead of the ζ-associated protein kinase (70 kDa). This rewiring, mediated by an increase of protein phosphatase 2A activity and high oxidative stress in T cells, leads to increased TCR sensitivity and downstream signaling.[4] Moreover, aberrant lipid raft formation and enhanced costimulatory signals from target organs such as the kidney all contribute to increased TCR and costimulatory signaling in SLE. Consequently, T-cell hyperactivation leads to increased production of reactive oxygen species (ROS) and evidence of oxidative stress in circulating immune cells of patients with SLE.[59]

Mammalian target of rapamycin (mTOR), a sensor of cell nutrient status and mitochondrial hyperpolarization, is activated by ROS. mTOR complex 1 (mTORC1) signaling is also increased in SLE. Multiple direct and indirect mechanisms have been implicated in mTORC1 hyperactivation, including oxidative stress, upregulation of the calcium/calmodulin-dependent protein kinase IV (CaMK4), pentose phosphate pathway metabolites, increased expression of the lipid phosphatase PTEN, and genetic factors.[4] This signaling pathway is crucial for CD8 and CD4 T-cell differentiation, including Th1, Tfh, and Th17 subsets.[60] In general, mTOR activation also has negative effects on Treg differentiation and function. mTOR blockade by rapamycin inhibits Th17 differentiation while promoting Treg generation, and has been shown to reduce SLE disease activity.[61] In addition, treatment with the reducing agent N-acetylcysteine, a precursor of glutathione and mTOR inhibitor, reverses the expansion of DNT cells and can decrease anti-dsDNA titers in patients with SLE.[62] Other therapeutic agents targeting mitochondrial and cell metabolism, including metformin, have corrected some of the dysfunctional phenotypes in T cells from lupus-prone mice and patients with SLE.[58] Given multiple lines of evidence suggesting metabolic abnormalities directly affect T-cell dysfunction in SLE, modulating these pathways in autoreactive T cells represents a promising therapeutic approach in SLE.

GENETICS AND EPIGENETICS OF T CELLS CONTRIBUTING TO SYSTEMIC LUPUS ERYTHEMATOSUS

Epigenetic and genome-wide association studies have identified multiple alterations that potentially contribute to T-cell dysregulation in SLE.[63] T-cell activation is highly dependent on the MHC, which is the first locus identified to have a strong genetic association with SLE.[64] CD8[+] T cells carrying a STAT4 risk allele, which is associated with a more severe SLE phenotype and an earlier onset of disease, show enhanced IL-12–induced IFN-γ production.[65] In addition, patients with SLE carrying the STAT4 risk allele have increased phosphorylation of STAT4 in response to IL-12 and IFN-α in CD8[+] T cells and are predisposed to have an earlier onset of disease, increased risk of stroke, and severe renal insufficiency.[65–67]

Lupus nephritis pathogenesis is attributed to multiple genes affecting T-cell signaling, including TNFSF4, which promotes Tfh cell responses via the OX40/OX40L pathway. Expression of TNFSF4 receptors is also associated with nephritis and disease activity in SLE.[51,66] The CD47 gene, which regulates T-cell production of vascular endothelial growth factor, is downregulated in SLE T cells and is associated with renal disease.[68] Lower expression of SRSF1 in T cells of patients with SLE is associated with lymphopenia.[69] Although genetic risk factors contribute to the development of SLE, this does not solely explain the heterogeneity of the disease.

Alteration of epigenetic modifications such as DNA methylation, histone modifications, and microRNA (miRNA) can also contribute to dysregulated T-cell phenotypes.[70] DNA methylation results in the silencing of gene expression and is regulated by DNA methyltransferase (DNMT) enzymes and methyl CpG–binding proteins, which function to enlist the help of histone deacetylases and other remodeling factors.[3,70,71] Interestingly, mTOR activation and oxidative stress, which are commonly found in T cells from patients with SLE, contribute to hypomethylation in these cells via inhibition of DNMT1.[3] Hypomethylation of CpG22 in CD4[+] T cells in patients with SLE is associated with increase in SLEDAI score, whereas hypomethylation of CpG15 is associated with an increase in anti-dsDNA.[72] Similarly, hypomethylation and consequent upregulation of the perforin (PRF) and granzyme B (GZMB) genes has been described in CD8[+] T cells, which is associated with production of autoantigens and increased disease activity.[3] DNA methylation also decreases in a dose-dependent manner in CD4[+] T cells exposed to ultraviolet B in patients with SLE.[73]

Specific SLE disease manifestations have been linked to hypomethylation and hypermethylation patterns. Renauer and colleagues[74] identified specific regions of hypomethylation and hypermethylation in naive T cells that correspond with cell proliferation and apoptotic pathways in subjects with active or past cutaneous manifestations, including malar and discoid rash. In all patients with SLE, irrespective of presence of cutaneous manifestation or renal involvement, hypomethylation was observed in IFN-regulated genes.[74,75] Coit and colleagues[75] identified 64 hypomethylated sites in naive CD4[+] T cells that are unique to lupus nephritis and patients with SLE with a history of renal involvement. DNA hypomethylation is also observed in the CD40LG and genes related to arthritis and development of connective tissue in CD4[+] T cells, whereas hypermethylation is observed in genes that correspond with metabolic pathways such as folate biosynthesis and the pentose phosphate pathway.[76]

In addition to DNA methylation, posttranscriptional mRNA modifications can also modulate gene expression. For example, the levels of 5-methylcytosine (m5C), a form of mRNA epigenetic modification, are decreased in $CD4^+$ T cells from patients with SLE compared with healthy controls. Moreover, lower m5C levels are associated with more severe SLE disease activity.[77]

miRNAs regulate expression of multiple gene targets through repression or degradation of mRNA. Aberrant expression of miRNAs in T cells can affect the downstream expression of target molecules implicated in SLE pathogenesis.[78] Mean expression of 6 types of miRNAs in T cells was found to be lower in patients with SLE than in healthy controls, and was positively correlated with serum vitamin D concentration. Interestingly, a vitamin D concentration of less than 20 ng/mL was identified as a potential risk factor for SLE via dysregulation of miRNA expression.[78]

Histone acetylation has also been implicated in SLE pathogenesis. Reduced histone H3 acetylation and H3K9 methylation is observed in SLE $CD4^+$ T cells, and histone marks are observed at the IL-17 and IL-10 gene clusters, suggesting increased gene expression. In contrast, histone condensation is seen in the IL-2 clusters.[79] This finding could relate to the Treg defects observed in patients with SLE.[80]

T-CELL BIOMARKERS AND THERAPEUTICS IN DEVELOPMENT

Because T cells play a central role in promoting B-cell differentiation and enhancing production of autoantibodies, efforts focused on targeting T-cell pathways in SLE have emerged.[81] However, many drugs have not progressed in development (**Table 1**).[82] Despite some early failures, next-generation therapeutics have been developed and are in different phases of clinical trials (**Table 2**). Dapirolizumab pegol (DZP), a CD40 ligand antagonist, showed improvement in immunologic and clinical outcomes in the DZP-receiving group in a phase 2B trial, and a phase 3 trial is currently underway.[82] Over the past decade, the voltage-gated Kv1.3 potassium channels in T lymphocytes have garnered attention as a therapeutic target because these are highly expressed in macrophages and effector memory T cells (Tem) of patients with autoimmune diseases.[83] Dalazatide, an inhibitor of T_{em} Kv1.3 channels, decreases the percentage of $CD4^+$ Tem cells expressing HLA-DR.[83,84] In an ex vivo study, dalazatide use led to inhibition of IFN-γ, IL-17, and tumor necrosis factor alpha (TNF-α) production by $CD4^+$ and $CD8^+$ T cells in SLE; a phase 2 trial is underway.[68] CaMK4 has also emerged as a potential target, given its role in Th17 cell differentiation and IL-17 production.[85]

Tacrolimus (TAC), a calcineurin inhibitor, blocks IL-2 expression in T cells, and suppress Th1, Th2, and Th17 cytokine production.[86] In addition, tacrolimus in

Table 1
Clinical trials of biologics targeting T-cell pathways that did not progress

T Cell–directed Therapeutic	Mechanistic Target	Clinical Trials Identifier	Last Study Phase in SLE Before Discontinuation
Ustekinumab	Monoclonal antibody targeting IL-12 and IL-23	NCT03517722	Phase 3
Abatacept	CTLA-4 agonist that inhibits CD28 binding to CD80/CD86	NCT01714817	Phase 3
Lulizumab	Anti-CD28 domain antibody	NCT02265744	Phase 2
Theralizumab (TAB08)	Anti-CD28 superagonist	NCT02711813	Phase 2

Table 2
T-cell pathway–targeting drugs that are currently being studied or developed for systemic lupus erythematosus

T Cell–directed Therapeutic	Mechanistic Target	NCT Trial Number	Target Patient Population	Most Recent Phase Study Completed in SLE	Notable Outcomes
Dalazatide	Kv1.3 channel inhibitor	NCT02446340	Healthy control and ex vivo pediatric and adult SLE	Phase 1b	• Dalazatide inhibited cytokine production by CD4$^+$ and CD8$^+$ Tem • CD8$^+$ Tem cell expression of Kv1.3 is higher in active lupus nephritis • Kv1.3 may be a useful biomarker for SLE disease activity
DZP	CD40 ligand antagonist	NCT02804763	Moderate to severely active patients with SLE	Phase 2b	• Did not meet the primary end point • No differences in treatment adverse reactions between placebo-controlled and DZP-receiving subjects; drug seems to be well tolerated • Consistent improvement in DZP group in anti-dsDNA antibody levels, and pharmacodynamics markers
TAC and STA-21 combination therapy	Calcineurin inhibitor and STA-21 inhibits STAT3 signaling	NA	SLE	Preclinical	• TAC suppresses Th1, Th2, and Th17 cells and reduces Treg expression • In combination with STA-21, TAC suppresses GC B cells, plasma cells, and the production of TNF-α
Sirolimus	mTOR pathway inhibition	NCT00779194	Patients with active SLE that are unresponsive to conventional medications	Phase 1/2	• Reduction in SLEDAI and British Isles Lupus Assessment Group (BILAG) score was observed after 12 mo on treatment • CD4$^+$FoxP3$^+$ Treg expansion in patients with SLE when comparing baseline with 6-mo data • Sirolimus was safe and efficacious in most trial participants

Abbreviations: DZP, dapirolizumab pegol; GC, germinal center; NA, not available; TAC, tacrolimus; Tem, T effector memory; TNF, tumor necrosis factor.

combination with STA-21, an STAT3 inhibitor, can increase the population of Treg and provide potential beneficial to patients with SLE.[86] Sirolimus (rapamycin), an mTOR inhibitor, prevents the development of lupus nephritis in lupus-prone murine models.[87] Results from the phase 1/2 trial determined that the therapeutic was safe and efficacious for patients with active SLE. Use of sirolimus increased CD4[+] memory T cells in patients with SLE and resulted in the expansion of CD8[+] T cells in those with an increase in mean SLEDAI score.[88] Off-label use of sirolimus also showed benefit in patients with SLE with musculoskeletal involvement, further supporting results from previous studies.[87] Recently, the next-generation calcineurin inhibitor voclosporin was US Food and Drug Administration approved for the treatment of lupus nephritis.[89] This result was highly encouraging regarding T-cell–suppressive therapy in SLE and suggests that some of the other T cell–directed therapies in earlier stages of development could be successful.

T cells are also being investigated as prognostic biomarkers to pave the way for precision medicine in SLE. A human immunophenotyping SLE study showed that patients can be stratified into T cell–independent, Tfh-dominant, and Treg-dominant groups. Although these groups could not be differentiated based on clinical differences, Tfh-dominant patients were more resistant to standard SLE therapy.[90,91] In addition, hypomethylation of CHST12 in CD4[+] T cells of patients with SLE was observed to be 86% sensitive and 64% specific for lupus nephritis, proving to be a potential biomarker.[68]

SUMMARY

T-cell dysregulation has been increasingly recognized as central to SLE pathogenesis and is manifested by an imbalance between populations with immunosuppressive functions and pathogenic T-cell subsets, which contribute to the break in immune tolerance and ongoing inflammation. Growing recognition of the role of T cells in SLE has led to findings of abnormalities in metabolism, epigenetics, and genetic factors contributing to the dysfunctional phenotypes observed in SLE. Greater understanding of T-cell dysregulation in SLE is crucial for therapeutic development designed to correct the aberrant phenotypes. Identification of biomarkers related to T-cell dysfunction as predictors of disease course or treatment response would also be of great benefit for optimal management of patients with SLE.

CLINICS CARE POINTS

- Various T-cell subsets are pathogenic in SLE, promoting systemic autoimmunity and end-organ damage.
- Epigenetic modifications, such as differential DNA and mRNA methylation patterns, could represent novel biomarkers to better characterize and stratify patients with SLE.
- Novel and repurposed therapeutic agents targeting T cell–related pathways could be beneficial to at least a subset of patients with SLE.

DISCLOSURE STATEMENT AND FUNDING

T.B. Niewold: grants from the Colton Center for Autoimmunity, NIH (AR060861, AR057781, AR065964, AI071651), the Lupus Research Foundation, and the Lupus Research Alliance; T.B. Niewold has received research grants from EMD Serono and Janssen, Inc, and has consulted for Thermo Fisher, Toran, Ventus, Roivant Sciences, and Inova, all unrelated to the current article. R. Fernandez-Ruiz and J.L. Paredes have nothing to disclose.

REFERENCES

1. Suárez-Fueyo A, Bradley SJ, Tsokos GC. T cells in systemic lupus erythematosus. Curr Opin Immunol 2016;43:32–8.
2. Katsuyama T, Tsokos GC, Moulton VR. Aberrant T cell signaling and subsets in systemic lupus erythematosus. Front Immunol 2018;9:1088.
3. Deng Q, Luo Y, Chang C, et al. The emerging epigenetic role of cd8+t cells in autoimmune diseases: a systematic review. Front Immunol 2019;10:856.
4. Sharabi A, Tsokos GC. T cell metabolism: new insights in systemic lupus erythematosus pathogenesis and therapy. Nat Rev Rheumatol 2020;16(2):100–12.
5. Raphael I, Nalawade S, Eagar TN, et al. T cell subsets and their signature cytokines in autoimmune and inflammatory diseases. Cytokine 2015;74(1):5–17.
6. Lee SK, Silva DG, Martin JL, et al. Interferon-γ excess leads to pathogenic accumulation of follicular helper T cells and germinal centers. Immunity 2012;37(5): 880–92.
7. Torell F, Eketjäll S, Idborg H, et al. Cytokine profiles in autoantibody defined subgroups of systemic lupus erythematosus. J Proteome Res 2019;18(3):1208–17.
8. Shah D, Kiran R, Wanchu A, et al. Oxidative stress in systemic lupus erythematosus: relationship to Th1 cytokine and disease activity. Immunol Lett 2010; 129(1):7–12.
9. Nakajima A, Hirose S, Yagita H, et al. Roles of IL-4 and IL-12 in the development of lupus in NZB/W F1 mice. J Immunol 1997;158(3):1466–72.
10. Sugimoto K, Morimoto S, Kaneko H, et al. Decreased IL-4 producing CD4+ T cells in patients with active systemic lupus erythematosus-relation to IL-12R expression. Autoimmunity 2002;35(6):381–7.
11. Mao YM, Zhao CN, Leng J, et al. Interleukin-13: a promising therapeutic target for autoimmune disease. Cytokine Growth Factor Rev 2019;45:9–23.
12. Spadaro A, Rinaldi T, Riccieri V, et al. Interleukin-13 in autoimmune rheumatic diseases: relationship with the autoantibody profile. Clin Exp Rheumatol 2002;20(2): 213–6.
13. Brugos B, Vincze Z, Sipka S, et al. Serum and urinary cytokine levels of SLE patients. Pharmazie 2012;67(5):411–3.
14. Carneiro JR, Fuzii HT, Kayser C, et al. IL-2, IL-5, TNF-α and IFN-γ mRNA expression in epidermal keratinocytes of systemic lupus erythematosus skin lesions. Clinics (Sao Paulo) 2011;66(1):77–82.
15. Zhu H, Mi W, Luo H, et al. Whole-genome transcription and DNA methylation analysis of peripheral blood mononuclear cells identified aberrant gene regulation pathways in systemic lupus erythematosus. Arthritis Res Ther 2016;18:162.
16. López P, Rodríguez-Carrio J, Caminal-Montero L, et al. A pathogenic IFNα, BLyS and IL-17 axis in systemic lupus erythematosus patients. Sci Rep 2016;6:20651.
17. Yang XY, Wang HY, Zhao XY, et al. Th22, but not Th17 might be a good index to predict the tissue involvement of systemic lupus erythematosus. J Clin Immunol 2013;33(4):767–74.
18. Zickert A, Amoudruz P, Sundström Y, et al. IL-17 and IL-23 in lupus nephritis - association to histopathology and response to treatment. BMC Immunol 2015; 16(1):7.
19. Fischer K, Przepiera-Będzak H, Sawicki M, et al. Serum interleukin-23 in polish patients with systemic lupus erythematosus: association with lupus nephritis, obesity, and peripheral vascular disease. Mediators Inflamm 2017;2017: 9401432.

20. Dai H, He F, Tsokos GC, et al. IL-23 limits the production of IL-2 and promotes autoimmunity in lupus. J Immunol 2017;199(3):903–10.
21. Bird L. Mucosal immunology: IL-22 keeps commensals in their place. Nat Rev Immunol 2012;12(8):550–1.
22. Qin WZ, Chen LL, Pan HF, et al. Expressions of IL-22 in circulating CD4+/CD8+ T cells and their correlation with disease activity in SLE patients. Clin Exp Med 2011;11(4):245–50.
23. Lin J, Yue LH, Chen WQ. Decreased plasma IL-22 levels and correlations with IL-22-producing T helper cells in patients with new-onset systemic lupus erythematosus. Scand J Immunol 2014;79(2):131–6.
24. Zhong W, Jiang Y, Ma H, et al. Elevated levels of CCR6(+) T helper 22 cells correlate with skin and renal impairment in systemic lupus erythematosus. Sci Rep 2017;7(1):12962.
25. Cheng F, Guo Z, Xu H, et al. Decreased plasma IL22 levels, but not increased IL17 and IL23 levels, correlate with disease activity in patients with systemic lupus erythematosus. Ann Rheum Dis 2009;68(4):604–6.
26. Pan HF, Zhao XF, Yuan H, et al. Decreased serum IL-22 levels in patients with systemic lupus erythematosus. Clin Chim Acta 2009;401(1–2):179–80.
27. Dolff S, Scharpenberg C, Specker C, et al. IL-22 production of effector CD4(+) T cells is altered in SLE patients. Eur J Med Res 2019;24(1):24.
28. Luk CC, Tam LS, Kwan BC, et al. Intrarenal and urinary Th9 and Th22 cytokine gene expression in lupus nephritis. J Rheumatol 2015;42(7):1150–5.
29. Deng Y, Wang Z, Chang C, et al. Th9 cells and IL-9 in autoimmune disorders: Pathogenesis and therapeutic potentials. Hum Immunol 2017;78(2):120–8.
30. Yang J, Li Q, Yang X, et al. Interleukin-9 is associated with elevated anti-double-stranded DNA antibodies in lupus-prone mice. Mol Med 2015;21(1):364–70.
31. Dantas AT, Marques CD, da Rocha Junior LF, et al. Increased serum interleukin-9 levels in rheumatoid arthritis and systemic lupus erythematosus: pathogenic role or just an epiphenomenon? Dis Markers 2015;2015:519638.
32. Yadav M, Stephan S, Bluestone JA. Peripherally induced tregs - role in immune homeostasis and autoimmunity. Front Immunol 2013;4:232.
33. Dominguez-Villar M, Hafler DA. Regulatory T cells in autoimmune disease. Nat Immunol 2018;19(7):665–73.
34. Bonelli M, Savitskaya A, von Dalwigk K, et al. Quantitative and qualitative deficiencies of regulatory T cells in patients with systemic lupus erythematosus (SLE). Int Immunol 2008;20(7):861–8.
35. Alexander T, Sattler A, Templin L, et al. Foxp3+ Helios+ regulatory T cells are expanded in active systemic lupus erythematosus. Ann Rheum Dis 2013;72(9):1549–58.
36. La Cava A. Tregs in SLE: an update. Curr Rheumatol Rep 2018;20(2):6.
37. Yu Y, Liu Y, Shi FD, et al. Tolerance induced by anti-DNA Ig peptide in (NZB×NZW)F1 lupus mice impinges on the resistance of effector T cells to suppression by regulatory T cells. Clin Immunol 2012;142(3):291–5.
38. Craft JE. Follicular helper T cells in immunity and systemic autoimmunity. Nat Rev Rheumatol 2012;8(6):337–47.
39. Chen PM, Tsokos GC. T cell abnormalities in the pathogenesis of systemic lupus erythematosus: an update. Curr Rheumatol Rep 2021;23(2):12.
40. Liarski VM, Kaverina N, Chang A, et al. Cell distance mapping identifies functional T follicular helper cells in inflamed human renal tissue. Sci Transl Med 2014;6(230):230ra246.

41. Kim SJ, Lee K, Diamond B. Follicular helper T cells in systemic lupus erythematosus. Front Immunol 2018;9:1793.
42. Zhang N, Bevan MJ. CD8(+) T cells: foot soldiers of the immune system. Immunity 2011;35(2):161–8.
43. Comte D, Karampetsou MP, Yoshida N, et al. Signaling lymphocytic activation molecule family member 7 engagement restores defective effector CD8+ T cell function in systemic lupus erythematosus. Arthritis Rheum 2017;69(5):1035–44.
44. McKinney EF, Lee JC, Jayne DR, et al. T cell exhaustion, co-stimulation and clinical outcome in autoimmunity and infection. Nature 2015;523(7562):612–6.
45. Katsuyama E, Suarez-Fueyo A, Bradley SJ, et al. The CD38/NAD/SIRTUIN1/EZH2 axis mitigates cytotoxic CD8 T cell function and identifies patients with SLE prone to infections. Cell Rep 2020;30(1):112–23.e114.
46. Tilstra JS, Avery L, Menk AV, et al. Kidney-infiltrating T cells in murine lupus nephritis are metabolically and functionally exhausted. J Clin Invest 2018; 128(11):4884–97.
47. Arazi A, Rao DA, Berthier CC, et al. The immune cell landscape in kidneys of patients with lupus nephritis. Nat Immunol 2019;20(7):902–14.
48. Li H, Adamopoulos IE, Moulton VR, et al. Systemic lupus erythematosus favors the generation of IL-17 producing double negative T cells. Nat Commun 2020; 11(1):2859.
49. Crispín JC, Oukka M, Bayliss G, et al. Expanded double negative T cells in patients with systemic lupus erythematosus produce IL-17 and infiltrate the kidneys. J Immunol 2008;181(12):8761–6.
50. Alexander JJ, Jacob A, Chang A, et al. Double negative T cells, a potential biomarker for systemic lupus erythematosus. Precision Clin Med 2020;3(1): 34–43.
51. Song K, Liu L, Zhang X, et al. An update on genetic susceptibility in lupus nephritis. Clin Immunol 2020;210:108272.
52. Bank I. The role of gamma delta T cells in autoimmune rheumatic diseases. Cells 2020;9(2):462.
53. Lawand M, Déchanet-Merville J, Dieu-Nosjean MC. Key Features of Gamma-Delta T cell Subsets in Human Diseases and Their Immunotherapeutic Implications. Front Immunol 2017;8:761.
54. Huang Y, Getahun A, Heiser RA, et al. γδ T cells shape preimmune peripheral B cell populations. J Immunol 2016;196(1):217–31.
55. Rampoldi F, Ullrich L, Prinz I. Revisiting the interaction of γδ T cells and B-cells. Cells 2020;9(3):743.
56. Li X, Kang N, Zhang X, et al. Generation of human regulatory gammadelta T cells by TCRgammadelta stimulation in the presence of TGF-beta and their involvement in the pathogenesis of systemic lupus erythematosus. J Immunol 2011; 186(12):6693–700.
57. Robak E, Niewiadomska H, Robak T, et al. Lymphocyctes Tgammadelta in clinically normal skin and peripheral blood of patients with systemic lupus erythematosus and their correlation with disease activity. Mediators Inflamm 2001;10(4): 179–89.
58. Vukelic M, Kono M, Tsokos GC. T cell metabolism in lupus. Immunometabolism 2020;2(2):e200009.
59. Perl A, Hanczko R, Lai ZW, et al. Comprehensive metabolome analyses reveal N-acetylcysteine-responsive accumulation of kynurenine in systemic lupus erythematosus: implications for activation of the mechanistic target of rapamycin. Metabolomics 2015;11(5):1157–74.

60. Delgoffe GM, Pollizzi KN, Waickman AT, et al. The kinase mTOR regulates the differentiation of helper T cells through the selective activation of signaling by mTORC1 and mTORC2. Nat Immunol 2011;12(4):295–303.
61. Kato H, Perl A. Mechanistic target of rapamycin complex 1 expands Th17 and IL-4+ CD4-CD8- double-negative T cells and contracts regulatory T cells in systemic lupus erythematosus. J Immunol 2014;192(9):4134–44.
62. Lai ZW, Hanczko R, Bonilla E, et al. N-acetylcysteine reduces disease activity by blocking mammalian target of rapamycin in T cells from systemic lupus erythematosus patients: a randomized, double-blind, placebo-controlled trial. Arthritis Rheum 2012;64(9):2937–46.
63. Su C, Johnson ME, Torres A, et al. Mapping effector genes at lupus GWAS loci using promoter capture-C in follicular helper T cells. Nat Commun 2020;11(1): 3294.
64. Tsokos GC, Lo MS, Costa Reis P, et al. New insights into the immunopathogenesis of systemic lupus erythematosus. Nat Rev Rheumatol 2016;12(12):716–30.
65. Hagberg N, Joelsson M, Leonard D, et al. The STAT4 SLE risk allele rs7574865[T] is associated with increased IL-12-induced IFN-γ production in T cells from patients with SLE. Ann Rheum Dis 2018;77(7):1070–7.
66. Iwamoto T, Niewold TB. Genetics of human lupus nephritis. Clin Immunol 2017; 185:32–9.
67. Kariuki SN, Kirou KA, MacDermott EJ, et al. Cutting edge: autoimmune disease risk variant of STAT4 confers increased sensitivity to IFN-alpha in lupus patients in vivo. J Immunol 2009;182(1):34–8.
68. Weeding E, Sawalha AH. Deoxyribonucleic acid methylation in systemic lupus erythematosus: implications for future clinical practice. Front Immunol 2018;9:875.
69. Katsuyama T, Martin-Delgado IJ, Krishfield SM, et al. Splicing factor SRSF1 controls T cell homeostasis and its decreased levels are linked to lymphopenia in systemic lupus erythematosus. Rheumatology 2020;59(8):2146–55.
70. Hedrich CM. Epigenetics in SLE. Curr Rheumatol Rep 2017;19(9):58.
71. Liao W, Li M, Wu H, et al. Down-regulation of MBD4 contributes to hypomethylation and overexpression of CD70 in CD4(+) T cells in systemic lupus erythematosus. Clin Epigenetics 2017;9:104.
72. Vordenbäumen S, Rosenbaum A, Gebhard C, et al. Associations of site-specific CD4(+)-T cell hypomethylation within CD40-ligand promotor and enhancer regions with disease activity of women with systemic lupus erythematosus. Lupus 2021;30(1):45–51.
73. Zhang M, Fang X, Wang GS, et al. Ultraviolet B decreases DNA methylation level of CD4+ T cells in patients with systemic lupus erythematosus. Inflammopharmacology 2017;25(2):203–10.
74. Renauer P, Coit P, Jeffries MA, et al. DNA methylation patterns in naïve CD4+ T cells identify epigenetic susceptibility loci for malar rash and discoid rash in systemic lupus erythematosus. Lupus Sci Med 2015;2(1):e000101.
75. Coit P, Renauer P, Jeffries MA, et al. Renal involvement in lupus is characterized by unique DNA methylation changes in naïve CD4+ T cells. J Autoimmun 2015; 61:29–35.
76. Jeffries MA, Dozmorov M, Tang Y, et al. Genome-wide DNA methylation patterns in CD4+ T cells from patients with systemic lupus erythematosus. Epigenetics 2011;6(5):593–601.
77. Guo G, Wang H, Shi X, et al. Disease activity-associated alteration of mRNA m(5) C methylation in CD4(+) T cells of systemic lupus erythematosus. Front Cell Dev Biol 2020;8:430.

78. Chen DJ, Li LJ, Yang XK, et al. Altered microRNAs expression in T cells of patients with SLE involved in the lack of vitamin D. Oncotarget 2017;8(37): 62099–110.
79. Hedrich CM. Mechanistic aspects of epigenetic dysregulation in SLE. Clin Immunol 2018;196:3–11.
80. Lever E, Alves MR, Isenberg DA. Towards precision medicine in systemic lupus erythematosus. Pharmacogenomics Pers Med 2020;13:39–49.
81. Nandkumar P, Furie R. T cell-directed therapies in systemic lupus erythematosus. Lupus 2016;25(10):1080–5.
82. Klavdianou K, Lazarini A, Fanouriakis A. Targeted biologic therapy for systemic lupus erythematosus: emerging pathways and drug pipeline. BioDrugs 2020; 34(2):133–47.
83. Oliveira IS, Ferreira IG, Alexandre-Silva GM, et al. Scorpion toxins targeting Kv1.3 channels: insights into immunosuppression. J Venom Anim Toxins Incl Trop Dis 2019;25:e148118.
84. Tarcha EJ, Olsen CM, Probst P, et al. Safety and pharmacodynamics of dalazatide, a Kv1.3 channel inhibitor, in the treatment of plaque psoriasis: a randomized phase 1b trial. PLoS One 2017;12(7):e0180762.
85. Koga T, Hedrich CM, Mizui M, et al. CaMK4-dependent activation of AKT/mTOR and CREM-α underlies autoimmunity-associated Th17 imbalance. J Clin Invest 2014;124(5):2234–45.
86. Park JS, Kim SM, Hwang SH, et al. Combinatory treatment using tacrolimus and a STAT3 inhibitor regulate Treg cells and plasma cells. Int J Immunopathol Pharmacol 2018;32. 2058738418778724.
87. Eriksson P, Wallin P, Sjöwall C. Clinical experience of sirolimus regarding efficacy and safety in systemic lupus erythematosus. Front Pharmacol 2019;10:82.
88. Lai ZW, Kelly R, Winans T, et al. Sirolimus in patients with clinically active systemic lupus erythematosus resistant to, or intolerant of, conventional medications: a single-arm, open-label, phase 1/2 trial. Lancet 2018;391(10126):1186–96.
89. Rovin BH, Solomons N, Pendergraft WF 3rd, et al. A randomized, controlled double-blind study comparing the efficacy and safety of dose-ranging voclosporin with placebo in achieving remission in patients with active lupus nephritis. Kidney Int 2019;95(1):219–31.
90. Tanaka Y, Kubo S, Miyagawa I, et al. Lymphocyte phenotype and its application to precision medicine in systemic autoimmune diseases(☆). Semin Arthritis Rheum 2019;48(6):1146–50.
91. Nagafuchi Y, Shoda H, Fujio K. Immune profiling and precision medicine in systemic lupus erythematosus. Cells 2019;8(2):140.

B Cells in Systemic Lupus Erythematosus

From Disease Mechanisms to Targeted Therapies

Susan P. Canny, MD, PhD[a,b], Shaun W. Jackson, MBChB, MD[a,c],*

KEYWORDS

- Systemic lupus erythematosus • B cells • Autoantibodies • BAFF • Belimumab
- B cell depletion

KEY POINTS

- Dysregulated B cell receptor and Toll-like receptor signals promote breaks in B cell tolerance in systemic lupus erythematosus (SLE).
- In addition to pathogenic autoantibody production, B cells initiate breaks in T cell tolerance via antigen presentation and cytokine production.
- Germinal center and extrafollicular activation pathways drive generation of pathogenic plasma cells in SLE.
- Recent clinical trials suggest clinical benefit for B cell–targeted therapies in human SLE.

In 1957, Holborow and colleagues[1] identified antibodies targeting cell nuclei in lupus sera, thereby linking B cells to the pathogenesis of human systemic lupus erythematosus (SLE). In the ensuing decades, we have gained a greater appreciation for the myriad roles for autoreactive B cells in lupus. These basic immunologic insights ultimately informed the development of belimumab, a monoclonal antibody targeting the B cell survival cytokine BAFF (B cell activating factor), as the first Food and Drug Administration (FDA)-approved therapy for human SLE in the modern era. Despite this regulatory success, the overall clinical efficacy of belimumab in SLE is relatively modest.[2,3] Thus, a greater understanding of B cell roles in human lupus, as well as the ability to specifically target pathogenic B cell clones, is necessary for the development of highly efficacious therapies for this complex autoimmune disease. In the current review, we first discuss the immune mechanisms by which B cells drive the initiation and propagation of human lupus. Second, we review B cell–directed treatments for human SLE.

[a] Department of Pediatrics, University of Washington School of Medicine, Seattle, WA, USA; [b] Benaroya Research Institute, 1201 Ninth Avenue, Seattle, WA 98101, USA; [c] Seattle Children's Research Institute, Seattle, WA, USA
* Corresponding author. Seattle Children's Research Institute, 1900 9th Avenue, Seattle, WA 98101.
E-mail address: shaun.jackson@seattlechildrens.org

Rheum Dis Clin N Am 47 (2021) 395–413
https://doi.org/10.1016/j.rdc.2021.04.006
0889-857X/21/© 2021 Elsevier Inc. All rights reserved.

MECHANISMS UNDERPINNING B CELL TOLERANCE BREAKS IN SYSTEMIC LUPUS ERYTHEMATOSUS

B Cell Autoreactivity Is an Inherent Feature of the Naïve Human B Cell Repertoire

To generate a broad antigen receptor repertoire able to recognize diverse pathogens, B cell receptors (BCR) are generated by the random recombination of germline-encoded gene segments. An inherent tradeoff in this process is the development of self-reactive B cells that may facilitate the development of autoimmunity. Despite layered tolerance mechanisms, including clonal deletion, receptor editing, and induction of functional anergy, a prominent subset of peripheral naïve B cells in healthy individuals exhibits autoreactivity across a continuum of self-antigen affinity.[4,5] SLE is an obvious example of the risks inherent in self-reactive B cells persisting within the naïve repertoire, raising the question as to why these potentially pathogenic anergic clones are not simply deleted during development. However, from an evolutionary standpoint, effective humoral responses against diverse pathogens require a broad repertoire. Thus, complete elimination of all self-reactive B cells would result in "holes" in the naïve repertoire that could be exploited by pathogens. Consistent with this hypothesis, self-reactive anergic B cells can be recruited into an adaptive immune response, via a process that has been termed "clonal redemption."[6] Ultimately, these observations indicate that B cell response thresholds must be carefully tuned to balance protective responses with the risk of humoral autoimmunity.

The B Cell Activating Factor Family of Cytokines and Receptors Exerts Diverse Impacts on the Pathogenesis of Systemic Lupus Erythematosus

BAFF and A proliferation-inducing ligand (APRIL) are homologous tumor necrosis factor (TNF) ligand family cytokines that exert distinct impacts on B cell differentiation and survival during development. The observation that transgenic BAFF overexpression promotes lupuslike disease in murine models[7,8] and that a subset of human patients with lupus exhibits elevated serum BAFF[9,10] fueled efforts to therapeutically target BAFF in SLE. As discussed in detail later in this article, these endeavors resulted in successful clinical trials of the BAFF inhibitor, belimumab.[2,3] However, although a subset of belimumab-treated patients exhibits durable remission,[11] the overall efficacy of BAFF inhibition in SLE is relatively modest; an observation that may be explained, in part, by the complex roles for BAFF family molecules in lupus pathogenesis.

Given this complexity, we refer the readers to more comprehensive reviews of the physiologic and pathogenic roles for BAFF in B cell immunity.[12,13] Briefly, BAFF signals are required for B cell survival and maturation beyond the transitional stage of B cell development. In contrast, APRIL is redundant for normal B cell differentiation, but supports class-switch recombination to immunoglobulin (Ig) A and facilitates the survival of long-lived plasma cells (LLPCs) in the bone marrow.[14,15] BAFF and APRIL exert these functions via distinct B cell surface receptors. For example, soluble BAFF circulates as trimers and in 60-subunit multimers, which preferentially activate the BAFF receptor (BAFF-R) and Transmembrane Activator and CAML Interactor (TACI), respectively. In contrast, APRIL binds TACI and the plasma cell receptor B cell maturation antigen (BCMA), the latter receptor facilitating LLPC persistence within bone marrow survival niches[12] (**Fig. 1**).

In keeping with the development of spontaneous lupus in transgenic BAFF overexpression models,[7,8] a genetic polymorphism in human *TNFSF13B* (encoding BAFF) that increases circulating BAFF levels is linked with an increased risk of SLE.[16] Thus, an important avenue of ongoing research aims to understand how elevated BAFF promotes breaks in B cell tolerance. Studies using autoreactive BCR transgenic

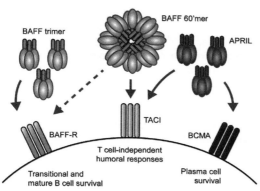

Fig. 1. BAFF, APRIL, and their receptors. Graphic representation of BAFF (trimeric and multimeric forms) and APRIL binding to respective BAFF family receptors to support different B cell functions.

models demonstrate that BAFF overexpression does not impact central tolerance.[17] Rather, supraphysiologic BAFF exerts a more subtle impact on transitional B cell selection and the survival of low-affinity autoreactive B cells.[17–19] In parallel, excess BAFF drives breaks in peripheral B cell tolerance by promoting T cell–independent activation of autoreactive B cell clones.[20] As described in detail later in this article, these events depend on engagement of the endosomal RNA-sensor TLR7 and downstream MyD88 signals.[20,21] Mechanistically, BAFF signals resulting in the generation of pathogenic plasmablasts are transduced by both BAFF-R,[21] the canonical B cell survival receptor, and TACI,[22–24] the surface receptor driving humoral responses to T cell–independent antigens.[25]

Dysregulated Signals Downstream of B Cell Receptor and Toll-like Receptors Initiate Breaks in B Cell Tolerance to Nuclear Autoantigens

Despite a theoretically unlimited number of potential autoantigens, SLE is characterized by relatively restricted autoantibody repertoire predominantly targeting nuclear antigens. This is likely explained by B cell expression of both clonally rearranged antigen receptors (BCRs) and innate pattern recognition receptors (including toll-like receptors [TLRs]). Dual engagement of these pathways promotes robust B cell activation.[26] The evolutionary logic behind this arrangement is that, during an acute viral infection, antigen-specific B cells traffic viral nucleic acid to endosomal compartments, resulting in MyD88-dependent TLR signaling and induction of protective antibody responses. However, because TLRs can also respond to endogenous nucleic acid–containing particles derived from apoptotic cells, this propensity toward integrated BCR and TLR activation also increases the risk of autoimmunity.[26–28] Of the MyD88-dependent TLRs, the endosomal receptors TLR7 and TLR9, have been most closely linked with lupus pathogenesis with TLR9 promoting autoantibodies to double-stranded DNA (dsDNA) and chromatin, whereas TLR7 facilitates reactivity to RNA-associated autoantigens.[29–32]

Importantly, dysregulated TLR signals can theoretically promote SLE via cell-intrinsic impacts on both B cells and myeloid lineages. In a feed-forward model for lupus progression, BCR/TLR-driven breaks in B cell tolerance result in the production of circulating immune complexes that promote TLR-dependent cytokine production (including type 1 interferons) by plasmacytoid dendritic cell and other myeloid lineages.[31,33] Interestingly, although TLR expression is higher in the myeloid compartment, multiple animals studies have demonstrated that B cell–intrinsic deletion of *Myd88*,[20,34–36] *Tlr7*,[37–40] or *Tlr9*[37,41] recapitulates the phenotype of global gene deletion in murine lupus.[29–32,42] Conversely, TLR7 overexpression in transgenic models or in male mice carrying the *Y-linked autoimmune accelerator* (Yaa) translocation (containing the *Tlr7* gene) is sufficient to promote spontaneous germinal centers (GCs) and murine lupus in a B cell–intrinsic manner.[38,39]

For these reasons, BCR and TLR signaling thresholds must be tightly regulated to balance effective pathogen responses with the risk of autoimmunity. Consistent with this model, genome-wide association studies of human lupus have identified multiple risk polymorphisms modulating BCR and TLR signaling pathways. These include genes impacting downstream BCR signaling cascades, such as *PTPN22*, *BANK1*, *BLK*, *LYN*, *GRB2*,[43] and *RASGRP3*, as well as variants in the *PXK* locus impacting BCR internalization.[44] Similarly, variants regulating endosomal TLR signaling pathways have been linked with lupus risk, including *TLR7*[45,46], *TNFAIP3*, *TNIP1,* and *UBE2L3* (modulating TLR-induced nuclear factor–κB activation)[47,48]; the TLR signaling kinase *IRAK1*[47]; *SLC15A4* and *CXORF21* (encoding the protein TASL[49]), which promote TLR-dependent interferon regulatory factor (IRF) activation[50]; and *IRF5* and *IRF7* (required for TLR-driven type 1 interferon production).[47,51] Importantly, individual immune variants show evidence of population-specific evolution, indicating that selection for efficient pathogen response has likely contributed to the risk of multiple autoimmune diseases, including SLE.[52,53] These human genetic data indicate that BCR and TLR signals are finely tuned and even modest alterations in activation thresholds can promote autoimmunity in the appropriate environmental context.

Parallel Germinal Center and Extrafollicular B Cell Activation Pathways in Systemic Lupus Erythematosus

Although serum antinuclear antibodies (ANA) are a characteristic feature of SLE, it has been challenging to define the cellular pathways responsible for the production of pathogenic plasma cells in humans. During the initial phase of a humoral immune response, short-lived, lower-affinity plasmablasts are generated via an extrafollicular (EF) B cell activation pathway. Subsequently, iterative interactions between antigen-specific B cells and cognate CD4$^+$ T cells within germinal centers (GCs) facilitate the production of high-affinity plasma cells that traffic to bone marrow survival niches to set up residence as LLPCs.[54]

Whereas these parallel B cell activation pathways can be more easily studied in the context of vaccination or pathogen response, SLE is a stochastic process characterized by the steady accumulation of autoreactive clones over a period of years.[55] Thus, identifying the source of individual plasma cell clones in human lupus is technically challenging. However, cloned autoantibodies from patients with lupus frequently exhibit extensive somatic hypermutation (SHM), implicating (but not proving[56]) a GC origin.[57] In addition, spontaneous GC formation is a characteristic feature of both murine and human SLE.[58]

In contrast with these studies linking dysregulated GCs to lupus pathogenesis, parallel data highlight a prominent role for EF B cell activation in pathogenic antibody secreting cell (ASC) expansion. In animal models, class-switched autoantibodies in BAFF-Tg mice can develop in a T cell–independent manner,[20] whereas in MRL.Fas^{lpr} mice, both the initial activation and somatic hypermutation of autoreactive B cells occurs outside the follicle.[56] In addition, human lupus flares are characterized by the expansion of a B cell subset, termed "activated naïve" cells (aNAV), defined by IgD$^+$CD27$^-$ surface phenotype and downregulation of CD21 and CD23. Using repertoire-sequencing approaches, aNAVs were shown to contribute to most circulating lupus ASCs.[59] Subsequently, the developmental "link" between aNAV and ASCs was provided by the identification of the class-switched IgD-, CD27-double negative DN2 cells (IgD⁻CD27⁻CXCR5⁻CD11c⁺). Because recombinant monoclonal antibodies cloned from aNAV cells showed lupuslike autoreactivity in the absence of somatic hypermutation,[59] these findings implicate a GC-independent EF activation pathway in which aNAV differentiates into DN2, which are precursors for pathogenic ASCs (**Fig. 2**).

In addition to reduced CD21/CD23 expression, lupus DN2 cells are characterized by increased expression of CD11c, SLAMF7, and the transcription factor T-bet.[60,61] These phenotypic characteristics thus mirror the phenotype of the "age/

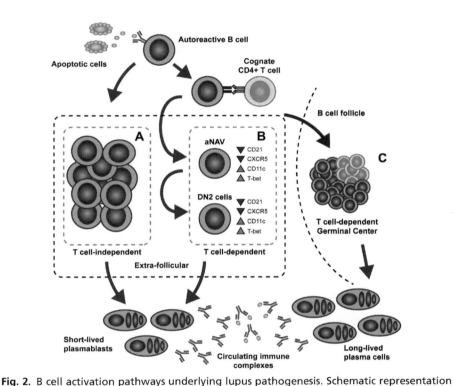

Fig. 2. B cell activation pathways underlying lupus pathogenesis. Schematic representation of the 3 known activation pathways resulting in the generation of pathogenic effector B cells in SLE. (A) Pathogenic plasmablasts can be generated without T cell help, most notably in the BAFF-Tg model. (B, C) Following initial autoantigen recognition, autoreactive B cells and CD4⁺ T cells interact at the T cell:B cell border. Subsequently, costimulatory signals and cytokine crosstalk promote B cell activation and autoantibody production via either a T cell–dependent EF pathway (B) or within spontaneous, autoimmune GCs (C). Recent studies in human lupus have uncovered a prominent contribution for EF B cell activation in the generation of autoantibody-producing ASCs via the sequentially defined aNAV and DN2 differentiation stages. (*Adapted from* Jenks SA, Cashman KS, Zumaquero E, et al. Distinct effector B cells induced by unregulated toll-like receptor 7 contribute to pathogenic responses in systemic lupus erythematosus. Immunity 2018;49(4):725-739 e726; Hale M, Rawlings DJ, Jackson SW. The long and the short of it: insights into the cellular source of autoantibodies as revealed by B cell depletion therapy. Curr Opin Immunol 2018;55:81-88; Jenks SA, Cashman KS, Woodruff MC, et al. Extrafollicular responses in humans and SLE. Immunol Rev 2019;288(1):136-148).

autoimmunity-associated B cells" (ABCs) reported in murine lupus models.[62,63] Although individual studies differ based on the gating strategies used to identify this subset, emerging data indicate that these B cell populations are likely functionally equivalent. For example, murine and human "ABC-like" cells similarly develop following TLR7, interferon (IFN)-γ, and interleukin (IL)-21 stimulation,[60,61,64,65] express the atypical memory marker Fc receptorlike protein 5 (FcRL5),[60,61] and rapidly differentiate into autoantibody-secreting plasmablasts ex vivo following cytokine and/or TLR stimulation.[60–63,66] The importance of these cells to human disease is further emphasized by the observation that CD11c$^+$T-bet$^+$ B cells comprise a significant proportion of B cells within inflamed lupus nephritis kidneys.[60,67] Together, these combined data suggest an important role for CD11c$^+$T-bet$^+$ B cells, and by inference EF B cell activation, in driving lupus pathogenesis.

Importantly, this EF B cell activation pathway is not unique to SLE or other humoral autoimmune diseases. *Salmonella typhimurium* infection in mice results in a massive EF B cell response yielding affinity mature anti-pathogen antibodies in the absence of GCs.[68] Moreover, and of particular current interest, patients with severe severe acute respiratory syndrome coronavirus 2 (SARS-CoV2) infection exhibit robust EF B cell activation that mirrors human SLE,[69] an observation that is supported by absent or limited GC formation in secondary lymphoid organs from subjects with fatal Coronavirus Disease 2019 (COVID 19).[70] Thus, imbalanced GC versus EF activation may be a general feature of dysregulated B cell responses in infectious and autoimmune contexts.

B CELL EFFECTOR FUNCTIONS IN SYSTEMIC LUPUS ERYTHEMATOSUS
B Cell Antigen Presentation and Cytokine Production Promotes Lupus T Cell Activation

Seminal studies in the late 1990s confirmed that B cell functions in SLE extend beyond the production of pathogenic autoantibodies. Specifically, B cell–deficient MRL/MpJ-Fas^{lpr} (MRL/*lpr*) lupus-prone mice exhibit markedly reduced T cell activation and interstitial nephritis.[71] Strikingly, these inflammatory T cell foci were restored in animals expressing B cells unable to secrete immunoglobulin.[72] These studies implicated antibody-independent B cell functions, including antigen presentation and cytokine production, in lupus development. Consistent with this model, T cell activation is preserved in MRL/*lpr* mice lacking CD11c$^+$ dendritic cells,[73] whereas genetic ablation of B cell antigen-presenting cell function prevented CD4$^+$ T cell activation, differentiation into effector memory and T follicular helper (Tfh) subsets, and progressive autoimmunity in separate murine lupus models.[34,74]

These events are also affected by cell-intrinsic cytokine crosstalk. For example, both type 1 (IFN-α, -β, -ϵ, -ω) and type 2 (IFN-γ) IFNs have been linked to murine and human lupus pathogenesis.[75–81] In contrast to the prevailing model in which type 1 IFN signals drive breaks in tolerance, independent studies demonstrated that IFN-γ receptor (IFN-γR) activation promotes murine lupus via cell-intrinsic activation of CD4$^+$ T cells and B cells, respectively.[81–83] Mechanistically, we showed that IFN-γ signals enhanced B cell IL-6 production, which facilitated autoimmune GC formation by promoting the differentiation of Tfh cells.[84] Importantly, although B cell–intrinsic type 1 IFN receptor (IFNAR) signals also accelerated autoantibody production, the absolute requirement for type 1 IFN signals in initiating B cell tolerance breaks varied between murine lupus models.[82,85]

Together, these studies implicate a critical role for B cells in orchestrating immunologic events leading to SLE development. Following initial BCR/TLR-dependent activation by nuclear self-antigens, B cells present autoantigens to cognate T cells and provide critical cytokine signals necessary for T cell activation and Tfh differentiation. Subsequently, the production of pathogenic autoantibodies results in circulating nucleic acid–containing immune complexes, which promote TLR7/TLR9-dependent type 1 IFN production by plasmacytoid dendritic cells (pDCs), further propagating an inflammatory feed-forward loop.[86–88] This model is strikingly consistent with data from longitudinal cohort studies of preclinical SLE, in which elevated serum IFN-γ and IL-6 is first observed at the time of initial autoantibody positivity, whereas the type 1 IFN signature develops shortly before clinical disease onset.[89,90]

Evidence for Pathogenic Roles for Autoantibodies in Systemic Lupus Erythematosus

Although ANA are first detected years before lupus diagnosis, circulating autoantibodies may play an underappreciated role in the clinical manifestations of SLE. First, several hematologic manifestations are directly autoantibody-driven, including Coombs+ hemolytic anemia and immune thrombocytopenia. Second, a consistent histopathologic feature of lupus nephritis is the identification of prominent glomerular immune complexes containing multiple immunoglobulin isotypes. As early as the 1960s, anti-dsDNA antibodies could be directly eluted from lupus nephritis kidneys,[91] placing this specificity at the "scene of the crime." Consistent with these data, transfer of certain anti-DNA monoclonal antibodies induced proteinuria in non-autoimmune animals.[92] Importantly, subsequent studies demonstrated that multiple autoantibodies (not only dsDNA) can be eluted from the glomeruli of lupus nephritis kidneys.[93] Finally, perhaps the most direct evidence that lupus autoantibodies can cause systemic inflammation derives from neonatal lupus erythematosus (NLE), which develops following passive transfer of maternal autoAb across the placenta. Because cellular lineages do not cross the placenta, these data suggest a direct role for autoantibodies in NLE; data further supported by the resolution of cutaneous lesions with clearance of maternal IgG. Interestingly, most mothers of infants with NLE do not have lupus, but rather are ANA+ in the absence of clinical symptoms.[94] These data imply that, although not necessarily sufficient for disease development, circulating autoantibodies can contribute to the clinical manifestations of SLE.

B CELL–TARGETED THERAPIES FOR HUMAN LUPUS

The diverse contributions of B cells to lupus pathogenesis strongly support B cell–targeted therapies as effective treatments for human SLE. This premise was further supported by clinical benefit and acceptable safety profile of anti-CD20 B cell depletion (rituximab) in a separate humoral autoimmune disease, rheumatoid arthritis.[95] However, this enthusiasm was dampened by a negative phase II/III randomized clinical trial study of rituximab in SLE (EXPLORER trial).[96] This study, together with other clinical failures, tempered the belief that B cell–directed approaches would ultimately prove successful. In a later article in this series, Dr Morand will provide a review of recent advances in lupus therapies. For this reason, we focus here on a broad overview of strategies used to target B cells in SLE (**Fig. 3**), including (1) newer B cell–depletion agents; (2) BAFF family blockade; (3) inhibitors of B cell signaling; and (4) plasma-cell–directed therapies. Informed by improved trial design, greater understanding of disease mechanisms, and better pharmacology, these strategies are beginning to show promise.

B Cell Depletion in Systemic Lupus Erythematosus

B cells express CD19, CD20, and CD22 on their cell surface, which render them susceptible to depletion using monoclonal antibodies to these cell surface markers.

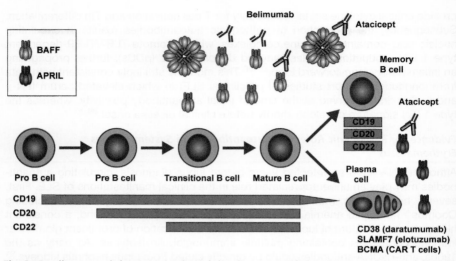

Fig. 3. B cell–targeted therapies in clinical development. Schematic representation of B cell development showing targets for B cell–directed therapies, including monoclonal antibodies targeting B cell surface antigens (CD19, CAR T cells; CD20, rituximab, ocrelizumab, obinutuzumab; and CD22, epratuzumab); BAFF family directed therapies (belimumab and atacicept); and plasma cell depletion strategies (APRIL, atacicept; CD38, daratumumab; SLAMF7, elotuzumab; BCMA CAR T cells).

Despite strong clinical rationale underpinning CD20 as a therapeutic target in human SLE, rituximab, a chimeric anti-CD20 monoclonal antibody, failed to meet primary endpoints in large clinical trials in human SLE (EXPLORER)[96] and lupus nephritis (LUNAR).[97] Similarly, epratuzumab, a nondepleting monoclonal antibody targeting the B cell inhibitory receptor CD22, also failed to improve response rates beyond standard therapy.[98] Each clinical trial failure in human lupus can be attributed to incorrect trial design, patient heterogeneity, or incorrect drug target.[99,100] In keeping with this, rituximab-treated patients exhibited improvements in proteinuria at later time points in the LUNAR trial,[97] and subgroup analysis of African American and Hispanic individuals suggested a clinical benefit in the EXPLORER study.[96] However, an additional important consideration is whether inefficient depletion of CD20[+] tissue-resident B cells following rituximab treatment accounted for some of the variability in treatment response. Although circulating B cells are rapidly depleted, persistence of B cells within inflamed target organs have been observed in patients with rituximab-treated rheumatoid arthritis or Sjögren syndrome.[101,102] Moreover in murine lupus models, the development of systemic autoimmunity limits the depth and durability of anti-CD20 B cell depletion,[103] whereas complete B cell ablation using anti-CD19 chimeric antigen receptor (CAR) T cells provides durable disease remission.[104] In keeping with this model, "complete peripheral B cell depletion" correlated with renal response in a post hoc analysis of LUNAR trial data.[105]

For this reason, newer anti-CD20 agents designed for more efficient B cell ablation and reduced infusion reactions are being tested in human lupus.[106] For example, ocrelizumab exhibited a trend toward improved renal response in subjects with active class III/IV lupus nephritis (Δ −12.7% vs placebo; $P = .065$), although infectious complications limited clinical development of this agent.[107] Obinutuzumab, a Type II monoclonal antibody that exhibits more effective B cell depletion than rituximab,[106,108] is being tested in an ongoing trial in class III/IV lupus nephritis (NOBILITY trial).

Promisingly, interim week 52 data from this study met both primary and secondary clinical endpoints (complete renal response: 34.9% obinutuzumab vs 22.6% placebo, P = .115; overall renal response: 55.6% obinutuzumab versus 35.5% placebo, P = .025).[109] Although B cell depletion as a lupus treatment strategy will undoubtably require further optimization to select appropriate clinical subsets, these data suggest that newer anti-CD20 agents, engineered for improved B cell ablation, may yet form part of the SLE armamentarium.

B Cell Activating Factor Family Targeted Therapies

Belimumab, a monoclonal antibody binding soluble BAFF, received FDA approval based on 2 pivotal phase III lupus trials. In the BLISS-52 and BLISS-76 trials, belimumab-treated patients exhibited significantly improved SLE Responder Index (SRI) at week 52 (placebo 44% vs belimumab 1 mg/kg 51%, P = .0129; and 10 mg/kg 55%, P = .0006) and week 76 (32.4% [placebo], 39.1% [1 mg/kg], and 38.5% [10 mg/kg]).[2,3] Similarly, a phase III trial conducted in China, Japan, and South Korea confirmed greater SRI (placebo 40.1% vs belimumab 53.8%; P = .0001), reduced rates of severe flares, and lower prednisone requirements.[110] Because of these clinical successes, several additional BAFF-targeted molecules have been developed. For example, the monoclonal antibody tabalumab and fusion protein blisibimod, which each inhibit both soluble and membrane-bound BAFF, have been studied for the treatment of human lupus. Although primary endpoints were only met in a subset of these trials, improvements in secondary endpoints such as lower corticosteroid use further supported the benefit of BAFF blockade in SLE.[111–113]

Although the 3 major belimumab clinical trials in general lupus each reached primary clinical endpoints, patients with severe renal disease were excluded from earlier studies. However, a pooled post hoc analysis of the BLISS studies uncovered a trend toward greater reductions in proteinuria and decreased lupus nephritis flares in subjects with renal disease at baseline, suggesting a potential role for BAFF inhibition in the management of lupus nephritis.[114] Consistent with this hypothesis, a recent high-profile study confirmed therapeutic benefit for belimumab in active lupus nephritis. Subjects treated with intravenous belimumab in addition to standard induction therapy (mycophenolate mofetil or cyclophosphamide) exhibited greater renal response (43% vs 32%; P = .03) or complete renal response (30% vs 20%; P = .02), with no unexpected safety signals.[115] As with all lupus trials, patient heterogeneity and a high response rate in the placebo arm results in modest overall clinical benefits. However, the durability of treatment response and large number of patients enrolled in pivotal studies (>2500 subjects in phase III clinical trials) speaks to the overall clinical benefit of BAFF blockade in SLE. In addition, although naïve B cells are reduced by ~95% following BAFF inhibition, belimumab has an excellent long-term safety profile and treatment feasibility has been enhanced by the development of an effective subcutaneous formulation.[116]

Despite these clinical successes, a prominent subset of belimumab-treated patients fails to respond to BAFF blockade. For this reason, investigators are testing whether the combination of anti-CD20 B cell depletion and BAFF blockade provides synergistic benefits. Although an initial trial of rituximab plus belimumab failed in lupus nephritis,[117] a phase 3 clinical trial of combination therapy in nonrenal SLE (BLISS-BELIEVE; NCT03312907) is ongoing and these data are eagerly awaited. An additional strategy currently being pursued to enhance the efficacy of BAFF blockade, is dual inhibition of BAFF and APRIL using recombinant fusion proteins incorporating the receptor TACI. Theoretically, this approach may confer greater clinical benefits in SLE via blockade of multimeric BAFF and improved plasma cell targeting, with the caveat of possible increased infectious complications. In this regard, an initial trial of atacicept in lupus nephritis was prematurely terminated because of hypogammaglobulinemia and serious pneumonia in the treatment arm,[118] although it should be noted that a decline in serum IgG was observed in several subjects before administration of study drug.[119] Subsequently, a trial of lupus flare prevention reported beneficial effects for atacicept, although 2 infectious deaths prompted premature termination of the more effective high-dose arm.[120] Finally, the ADDRESS II study reported positive efficacy data for atacicept, especially in subjects with high clinical and serologic disease activity, without overt safety signals.[121] In addition, telitacicept, a related BAFF/APRIL binding compound, exhibited remarkable efficacy in a phase 2b lupus clinical trial resulting in fast-track designation by the FDA.[122]

Together, these studies demonstrate that BAFF blockade provides reproducible clinical benefit in both SLE and lupus nephritis, albeit with an overall modest effect size, whereas combined BAFF/APRIL inhibition holds the promise of greater treatment efficacy at the potential cost of more frequent infectious complications.

Inhibition of B Cell Signaling

An alternate strategy to broad B cell depletion is to specifically target the B cell signaling pathways underlying lupus pathogenesis. For example, several pharmaceutical companies are developing inhibitors of Bruton's tyrosine kinase (BTK), a tyrosine-protein kinase required for BCR signaling. However, fenebrutinib, an oral highly selective BTK inhibitor, failed to meet clinical targets in a phase II lupus clinical trial, despite an expected decline in total peripheral B cells, anti-dsDNA titers, and circulating plasmablasts.[123] A separate approach is to inhibit endosomal TLR activation or downstream TLR signaling cascades. In support of this hypothesis, the long-appreciated benefits for hydroxychloroquine in SLE have been linked to reduced endosomal acidification and subsequent TLR7/TLR9 inhibition. Although drugs targeting this pathway are currently in early development, inhibition of key components of the endosomal TLR signaling pathway (TLR7, TLR9, MYD88, IRAK1, IRAK4, TAK1, IRF5) may prove an effective strategy in human SLE.[124,125]

Plasma Cell Targeting

Whether lupus-associated autoantibodies are pathogenic or merely biomarkers for this disease is an ongoing source of controversy. Because plasma cells downregulate surface expression of the targets of therapeutic B cell depletion (CD19, CD20) and do not require BAFF for long-term survival,[126] LLPCs are resistant to available B cell–targeted therapies, such as rituximab and belimumab. This observation, together with the evidence described previously implicating autoantibodies in lupus pathogenesis, support efforts to directly target plasma cells in SLE. Thus, we briefly describe various plasma cell ablation strategies that are currently in development.

Proteosome inhibition

The ubiquitin proteasome pathway is required for degradation of misfolded proteins. Because plasma cells produce large quantities of monoclonal immunoglobulin, proteosome inhibition has been pursed as a strategy to target plasma cells in SLE. In animal models, bortezomib depleted plasma cells and prolonged survival in lupus-prone mice.[127] However, in a small, randomized trial in human SLE, potential clinical benefits were complicated by high rates of treatment discontinuation and minimal impact on dsDNA titers.[128] The dose-limiting side effect profile for bortezomib, including painful neuropathy, infusion reactions, and hepatic dysfunction, has driven interest in immune cell–specific inhibition of the immunoproteasome. Unfortunately, compensatory upregulation of constitutive proteasome components may protect against plasma cell death and limit the long-term feasibility of this approach.[129]

Biologic plasma cell targeting

Lessons from multiple myeloma therapies: The oncology community has made remarkable progress in the treatment of multiple myeloma, an intractable plasma cell malignancy.[130] These clinical successes suggest feasibility of directly targeting pathogenic plasma cells using FDA-approved myeloma therapies, with the caveat that loss of protective antibodies following plasma cell depletion may necessitate intravenous immunoglobulin replacement. Daratumumab, an anti-CD38 monoclonal antibody, was recently reported to induce striking clinical benefits in severe refractory SLE. In this small case series, disease remission was preceded by a rapid decline in both pathogenic anti-dsDNA and vaccine-induced antibodies, supporting depletion of CD38+ LLPC as the likely therapeutic mechanism.[131] However, because CD38 is expressed on other immune lineages, including natural killer cells, plasmacytoid dendritic cells, and CD38+ regulatory T cells, alternate plasma cell targeting strategies should be pursued in SLE. For example, the FDA-approved myeloma therapy elotuzumab targets SLAMF7, expressed on myeloma cells and nonmalignant plasma cells, as well as activated DN2 cells and circulating ASCs in human SLE.[61] Alternatively, CAR T cells targeting BCMA, a surface marker expressed by malignant and normal plasma cells, has resulted in long-term remission and rapid declines in paraprotein in patients with treatment-refractory myeloma.[132] Although these agents have not yet been tested in nonmalignant disorders, these novel approaches may prove efficacious in SLE and other humoral autoimmune diseases.

SUMMARY

Recent research has advanced our understanding of the cellular and immunologic mechanisms by which B cells drive the initiation and progression of human SLE. This knowledge led directly to FDA approval for belimumab, an agent with modest, yet durable, therapeutic efficacy in a subset of patients with lupus. In future years, a greater understanding of the B cell signals underlying breaks in tolerance, of the relative contributions of EF-dependent versus GC-dependent B cell activation in lupus pathogenesis, and of roles for B cell memory and LLPCs in disease chronicity may inform the development of safe and effective therapies for SLE. Ultimately, combined approaches targeting both innate and adaptive arms of the immune system and an improved understanding of disease heterogeneity may be needed to provide relief to patients with this intractable disease.

CLINICS CARE POINTS

- Belimumab, a monoclonal inhibitor of soluble BAFF, provides modest but durable clinical benefit in patients with lupus and lupus nephritis.

- Despite initial failures of randomized clinical trials of Rituximab in SLE and lupus nephritis, newer B cell targeted agents optimized for improved depletion have shown promise in ongoing trials.

- Direct plasma cell targeting may have additional benefits beyond those achieved by depleting CD20 B cells.

ACKNOWLEDGMENTS

This work was supported by the National Institutes of Health under award numbers: T32AR007108 and T32 HD007233 (S.P. Canny), K08AI112993 (S.W. Jackson), R03 AI139716 (S.W. Jackson), R01AR075813 (S.W. Jackson), and R01AR073938 (S.W. Jackson). The content is solely the responsibility of the authors and does not necessarily represent the official views of the National Institutes of Health. Additional support provided by The American College of Rheumatology, Rheumatology Research Foundation (ACR RRF) Career Development K Supplement (S.W. Jackson); by the Arthritis National Research Foundation (ANRF) Eng Tan Scholar Award (S.W. Jackson); and by a Lupus Research Alliance, Novel Research Grant (S.W. Jackson).

DISCLOSURE

The authors have no disclosures.

REFERENCES

1. Holborow EJ, Weir DM, Johnson GD. A serum factor in lupus erythematosus with affinity for tissue nuclei. Br Med J 1957;2(5047):732–4.
2. Furie R, Petri M, Zamani O, et al. A phase III, randomized, placebo-controlled study of belimumab, a monoclonal antibody that inhibits B lymphocyte stimulator, in patients with systemic lupus erythematosus. Arthritis Rheum 2011; 63(12):3918–30.
3. Navarra SV, Guzman RM, Gallacher AE, et al. Efficacy and safety of belimumab in patients with active systemic lupus erythematosus: a randomised, placebo-controlled, phase 3 trial. Lancet 2011;377(9767):721–31.
4. Nemazee D. Mechanisms of central tolerance for B cells. Nat Rev Immunol 2017;17(5):281–94.
5. Zikherman J, Parameswaran R, Weiss A. Endogenous antigen tunes the responsiveness of naive B cells but not T cells. Nature 2012;489(7414):160–4.
6. Burnett DL, Langley DB, Schofield P, et al. Germinal center antibody mutation trajectories are determined by rapid self/foreign discrimination. Science 2018; 360(6385):223–6.
7. Mackay F, Woodcock SA, Lawton P, et al. Mice transgenic for BAFF develop lymphocytic disorders along with autoimmune manifestations. J Exp Med 1999;190(11):1697–710.
8. Gavin AL, Duong B, Skog P, et al. deltaBAFF, a splice isoform of BAFF, opposes full-length BAFF activity in vivo in transgenic mouse models. J Immunol 2005; 175(1):319–28.
9. Petri M, Stohl W, Chatham W, et al. BLyS plasma concentrations correlate with disease activity and levels of anti-dsDNA autoantibodies and immunoglobulins (IgG) in a SLE patient observational study. Arthritis Rheum 2003;48:S655 (abstract).
10. Stohl W, Metyas S, Tan SM, et al. B lymphocyte stimulator overexpression in patients with systemic lupus erythematosus: longitudinal observations. Arthritis Rheum 2003;48(12):3475–86.
11. Urowitz MB, Ohsfeldt RL, Wielage RC, et al. Organ damage in patients treated with belimumab versus standard of care: a propensity score-matched comparative analysis. Ann Rheum Dis 2019;78(3):372–9.
12. Mackay F, Schneider P. Cracking the BAFF code. Nat Rev Immunol 2009;9(7): 491–502.

13. Jackson SW, Davidson A. BAFF inhibition in SLE-Is tolerance restored? Immunol Rev 2019;292(1):102–19.
14. Varfolomeev E, Kischkel F, Martin F, et al. APRIL-deficient mice have normal immune system development. Mol Cell Biol 2004;24(3):997–1006.
15. Castigli E, Scott S, Dedeoglu F, et al. Impaired IgA class switching in APRIL-deficient mice. Proc Natl Acad Sci U S A 2004;101(11):3903–8.
16. Steri M, Orrù V, Idda ML, et al. Overexpression of the cytokine BAFF and auto-immunity risk. N Engl J Med 2017;376(17):1615–26.
17. Thien M, Phan TG, Gardam S, et al. Excess BAFF rescues self-reactive B cells from peripheral deletion and allows them to enter forbidden follicular and marginal zone niches. Immunity 2004;20(6):785–98.
18. Lesley R, Xu Y, Kalled SL, et al. Reduced competitiveness of autoantigen-engaged B cells due to increased dependence on BAFF. Immunity 2004; 20(4):441–53.
19. Hondowicz BD, Alexander ST, Quinn WJ 3rd, et al. The role of BLyS/BLyS receptors in anti-chromatin B cell regulation. Int Immunol 2007;19(4):465–75.
20. Groom JR, Fletcher CA, Walters SN, et al. BAFF and MyD88 signals promote a lupuslike disease independent of T cells. J Exp Med 2007;204(8):1959–71.
21. Du SW, Jacobs HM, Arkatkar T, et al. Integrated B cell, toll-like, and BAFF receptor signals promote autoantibody production by transitional B cells. J Immunol 2018;201(11):3258–68.
22. Figgett WA, Deliyanti D, Fairfax KA, et al. Deleting the BAFF receptor TACI protects against systemic lupus erythematosus without extensive reduction of B cell numbers. J Autoimmun 2015;61:9–16.
23. Arkatkar T, Jacobs HM, Du SW, et al. TACI deletion protects against progressive murine lupus nephritis induced by BAFF overexpression. Kidney Int 2018;94(4): 728–40.
24. Jacobs HM, Thouvenel CD, Leach S, et al. Cutting edge: BAFF promotes auto-antibody production via TACI-dependent activation of transitional B cells. J Immunol 2016;196(9):3525–31.
25. von Bulow GU, van Deursen JM, Bram RJ. Regulation of the T-independent humoral response by TACI. Immunity 2001;14(5):573–82.
26. Rawlings DJ, Schwartz MA, Jackson SW, et al. Integration of B cell responses through Toll-like receptors and antigen receptors. Nat Rev Immunol 2012; 12(4):282–94.
27. Shlomchik MJ. Activating systemic autoimmunity: B's, T's, and tolls. Curr Opin Immunol 2009;21(6):626–33.
28. Green NM, Marshak-Rothstein A. Toll-like receptor driven B cell activation in the induction of systemic autoimmunity. Semin Immunol 2011;23(2):106–12.
29. Christensen SR, Shupe J, Nickerson K, et al. Toll-like receptor 7 and TLR9 dictate autoantibody specificity and have opposing inflammatory and regulatory roles in a murine model of lupus. Immunity 2006;25(3):417–28.
30. Berland R, Fernandez L, Kari E, et al. Toll-like receptor 7-dependent loss of B cell tolerance in pathogenic autoantibody knockin mice. Immunity 2006;25(3): 429–40.
31. Christensen SR, Kashgarian M, Alexopoulou L, et al. Toll-like receptor 9 controls anti-DNA autoantibody production in murine lupus. J Exp Med 2005;202(2): 321–31.
32. Lartigue A, Courville P, Auquit I, et al. Role of TLR9 in anti-nucleosome and anti-DNA antibody production in lpr mutation-induced murine lupus. J Immunol 2006;177(2):1349–54.

33. Yasuda K, Richez C, Maciaszek JW, et al. Murine dendritic cell type I IFN production induced by human IgG-RNA immune complexes is IFN regulatory factor (IRF)5 and IRF7 dependent and is required for IL-6 production. J Immunol 2007; 178(11):6876–85.

34. Becker-Herman S, Meyer-Bahlburg A, Schwartz MA, et al. WASp-deficient B cells play a critical, cell-intrinsic role in triggering autoimmunity. J Exp Med 2011;208(10):2033–42.

35. Teichmann LL, Schenten D, Medzhitov R, et al. Signals via the adaptor MyD88 in B cells and DCs make distinct and synergistic contributions to immune activation and tissue damage in lupus. Immunity 2013;38(3):528–40.

36. Hua Z, Gross AJ, Lamagna C, et al. Requirement for MyD88 signaling in B cells and dendritic cells for germinal center anti-nuclear antibody production in Lyn-deficient mice. J Immunol 2014;192(3):875–85.

37. Jackson SW, Scharping NE, Kolhatkar NS, et al. Opposing impact of B cell-intrinsic TLR7 and TLR9 signals on autoantibody repertoire and systemic inflammation. J Immunol 2014;192(10):4525–32.

38. Walsh ER, Pisitkun P, Voynova E, et al. Dual signaling by innate and adaptive immune receptors is required for TLR7-induced B-cell-mediated autoimmunity. Proc Natl Acad Sci U S A 2012;109(40):16276–81.

39. Hwang SH, Lee H, Yamamoto M, et al. B cell TLR7 expression drives anti-RNA autoantibody production and exacerbates disease in systemic lupus erythematosus-prone mice. J Immunol 2012;189(12):5786–96.

40. Soni C, Wong EB, Domeier PP, et al. B cell-intrinsic TLR7 signaling is essential for the development of spontaneous germinal centers. J Immunol 2014;193(9): 4400–14.

41. Tilstra JS, John S, Gordon RA, et al. B cell-intrinsic TLR9 expression is protective in murine lupus. J Clin Invest 2020;130(6):3172–87.

42. Lau CM, Broughton C, Tabor AS, et al. RNA-associated autoantigens activate B cells by combined B cell antigen receptor/Toll-like receptor 7 engagement. J Exp Med 2005;202(9):1171–7.

43. Julia A, Lopez-Longo FJ, Perez Venegas JJ, et al. Genome-wide association study meta-analysis identifies five new loci for systemic lupus erythematosus. Arthritis Res Ther 2018;20(1):100.

44. Vaughn SE, Foley C, Lu X, et al. Lupus risk variants in the PXK locus alter B-cell receptor internalization. Front Genet 2014;5:450.

45. Shen N, Fu Q, Deng Y, et al. Sex-specific association of X-linked Toll-like receptor 7 (TLR7) with male systemic lupus erythematosus. Proc Natl Acad Sci U S A 2010;107(36):15838–43.

46. Deng Y, Zhao J, Sakurai D, et al. MicroRNA-3148 modulates allelic expression of toll-like receptor 7 variant associated with systemic lupus erythematosus. PLoS Genet 2013;9(2):e1003336.

47. Sun C, Molineros JE, Looger LL, et al. High-density genotyping of immune-related loci identifies new SLE risk variants in individuals with Asian ancestry. Nat Genet 2016;48(3):323–30.

48. Adrianto I, Wen F, Templeton A, et al. Association of a functional variant downstream of TNFAIP3 with systemic lupus erythematosus. Nat Genet 2011;43(3): 253–8.

49. Heinz LX, Lee J, Kapoor U, et al. TASL is the SLC15A4-associated adaptor for IRF5 activation by TLR7-9. Nature 2020;581(7808):316–22.

50. Odhams CA, Roberts AL, Vester SK, et al. Interferon inducible X-linked gene CXorf21 may contribute to sexual dimorphism in systemic lupus erythematosus. Nat Commun 2019;10(1):2164.

51. Deng Y, Tsao BP. Updates in lupus genetics. Curr Rheumatol Rep 2017; 19(11):68.

52. Grossman SR, Andersen KG, Shlyakhter I, et al. Identifying recent adaptations in large-scale genomic data. Cell 2013;152(4):703–13.

53. Ramos PS, Shaftman SR, Ward RC, et al. Genes associated with SLE are targets of recent positive selection. Autoimmune Dis 2014;2014:203435.

54. Nutt SL, Hodgkin PD, Tarlinton DM, et al. The generation of antibody-secreting plasma cells. Nat Rev Immunol 2015;15(3):160–71.

55. Arbuckle MR, McClain MT, Rubertone MV, et al. Development of autoantibodies before the clinical onset of systemic lupus erythematosus. N Engl J Med 2003; 349(16):1526–33.

56. William J, Euler C, Christensen S, et al. Evolution of autoantibody responses via somatic hypermutation outside of germinal centers. Science 2002;297(5589): 2066–70.

57. Wellmann U, Letz M, Herrmann M, et al. The evolution of human anti-double-stranded DNA autoantibodies. Proc Natl Acad Sci U S A 2005;102(26):9258–63.

58. Vinuesa CG, Sanz I, Cook MC. Dysregulation of germinal centres in autoimmune disease. Nat Rev Immunol 2009;9(12):845–57.

59. Tipton CM, Fucile CF, Darce J, et al. Diversity, cellular origin and autoreactivity of antibody-secreting cell population expansions in acute systemic lupus erythematosus. Nat Immunol 2015;16(7):755–65.

60. Wang S, Wang J, Kumar V, et al. IL-21 drives expansion and plasma cell differentiation of autoreactive CD11c(hi)T-bet(+) B cells in SLE. Nat Commun 2018; 9(1):1758.

61. Jenks SA, Cashman KS, Zumaquero E, et al. Distinct effector B cells induced by unregulated toll-like receptor 7 contribute to pathogenic responses in systemic lupus erythematosus. Immunity 2018;49(4):725–739 e726.

62. Rubtsov AV, Rubtsova K, Fischer A, et al. Toll-like receptor 7 (TLR7)-driven accumulation of a novel CD11c(+) B-cell population is important for the development of autoimmunity. Blood 2011;118(5):1305–15.

63. Hao Y, O'Neill P, Naradikian MS, et al. A B-cell subset uniquely responsive to innate stimuli accumulates in aged mice. Blood 2011;118(5):1294–304.

64. Naradikian MS, Myles A, Beiting DP, et al. Cutting edge: IL-4, IL-21, and IFN-gamma interact to govern T-bet and CD11c expression in TLR-activated B cells. J Immunol 2016;197(4):1023–8.

65. Du SW, Arkatkar T, Jacobs HM, et al. Generation of functional murine CD11c(+) age-associated B cells in the absence of B cell T-bet expression. Eur J Immunol 2019;49(1):170–8.

66. Du SW, Arkatkar T, Al Qureshah F, et al. Functional characterization of CD11c(+) age-associated B cells as memory B cells. J Immunol 2019;203(11):2817–26.

67. Arazi A, Rao DA, Berthier CC, et al. The immune cell landscape in kidneys of patients with lupus nephritis. Nat Immunol 2019;20(7):902–14.

68. Di Niro R, Lee SJ, Vander Heiden JA, et al. Salmonella infection drives promiscuous B cell activation followed by extrafollicular affinity maturation. Immunity 2015;43(1):120–31.

69. Woodruff MC, Ramonell RP, Nguyen DC, et al. Extrafollicular B cell responses correlate with neutralizing antibodies and morbidity in COVID-19. Nat Immunol 2020;21(12):1506–16.

70. Kaneko N, Kuo HH, Boucau J, et al. Loss of Bcl-6-expressing t follicular helper cells and germinal centers in COVID-19. Cell 2020;183(1):143–57.e3.
71. Chan O, Shlomchik MJ. A new role for B cells in systemic autoimmunity: B cells promote spontaneous T cell activation in MRL-lpr/lpr mice. J Immunol 1998; 160(1):51–9.
72. Chan OT, Hannum LG, Haberman AM, et al. A novel mouse with B cells but lacking serum antibody reveals an antibody-independent role for B cells in murine lupus. J Exp Med 1999;189(10):1639–48.
73. Teichmann LL, Ols ML, Kashgarian M, et al. Dendritic cells in lupus are not required for activation of T and B cells but promote their expansion, resulting in tissue damage. Immunity 2010;33(6):967–78.
74. Giles JR, Kashgarian M, Koni PA, et al. B cell-specific MHC class II deletion reveals multiple nonredundant roles for B cell antigen presentation in murine lupus. J Immunol 2015;195(6):2571–9.
75. Baechler EC, Batliwalla FM, Karypis G, et al. Interferon-inducible gene expression signature in peripheral blood cells of patients with severe lupus. Proc Natl Acad Sci U S A 2003;100(5):2610–5.
76. Bennett L, Palucka AK, Arce E, et al. Interferon and granulopoiesis signatures in systemic lupus erythematosus blood. J Exp Med 2003;197(6):711–23.
77. Kirou KA, Lee C, George S, et al. Activation of the interferon-alpha pathway identifies a subgroup of systemic lupus erythematosus patients with distinct serologic features and active disease. Arthritis Rheum 2005;52(5):1491–503.
78. Pollard KM, Cauvi DM, Toomey CB, et al. Interferon-gamma and systemic autoimmunity. Discov Med 2013;16(87):123–31.
79. Haas C, Ryffel B, Le Hir M. IFN-gamma is essential for the development of autoimmune glomerulonephritis in MRL/lpr mice. J Immunol 1997;158(11):5484–91.
80. Schwarting A, Wada T, Kinoshita K, et al. IFN-gamma receptor signaling is essential for the initiation, acceleration, and destruction of autoimmune kidney disease in MRL-Fas(lpr) mice. J Immunol 1998;161(1):494–503.
81. Lee SK, Silva DG, Martin JL, et al. Interferon-gamma excess leads to pathogenic accumulation of follicular helper T cells and germinal centers. Immunity 2012;37(5):880–92.
82. Jackson SW, Jacobs HM, Arkatkar T, et al. B cell IFN-gamma receptor signaling promotes autoimmune germinal centers via cell-intrinsic induction of BCL-6. J Exp Med 2016;213(5):733–50.
83. Domeier PP, Chodisetti SB, Soni C, et al. IFN-gamma receptor and STAT1 signaling in B cells are central to spontaneous germinal center formation and autoimmunity. J Exp Med 2016;213(5):715–32.
84. Arkatkar T, Du SW, Jacobs HM, et al. B cell-derived IL-6 initiates spontaneous germinal center formation during systemic autoimmunity. J Exp Med 2017; 214(11):3207–17.
85. Domeier PP, Chodisetti SB, Schell SL, et al. B-cell-intrinsic type 1 interferon signaling is crucial for loss of tolerance and the development of autoreactive B cells. Cell Rep 2018;24(2):406–18.
86. Hall JC, Rosen A. Type I interferons: crucial participants in disease amplification in autoimmunity. Nat Rev Rheumatol 2010;6(1):40–9.
87. Jackson SW, Kolhatkar NS, Rawlings DJ. B cells take the front seat: dysregulated B cell signals orchestrate loss of tolerance and autoantibody production. Curr Opin Immunol 2015;33:70–7.
88. Rawlings DJ, Metzler G, Wray-Dutra M, et al. Altered B cell signalling in autoimmunity. Nat Rev Immunol 2017;17(7):421–36.

89. Lu R, Munroe ME, Guthridge JM, et al. Dysregulation of innate and adaptive serum mediators precedes systemic lupus erythematosus classification and improves prognostic accuracy of autoantibodies. J Autoimmun 2016;74:182–93.

90. Munroe ME, Lu R, Zhao YD, et al. Altered type II interferon precedes autoantibody accrual and elevated type I interferon activity prior to systemic lupus erythematosus classification. Ann Rheum Dis 2016;75(11):2014–21.

91. Koffler D, Schur PH, Kunkel HG. Immunological studies concerning the nephritis of systemic lupus erythematosus. J Exp Med 1967;126(4):607–24.

92. Ehrenstein MR, Katz DR, Griffiths MH, et al. Human IgG anti-DNA antibodies deposit in kidneys and induce proteinuria in SCID mice. Kidney Int 1995;48(3):705–11.

93. Mannik M, Merrill CE, Stamps LD, et al. Multiple autoantibodies form the glomerular immune deposits in patients with systemic lupus erythematosus. J Rheumatol 2003;30(7):1495–504.

94. Izmirly PM, Rivera TL, Buyon JP. Neonatal lupus syndromes. Rheum Dis Clin North Am 2007;33(2):267–85, vi.

95. Edwards JC, Szczepanski L, Szechinski J, et al. Efficacy of B-cell-targeted therapy with rituximab in patients with rheumatoid arthritis. N Engl J Med 2004;350(25):2572–81.

96. Merrill JT, Neuwelt CM, Wallace DJ, et al. Efficacy and safety of rituximab in moderately-to-severely active systemic lupus erythematosus: the randomized, double-blind, phase II/III systemic lupus erythematosus evaluation of rituximab trial. Arthritis Rheum 2010;62(1):222–33.

97. Rovin BH, Furie R, Latinis K, et al. Efficacy and safety of rituximab in patients with active proliferative lupus nephritis: the Lupus Nephritis Assessment with Rituximab study. Arthritis Rheum 2012;64(4):1215–26.

98. Clowse ME, Wallace DJ, Furie RA, et al. Efficacy and safety of epratuzumab in moderately to severely active systemic lupus erythematosus: results from two phase III randomized, double-blind, placebo-controlled trials. Arthritis Rheum 2017;69(2):362–75.

99. Merrill JT, Manzi S, Aranow C, et al. Lupus community panel proposals for optimising clinical trials: 2018. Lupus Sci Med 2018;5(1):e000258.

100. Wofsy D, Hillson JL, Diamond B. Comparison of alternative primary outcome measures for use in lupus nephritis clinical trials. Arthritis Rheum 2013;65(6):1586–91.

101. Teng YK, Levarht EW, Toes RE, et al. Residual inflammation after rituximab treatment is associated with sustained synovial plasma cell infiltration and enhanced B cell repopulation. Ann Rheum Dis 2009;68(6):1011–6.

102. Pijpe J, Meijer JM, Bootsma H, et al. Clinical and histologic evidence of salivary gland restoration supports the efficacy of rituximab treatment in Sjogren's syndrome. Arthritis Rheum 2009;60(11):3251–6.

103. Ahuja A, Shupe J, Dunn R, et al. Depletion of B cells in murine lupus: efficacy and resistance. J Immunol 2007;179(5):3351–61.

104. Kansal R, Richardson N, Neeli I, et al. Sustained B cell depletion by CD19-targeted CAR T cells is a highly effective treatment for murine lupus. Sci Transl Med 2019;11(482):eaav1648.

105. Gomez Mendez LM, Cascino MD, Garg J, et al. Peripheral blood B cell depletion after rituximab and complete response in lupus nephritis. Clin J Am Soc Nephrol 2018;13(10):1502–9.

106. Meyer S, Evers M, Jansen JHM, et al. New insights in Type I and II CD20 antibody mechanisms-of-action with a panel of novel CD20 antibodies. Br J Haematol 2018;180(6):808–20.

107. Mysler EF, Spindler AJ, Guzman R, et al. Efficacy and safety of ocrelizumab in active proliferative lupus nephritis: results from a randomized, double-blind, phase III study. Arthritis Rheum 2013;65(9):2368–79.

108. Marinov AD, Wang H, Bastacky SI, et al. The type II anti-CD20 antibody obinutuzumab (GA101) is more effective than rituximab at depleting B cells and treating disease in a murine lupus model. Arthritis Rheum 2021;73(5):826–36.

109. Furie R, Aroca G, Alvarez A, et al. A phase II randomized, double-blind, placebo-controlled study to evaluate the efficacy and safety of obinutuzumab or placebo in combination with mycophenolate mofetil in patients with active class III or IV lupus nephritis [abstract]. Paper presented at: 2019 ACR/ARP Annual Meeting Atlanta, GA: November 8-13, 2019.

110. Zhang F, Bae SC, Bass D, et al. A pivotal phase III, randomised, placebo-controlled study of belimumab in patients with systemic lupus erythematosus located in China, Japan and South Korea. Ann Rheum Dis 2018;77(3):355–63.

111. Isenberg DA, Petri M, Kalunian K, et al. Efficacy and safety of subcutaneous tabalumab in patients with systemic lupus erythematosus: results from ILLUMINATE-1, a 52-week, phase III, multicentre, randomised, double-blind, placebo-controlled study. Ann Rheum Dis 2016;75(2):323–31.

112. Merrill JT, van Vollenhoven RF, Buyon JP, et al. Efficacy and safety of subcutaneous tabalumab, a monoclonal antibody to B-cell activating factor, in patients with systemic lupus erythematosus: results from ILLUMINATE-2, a 52-week, phase III, multicentre, randomised, double-blind, placebo-controlled study. Ann Rheum Dis 2016;75(2):332–40.

113. Merrill JT, Shanahan WR, Scheinberg M, et al. Phase III trial results with blisibimod, a selective inhibitor of B-cell activating factor, in subjects with systemic lupus erythematosus (SLE): results from a randomised, double-blind, placebo-controlled trial. Ann Rheum Dis 2018;77(6):883–9.

114. Dooley MA, Houssiau F, Aranow C, et al. Effect of belimumab treatment on renal outcomes: results from the phase 3 belimumab clinical trials in patients with SLE. Lupus 2013;22(1):63–72.

115. Furie R, Rovin BH, Houssiau F, et al. Two-year, randomized, controlled trial of belimumab in lupus nephritis. N Engl J Med 2020;383(12):1117–28.

116. Stohl W, Schwarting A, Okada M, et al. Efficacy and safety of subcutaneous belimumab in systemic lupus erythematosus: a fifty-two-week randomized, double-blind, placebo-controlled study. Arthritis Rheum 2017;69(5):1016–27.

117. Atisha-Fregoso Y, Malkiel S, Harris KM, et al. Phase II randomized trial of rituximab plus cyclophosphamide followed by belimumab for the treatment of lupus nephritis. Arthritis Rheum 2020;73(1):121–31.

118. Ginzler EM, Wax S, Rajeswaran A, et al. Atacicept in combination with MMF and corticosteroids in lupus nephritis: results of a prematurely terminated trial. Arthritis Res Ther 2012;14(1):R33.

119. Isenberg DA. Meryl Streep and the problems of clinical trials. Arthritis Res Ther 2012;14(2):113.

120. Isenberg D, Gordon C, Licu D, et al. Efficacy and safety of atacicept for prevention of flares in patients with moderate-to-severe systemic lupus erythematosus (SLE): 52-week data (APRIL-SLE randomised trial). Ann Rheum Dis 2015; 74(11):2006–15.

121. Merrill JT, Wallace DJ, Wax S, et al. Efficacy and safety of atacicept in patients with systemic lupus erythematosus: results of a twenty-four-week, multicenter, randomized, double-blind, placebo-controlled, parallel-arm, phase IIb study. Arthritis Rheum 2018;70(2):266–76.
122. Wu D, Li J, Xu D, et al. A human recombinant fusion protein targeting B lymphocyte stimulator (BlyS) and a proliferation-inducing ligand (APRIL), telitacicept (RC18), in systemic lupus erythematosus (SLE): results of a phase 2b study. Arthritis Rheum 2019;71(suppl 10) [abstract].
123. Isenberg DFR, Jones N, Guibord P, et al. Efficacy, safety, and pharmacodynamic effects of the Bruton's tyrosine kinase inhibitor, fenebrutinib (GDC-0853), in moderate to severe systemic lupus erythematosus: results of a phase 2 randomized controlled trial. Arthritis Rheum 2019;71(suppl 10) [abstract].
124. Fillatreau S, Manfroi B, Dorner T. Toll-like receptor signalling in B cells during systemic lupus erythematosus. Nat Rev Rheumatol 2021;17(2):98–108.
125. Song S, De S, Nelson V, et al. Inhibition of IRF5 hyperactivation protects from lupus onset and severity. J Clin Invest 2020;130(12):6700–17.
126. Scholz JL, Crowley JE, Tomayko MM, et al. BLyS inhibition eliminates primary B cells but leaves natural and acquired humoral immunity intact. Proc Natl Acad Sci U S A 2008;105(40):15517–22.
127. Neubert K, Meister S, Moser K, et al. The proteasome inhibitor bortezomib depletes plasma cells and protects mice with lupus-like disease from nephritis. Nat Med 2008;14(7):748–55.
128. Ishii T, Tanaka Y, Kawakami A, et al. Multicenter double-blind randomized controlled trial to evaluate the effectiveness and safety of bortezomib as a treatment for refractory systemic lupus erythematosus. Mod Rheumatol 2018;28(6):986–92.
129. Ladi E, Everett C, Stivala CE, et al. Design and evaluation of highly selective human immunoproteasome inhibitors reveal a compensatory process that preserves immune cell viability. J Med Chem 2019;62(15):7032–41.
130. Anderson KC. Progress and paradigms in multiple myeloma. Clin Cancer Res 2016;22(22):5419–27.
131. Ostendorf L, Burns M, Durek P, et al. Targeting CD38 with daratumumab in refractory systemic lupus erythematosus. N Engl J Med 2020;383(12):1149–55.
132. Raje N, Berdeja J, Lin Y, et al. Anti-BCMA CAR T-cell therapy bb2121 in relapsed or refractory multiple myeloma. N Engl J Med 2019;380(18):1726–37.

Systemic Lupus Erythematosus Outcome Measures for Systemic Lupus Erythematosus Clinical Trials

Taraneh Tofighi, MD[a],*, Eric F. Morand, MBBS, FRACP, PhD[b],
Zahi Touma, MD, PhD[c]

KEYWORDS

- Lupus • Measures • Outcomes • Systemic lupus • SLEDAI • BILAG • SRI • BICLA

KEY POINTS

- SLE is a complex and heterogenous disease with ideal index equipped to capture active/inactive disease states, changes in disease activity, and magnitude/severity organ manifestations.
- Composite outcome measures such as the SRI and BICLA have been most commonly used as primary endpoints in phase II and III trials.
- Given many phase III RCTs unsuccessful in reaching primary outcome, several avenues for further exploration include dual endpoints, incorporating glucocorticoid reduction, and measuring partial improvement in global indices such as in S2K RI-50.

INTRODUCTION

Systemic lupus erythematosus (SLE) is a complex, multisystem disease with variability in disease course and progression among patients. As such, it can be challenging to evaluate disease activity in clinical and research settings, including in the measurement of treatment responses in clinical trials. This challenge lies in accounting for the wide range of organ manifestations and the ultimate heterogeneity of disease trajectory.[1]

In 1988, the outcome measures in rheumatology (OMERACT) group sought to identify a set of domains to be used for randomized clinical trials (RCTs) and longitudinal observation studies (LOS).[2] The group recommended assessment of patients in

[a] Department of Medicine, University of Toronto, 200 Elizabeth St, Toronto, ON M5G 2C4, Canada; [b] Centre for Inflammatory Disease, Monash University, Melbourne, Australia; [c] Centre for Prognosis Studies in the Rheumatic Diseases, Toronto Western Hospital, University of Toronto Lupus Clinic, EW, 1-412, 399 Bathurst Street, Toronto, ON, M5T 2S8, Canada
* Corresponding author.
E-mail address: tara.tofighi@mail.utoronto.ca

Rheum Dis Clin N Am 47 (2021) 415–426
https://doi.org/10.1016/j.rdc.2021.04.007
0889-857X/21/© 2021 Elsevier Inc. All rights reserved.

accordance with the following domains: disease activity, damage resulting from disease activity or related to treatment in all organ systems involved, adverse drug events, health-related quality of life, and economic impact. Years after the preceding domains were first identified, various organizations and scientists continue the development and assessment of response criteria pertaining to SLE disease state and changes. Core domains that are measured consistently, and validated instruments composed of these domains, are essential to effectively evaluating innovative drugs and treatment strategies. The domains mentioned previously were ratified with the understanding that in a heterogeneous, multisystem disease such as SLE, any validated instrument for a specific domain (eg, disease activity) will capture only one aspect of the disease. Nevertheless, we have learned from recent trials that it might require more than one instrument to accurately measure changes in SLE disease activity. For instance, the ideal tool for RCTs should be able to identify active and inactive SLE disease states (discriminative instrument) as well as changes, both improvement and worsening, over time (evaluative instrument). However, recent trials have adopted the use of historically reported composite indices in an attempt to measure all facets of SLE disease activity, but without validating that these goals are met. The challenge in the trial setting lies in identifying the appropriate instrument(s), and endpoint comprising these instruments, that address the question at hand.

Many promising SLE therapeutics have failed to achieve their primary outcome in phase III clinical trials, in part due to the challenges in selecting appropriate outcome measures and endpoints. To this day, there is no clear consensus on response criteria in SLE, although various organizations have identified disease activity indices for use in SLE RCTs.[3] In this article, we discuss the outcome measures and endpoints used in the clinical trial setting, weigh the strengths and gaps in these measures, and explore potential avenues for further development.

PRIMARY ENDPOINTS IN SYSTEMIC LUPUS ERYTHEMATOSUS RANDOMIZED CONTROLLED TRIALS
Starting at the Beginning: Single Outcome Measures

Early RCTs used single disease measures as their primary outcomes, although the more updated trials tend to use these disease indices as secondary outcomes and composite indices as the primary outcomes. The 2 most notable single disease indices, the Systemic Lupus Erythematosus Disease Activity Index (SLEDAI) and the British Isles Lupus Assessment Group Index (BILAG) have been shown to correlate with one another despite the fact the SLEDAI measures global disease activity while the BILAG measures organ-specific disease changes as well as the change within the organ systems affected by disease.[4,5]

Systemic Lupus Erythematosus Disease Activity Index
The SLEDAI is an example of a global disease activity index composed of 24 descriptors that are each weighted differently. It has undergone several iterations including SELENA-SLEDAI, and the SLEDAI-2000 (SLEDAI-2K), which is the iteration most often used in recent clinical trials.[6–9]

In 2002, SLEDAI-2K was validated against the original SLEDAI and incorporated modification in the definitions of 4 descriptors to allow the identification of persistent disease activity in mucocutaneous (skin rash, alopecia, oral ulcers) and renal (proteinuria >0.5 g in 24 hours) systems instead of solely new or recurrent activity.[10] Although the SLEDAI score descriptors are based on activity present in the 10 days preceding index administration, in 2011, the SLEDAI-2K-30 days was validated against SLEDAI-2K-10 days to make it more comparable with other tools measuring activity in the preceding 30 days.[11]

The SELENA-SLEDAI and SELENA flare index (SFI) were both primary outcome measures in the phase II intravenous belimumab trial.[12] The SFI complements the SLEDAI by accounting for severity in the form of mild/moderate or severe flares with a physician assessment and treatment decision component.[7]

The advantages of the SLEDAI and its derivates are largely their simplicity and ease of use. However, as activity in organ domain subscores are scored as simply present or absent, the index lacks the ability to measure different levels of disease activity within the same descriptors, and therefore lacks the capacity to identify changes such as improvement and worsening. For example, thrombocytopenia is assigned a weight of 1 in the index irrespective of the severity of the abnormality, although degree of thrombocytopenia has implications in clinical care and management.[13] To overcome this deficiency, Touma and colleagues[14] recently developed a novel index that addresses gaps in weighting scoring while accounting for disease activity.

Among global disease indices, SLEDAI-2K is most commonly used in clinical trials. In 2018, a modification to the SLEDAI was introduced in the form of the SLEDAI-2 KG, which incorporates a new descriptor: a weighted score ranging from 0 to 8 based on the dose of glucocorticoids at the assessment.[13] This is a promising tool for RCTs and LOS, as it includes a glucocorticoid reduction item. Touma and colleagues[14] showed recently that SLEDAI-2KG identifies additional responders among SLEDAI-2K nonresponders, which results from the ability of the new index to adjust for the decrease in glucocorticoid dose on follow-up. Given that a recent meta-analysis by Nikpour and colleagues[15] showed that most phase III SLE trial therapeutics, aside from EXPLORER and ILUMINATE-1, showed a glucocorticoid-sparing effect, the SLEDAI-2KG may serve as a useful index in future trials, although this has yet to be tested in the trial setting.[13]

British Isles Lupus Assessment Group Index

The BILAG has also gone through several iterations, such as the BILAG-2004 and BILAG-2009, the former of which is used in clinical trials.[16–18] The advantage of the BILAG over the SLEDAI lies in its ability to evaluate partial change over time in the various organ systems. The index includes 9 organ systems with a score in each domain. Changes over time are accounted for by the following scoring system: 0 (not present), 1 (improving), 2 (same), 3 (worse) or 4 (new), pertaining to activity in the past 4 weeks compared with the previous 4 weeks. The index also accounts for severity by computing organ domain activity into categories as follows: A (severe), B (moderate), C (mild), D (no activity), or E (no history). Although the ability to measure change within an organ system is an advantage compared with SLEDAI, the requirement to "look back" at the trajectory of disease can mean that 2 patients with the same features may receive different scores depending on the direction in which their disease activity has moved from the previous assessment. In addition, the comprehensive nature of the BILAG instrument also means it is more complex to complete than the SLEDAI-based measures.

In clinical trials using this index, the outcomes are classified as an improvement (BILAG response), flare (BILAG flares), or a combination. The original BILAG was used in several early RCTs from the past decade including the phase IIb abatacept in nonrenal SLE trial, the phase III rituximab in nonrenal SLE trial, and the phase II/III atacicept trial in SLE trial.[19–21] More recent trials from the past 5 years, such as the phase II rontalizumab trial, use the BILAG-2004, which is more sensitive.[22] However, the heterogeneity in defining endpoints makes comparisons across trials difficult.

Composite Outcome Measures

We now arrive at composite outcome measures, which are the most commonly used in recent phase II and III SLE trials. These composite measures have been designed to compensate for the weaknesses of individual measures, in that they incorporate different disease measures to capture improvement, and nonworsening, to identify responders in RCTs.

Systemic lupus erythematosus responder index

The systemic lupus erythematosus responder index (SRI) was developed after the phase II belimumab trial failed to meet its primary outcome measure endpoints: percentage change in SELENA-SLEDAI from baseline to 24 weeks and time to first disease flare as informed by the SFI.[12] The SRI incorporates 3 tools: the SELENA-SLEDAI for global improvement capture, the BILAG to catch any worsening in organ systems that is, missed in the SLEDAI, and a Physician Global Assessment (PGA) to capture any disease worsening the other 2 tools may have missed. The SRI was derived from a post hoc analysis of the same phase II belimumab trial, which led to its inception (**Fig. 1**).[3] In the study, SRI was defined as follows:

1. A prespecified reduction in the SELENA-SLEDAI score, with a ≥4-point reduction from baseline, SRI-4, most commonly used in RCTs
2. No new BILAG A or ≤1 new BILAG B domain score compared with baseline
3. No deterioration from baseline in the PGA by ≥0.3 points, on a 0 to 3 scale where 0 is no disease activity and 3 is maximum possible disease activity

Importantly, as improvement is based on changes in SLEDAI, complete resolution of activity in organ systems with weights of at least 4 is required to be designated a responder; improvement in all systems is not required. The SRI was first applied to as part of a post hoc analysis of a subset of patients in the belimumab phase II trial with positive ANA ≥1:80 and/or anti-dsDNA ≥30 IU/mL, with a significant difference noted between the placebo and belimumab groups using both an SRI-4 and SRI-5 definition (which uses a higher SLEDAI reduction of ≥5 points). When the analysis

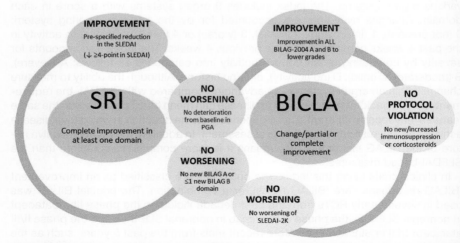

Fig. 1. BICLA and SRI component comparison. This figure captures the various lenses offered by the SRI and BICLA, in terms of areas of overlap and differences that result in capturing partial improvement through the BICLA.

was expanded to the larger trial population, there remained a higher week 52 response in the belimumab group compared with placebo (45.9% compared with 35.4%, $P = .045$).[3,12]

Since the belimumab trial, the SRI has been used as the primary endpoint in several trials including the phase III intravenous (BLISS-52 and BLISS-76) and subcutaneous (BLISS-SC) belimumab trials, which met the SRI-4 endpoint in all 3 trials at the 52-week mark.[23–25] It was also recently used in the EMBRACE trial, which did not meet its endpoint.[26] In addition, the SRI-5 was used as the endpoint in the ILLUMINATE 1 and ILLUMINATE 2 phase III trials of tabalumab, another anti-BAFF monoclonal antibody, only showing significance with the higher 120 mg twice weekly subcutaneous dose in ILLUMINATE 2.[26–28]

There are several trials using the SRI as the primary outcome, which did not achieve significance. Namely, SRI-6 was used as the primary endpoint in phase III blisibimod trial, which did not meet its outcome, which may be explained by the effects of higher glucocorticoid doses in the standard of care group.[29] In addition, SRI-4 was used as the primary outcome in the TULIP-1 anifrolumab trial, which also did not meet its endpoint.[30] That the companion TULIP-2 trial did demonstrate significant differences from placebo in SRI-4, in a trial with the same patient characteristics and treatment, casts additional doubt about the reliability of the SRI-4 as an outcome measure.[31]

BILAG-based combined lupus assessment
The BILAG-based combined lupus assessment (BICLA) is an interesting composite index in that it also captures partial improvements with its BILAG-2004 based component.

Response by BICLA criteria is defined as follows:

1. Improvement in moderate-severe BILAG-2004 activity (A scores at baseline to B/C/D, B scores to C/D)
2. No worsening in global and organ-specific disease activity (no new BILAG-2004 A or ≤1 new BILAG B score, no worsening of SLEDAI-2K score from baseline to endpoint, and no worsening in PGA (<10% worsening)
3. No treatment failure, defined as nonprotocol introduction of new/increased immunosuppressants or antimalarial, increased or parenteral corticosteroids, or early withdrawal from study group

In contrast to SRI, the BILAG is the primary way in which improvement is captured in BICLA, meaning that substantial but not total improvement is required in baseline organ systems, but importantly that all systems active at baseline must improve. In addition, organ systems are not weighted in BILAG, unlike in SLEDAI. The BICLA was first used in the EMBLEM epratuzumab phase IIb trial, which did not meet its endpoint for overall treatment with epratuzumab at week 12, although it did meet its endpoint for the 2400-mg dose at week 8.[32] BICLA was further applied in phase III EMBODY-1 and EMBODY-2 epratuzumab trials, which were negative trials at week 48, although it should be noted that a negative outcome was seen across various outcome measures and a post hoc analysis using an adjusted BICLA and modified SRI-4, 6, and 8.[33] Interestingly, the BICLA was used as the revised primary outcome in the TULIP-2 anifrolumab trial, which had initially been planned to use SRI-4 as the primary outcome.[30] TULIP-2 did show a highly significant difference in week 52 with 47.8% response in the anifrolumab group compared with 31.5% in placebo.

As there are identified weaknesses of the currently available disease activity instruments, the composite outcome measures may confer an advantage over single indices such as the SLEDAI and BILAG that have led to them being successfully applied in phase III clinical trials, and through incorporating various tools they may be getting closer to defining the desired outcome of separating responders and nonresponders in RCTs. Where the SRI and BICLA differ is in the picture they paint: as the SLEDAI is a binary assessment, it makes note of the presence or absence of activity in each organ domain, whereas the BILAG has the capability to note partial improvements or worsening in each organ system. As seen in the results of the TULIP-2 anifrolumab trial, the BILAG-based BICLA can capture partial improvement in addition to complete resolution of activity, suggesting it may be a more sensitive index than the SLEDAI-based SRI.

ORGAN-SPECIFIC OUTCOME MEASURES
Skin Disease

Both the SLEDAI and BILAG include several items that account for mucocutaneous disease, although neither do so as comprehensively as the Cutaneous Lupus Erythematosus Disease Area and Severity Index (CLASI) index, which was developed in 2005.[34,35] The index has proven good content validity and reliability, assigning a score to each area of the body and providing a measure of both cutaneous activity and damage.[34] Activity is captured by presence of erythema, scale, mucous membrane lesions, and alopecia, with points for the severity of these manifestations and greater weighting of lesions in more visible areas of the body. Damage is captured by the presence of scarring, atrophy, or panniculitis.

A subindex of the CLASI, limited to measurement of activity (CLASI-A) has been applied successfully in both TULIP-1 and -2 trials of anifrolumab. In fact, although the SRI-4 endpoint was not met in TULIP-1, there was a benefit of anifrolumab over placebo in proportion of patients who achieved at least 50% improvement in CLASI-A score at week 12 in individuals with a baseline score of at least 10 in both trials.[30,31]

In terms of strengths and weaknesses, the CLASI has been noted to take an average of 1 to 11 minutes to compile and has demonstrated intrarater and interrater reliability among both rheumatologists and dermatologists.[34,35] To date, CLASI has not been accepted by regulatory agencies such, as the US Food and Drug Administration, as a primary SLE trial outcome measures.

Arthritis Measures

Joint involvement occurs frequently among patients with SLE, affecting up to 90% of patients.[36] As such, all SLE disease activity indices include a descriptor on lupus arthritis, although there is no gold standard measure for assessment of joint involvement in SLE. Among the global indices, the SLEDAI-2K includes an item with a weight of 4, which defines the presence of arthritis as 2 or more painful joints with signs of inflammation as characterized by tenderness, edema, or effusion.[13] The SLEDAI arthritis domain was successfully used as a primary outcome measure, in combination with SLEDAI skin domain, in the Phase II trial of baricitinib.[37] The Systemic Lupus Erythematosus Disease Activity Index 2000 Responder Index-50 (S2K RI-50), which was based on the SLEDAI-2K, comprises the same descriptor for arthritis, requiring a minimum 50% improvement, defined as ≥50% reduction in the number of active joints compared with previous visit.[38]

In rheumatoid arthritis literature, the Disease Activity Score 28 (DAS28) has been validated and commonly used in clinical trials.[39] Based on the impact of this work, several SLE clinical trials have included arthritis as an exploratory or secondary endpoint captured as a 28 tender and swollen join count similar to those validated in rheumatoid arthritis. There are limits to this, as these endpoints typically do not include the hip, ankle or feet joints.[13] Indeed, a tool similar to the DAS28 may be better equipped to capture sensitive changes in arthritis compared with global indices, although further studies are needed to validate such tools in the SLE population. Simpler measures such as swollen and tender joint counts have been used as secondary outcome measures in the anifrolumab trials.

A new index known as the LARI (Lupus Arthritis Responder Index) was used in phase Ib of the AMG 557 trial with a trend toward response in the treatment group. Improved arthritis activity was defined as a 50% decrease in the combined tender and swollen joint counts, ≥ 1 letter improvement in the BILAG musculoskeletal system score, and incorporation of a glucocorticoid reduction component.[40]

Renal Indices

When it comes to renal indices, there is limited consensus on response endpoints. Earlier studies used renal flare as their primary endpoint, whereas more recent trials used composite endpoints of complete and partial response. However, it should be noted that there is no consistent definition of complete and partial remission used in clinical trials. For example, the LUNAR (phase III rituximab), ALMS (mycophenolate mofetil) and ACCESS (abatacept and cyclophosphamide combination) trials each had a unique definition of complete response in terms of the urine protein:creatinine ratio, serum creatinine and urinalysis cutoffs, as well as glucocorticoid taper parameters and number of consecutive visits needed to ascertain complete response.[41-45] Indeed, to test just how different results can be with the different definitions, an analysis of the IM101075 trial (phase II/III trial of abatacept in lupus nephritis) used criteria from the LUNAR, ALMS and ACCESS trials and showed a difference in response based on the different definition of complete response.[44]

Although the Euro-Lupus Nephritis Trial and MAINTAIN Nephritis Trial have identified proteinuria at 12 months as the best available predictor of long-term renal outcome in lupus nephritis (LN), urine erythrocyte counts continue to be used as an endpoint in trials, even though Houssiau and colleagues[46] and Fung and colleagues[45] demonstrated the low precision, lack of accuracy, and poor prognosticatory value for renal outcomes.[46,47] In trials that do consider proteinuria as the endpoint, there remains great heterogeneity in length of follow-up, although studies have demonstrated that proteinuria can be a slowly changing marker, with only 28% of patients showing recovery from proteinuria (0.5 g/d) at year 1 and 52% at year 2, compared with 74% at year 5.[47]

Most recently, a positive 2-year RCT of belimumab in lupus nephritis used 2 different renal endpoints with polymerase chain reaction cutoffs of ≤ 0.7 and ≤ 0.5 g/d, demonstrating a statistically significant difference between belimumab and placebo at week 104 with both cutoffs. Less stringent cutoffs may lend themselves to effectively powering a study; however, this may be a double-edged sword in conferring an advantage to the placebo group, although this was not the case in the belimumab trial.[48]

TREAT TO TARGET ENDPOINTS: THE LUPUS LOW DISEASE ACTIVITY STATE

There has been a movement toward using measures of low disease activity as endpoint in RCTs, with a promising index known as the Lupus Low Disease Activity State (LLDAS). This new index not only accounts for disease activity through incorporating the SLEDAI-2K and PGA but also for prednisone and immunosuppressive use.[49] A major point of difference from SRI and BICLA endpoints is that this records attainment of a target state, rather than change from baseline. The criteria that need to meet target in the LLDAS include the following:

1. SLEDAI-2K score ≤ 4, with no activity in the renal, central nervous system, and cardiopulmonary systems and absence of vasculitis and fever
2. No new disease activity compared with the last visit
3. PGA score ≤ 1
4. Current prednisolone-equivalent dosage ≤ 7.5 mg/d
5. Standard maintenance dosages of immunosuppressive drugs and approved biologics allowed

What do we know about the validity of the LLDAS? In terms of prognosis, multiple retrospective studies and a multicentre prospective study have demonstrated that LLDAS attainment is associated with improved prognosis including protection from damage accrual and mortality. The tool has not yet been used as a primary endpoint in RCTs; however, we do have promising results from post hoc analyses of phase II trial of anifrolumab (MUSE) and atacicept (ADDRESS II) studies.[50–53] In these trials the tool was shown to be positively associated with responder status but more discriminatory than the SRI-4 and BICLA. The LLDAS shows promise in that it can discern drug responders from nonresponders while being a more stringent tool with prognostic value.

SUMMARY AND FUTURE WORK

Given the complexity of disease and the vast heterogeneity in patient presentations, several groups been working to develop an index that will move us closer to measuring disease improvement in SLE and define responders in RCTs. With each iteration, we inch closer to a validated endpoint that will ideally measure active and inactive disease states, changes in disease activity, as well as magnitude and severity of organ manifestations.

As noted previously, composite outcome measures such as the SRI and BICLA have been most commonly used as primary endpoints in phase II and III trials. Although their roles are complementary, there remain gaps in each tool, for example, the SLEDAI-based SRI is unable to capture partial improvement outside of dichotomous disease activity, and the BICLA may be less sensitive to clinically significant global changes. With consideration of organ-specific indices that are often used as secondary endpoints, there is room for improvement in terms of increased use of standardized organ-specific measures and cutoffs to assess joint, skin, nephritis, and other manifestations.

Given many phase III RCTs have been unsuccessful in achieving their primary outcomes, there are several gaps to address, including standardizing cutoffs and endpoints through identifying an MCID for each tool, perhaps to be derived from RCT data rather than adopted MCIDs that were derived from cohort data. Avenues for further exploration include incorporating glucocorticoid reduction, such as is as captured in the SLEDAI-2KG, as a primary endpoint in future trials, given that many phase III trials have shown a steroid-sparing effect. In addition, there may be a role to new tools such as the S2K RI-50 to record partial improvements in global disease indices, adding further data on clinically significant improvements that may be otherwise uncaptured. The LLDAS shows great promise through accounting for activity and prednisone use, thereby capturing risk factors for damage accrual.

As demonstrated by the divergent results of the TULIP-1 and TULIP-2 studies, the way forward may lie in redesigning trials to evaluate multiple indices and different primary outcomes in studies of novel drugs, especially via the careful analysis of Phase 2 trial data before committing to an endpoint for Phase 3 trials. The potential for dual endpoints in Phase 3 studies has yet to be tested but may offer another way to reduce the lost opportunities that so many negative SLE trials represent.

CLINICS CARE POINTS

- Glucocorticoid reduction, which is captured in SLEDAI-2KG may be a useful endpoint in future trials given several phase III trials show steroid sparing effect.
- Role for indices that capture partial improvement such as in S2K RI-50.
- LLDAS shows great promise in accounting for activity and prednisone use, thereby capturing risk factors for damage accrual.
- Potential for dual endpoints to capture complexities and heterogeneities in SLE clinical course.

DISCLOSURE

The authors have nothing to disclose.

REFERENCES

1. Kaul A, Gordon C, Crow MK, et al. Systemic lupus erythematosus. Nat Rev Dis Primers 2016;2:16039.
2. Smolen JS, Strand VI, Cardiel M, et al. Randomized clinical trials and longitudinal observational studies in systemic lupus erythematosus: consensus on a preliminary core set of outcome domains. J Rheumatol 1999;26(2):504–7.
3. Furie R, Petri M, Wallace D, et al. Novel evidence-based systemic lupus erythematosus responder index. Arthritis Rheum 2009;61:1143–51.
4. Griffiths B, Mosca M, Gordon C. Assessment of patients with systemic lupus erythematous and the use of lupus disease activity indices. Best Pract Res Clin Rheumatol 2005;19:685–708.
5. Gladman DD, Goldsmith CH, Urowitz MB, et al. Crosscultural validation and reliability of 3 disease activity indices in systemic lupus erythematosus. J Rheumatol 1992;19:608–11.
6. Bombardier C, Gladman DD, Urowitz MB, et al. Derivation of the SLEDAI. A disease activity index for lupus patients. The Committee on Prognosis Studies in SLE. Arthritis Rheum 1992;35:630–40.
7. Petri M, Kim MY, Kalunian KC, et al, OC-SELENA Trial. Combined oral contraceptives in women with systemic lupus erythematosus. N Engl J Med 2005;353: 2550–8.
8. Gladman DD, Ibanez D, Urowitz MB. Systemic lupus erythematosus disease activity index 2000. J Rheumatol 2002;29:288–91.
9. Buyon JP, Petric MA, Kim MY, et al. The effect of combined estrogen and progesterone hormone replacement therapy on disease activity in systemic lupus erythematosus: a randomized trial. Ann Intern Med 2005;142:953–62.
10. Parker B, Bruce I. Clinical markers, metrics, indices and clinical trials. Dubois' Lupus Erythematosus and Related Syndromes. 9th edition, Wallace D and Hahn B eds: Elsevier, 2019.
11. Touma Z, Urowitz MB, Ibañez D, et al. SLEDAI-2K 10 days versus SLEDAI-2K 30 days in a longitudinal evaluation. Lupus 2011;20(1):67–70.

12. Wallace DJ, Stohl W, Furie RA, et al. A phase II, randomized, double-blind, pla-cebo-controlled, dose-ranging study of belimumab in patients with active sys-temic lupus erythematosus. Arthritis Rheum 2009;61:1168–78.

13. Metrics and Outcomes of SLE Clinical trials, Touma Z, Gladman DD, Su J, et al. A novel lupus activity index accounting for glucocorticoids: SLEDAI-2K glucocor-ticoid index. Rheumatology 2018;57(8):1370–6.

14. Touma Z, Gladman DD, Zandy M, et al. Identifying a response for the systemic lupus erythematosus disease activity glucocorticoid index (SLEDAI-2KG). Arthritis Care Res (Hoboken) 2020. https://doi.org/10.1002/acr.24261.

15. Oon S, Huq M, Nikpour M. Steroid sparing effect: an essential element in assess-ing therapeutic efficacy in SLE: response to 'Time to change the primary outcome of lupus trials' by Houssiau. Ann Rheum Dis 2019 Aug 16. https://doi.org/10.1136/annrheumdis-2019-216113.

16. Hay EM, Bacon PA, Gordon C, et al. The BILAG index: a reliable and valid instru-ment for measuring clinical disease activity in systemic lupus erythematosus. Q J Med 1993;86:447–58.

17. Isenberg DA, Rahman A, Allen E, et al. BILAG 2004. Development and initial vali-dation of an updated version of the British Isles Lupus Assessment Group's dis-ease activity index for patients with systemic lupus erythematosus. Rheumatology (Oxford) 2005;44:902–6.

18. Yee CS, Farewell V, Isenberg DA, et al. The BILAG-2004 index is sensitive to change for assessment of SLE disease activity. Rheumatology (Oxford) 2009; 48:691–5.

19. Merrill JT, Burgos-Vargas R, Westhovens R, et al. The efficacy and safety of aba-tacept in patients in non-life threatening manifestations of systemic lupus erythe-matosus: results of a twelve-month, multicentre, exploratory, phase IIb, randomized, double-blind, placebo-controlled trial. Arthritis Rheum 2010;62: 3077–87.

20. Merrill JT, Neuwelt CM, Wallace DJ, et al. Efficacy and safety of rituximab in moderately-to-severely active systemic lupus erythematosus: the randomized, double-blind, phase II/III systemic lupus erythematosus evaluation of rituximab trial. Arthritis Rheum 2010;62:222–33.

21. Isenberg D, Gordon C, LIcu D, et al. Efficacy and safety of atacicept for preven-tion of flares in patients with moderate-to-severe systemic lupus erythematosus (SLE): 52-week data (APRIL-SLE randomised trial). Ann Rheum Dis 2015;74: 2006–15.

22. Kalunian KC, Merrill JT, Maciuca R, et al. A phase II study of the efficacy and safety of rontalizumab (rhuMAb interferon-a) in patients with systemic lupus ery-thematosus (ROSE). Ann Rheum Dis 2016;75:196–202.

23. Furie R, Petri M, Zamani O, et al. A phase III, randomized, placebo-controlled study of belimumab, a monoclonal antibody that inhibits B lymphocyte stimulator, in patients with systemic lupus erythematosus. Arthritis Rheum 2011;63(12): 3912–30.

24. Navarra S, Guzmán R, Gallacher A, et al. Efficacy and safety of belimumab in pa-tients with active systemic lupus erythematosus: a randomised, placebo-controlled, phase 3 trial. Lancet 2011;377:721–31.

25. Stohl W, Schwarting A, Okada M, et al. Efficacy and safety of subcutaneous be-limumab in systemic lupus erythemaosus: a fifty-two-week randomized, double-blind, placebo-controlled study. Arthritis Rheumatol 2017;69(5):1016–27.

26. D'Cruz D, Maksimowicz-McKinnon K, Oates J, et al. 200 Efficacy and safety of belimumab in patients of black race with systemic lupus erythematosus: results

from the EMBRACE study. Lupus Sci Med 2019;6. https://doi.org/10.1136/lupus-2019-lsm.200.

27. Isenberg DA, Petri M, Kalunian K, et al. Efficacy and safety of subcutaneous ta-balumab in patients with systemic lupus erythematosus: results from ILLUMINATE-1, a 52-week, phase III, multicentre, randomised, double-blind, pla-cebo-controlled study. Ann Rheum Dis 2016;75:323–31.

28. Merrill JT, van Vollenhoven RF, Buyon JP, et al. Efficacy and safety of subcutane-ous tabalumab, a monoclonal antibody to B-cell activating factor, in patients with systemic lupus erythematosus: results from ILLUMINATE-2, a 52-week, phase III, multicentre, randomised, double-blind, placebo-controlled study. Ann Rheum Dis 2016;75:332–40.

29. Merrill JT, Shanahan WR, Scheinberg M, et al. Phase III trial results with blisibi-mod, a selective inhibitor of B-cell activating factor, in subjects with systemic lupus erythematosus (SLE): results from a randomised, double-blind, placebo-controlled trial. Ann Rheum Dis 2018;77:883–9.

30. Furie RA, Morand EF, Bruce IN, et al. Type 1 interferon inhibitor anifrolumab in active systemic lupus erythematosus (TULIP-1): a randomised, controlled, phase 3 trial. Lancet Rheumatol 2019;1:e208–19.

31. Morand EF, Furie R, Tanaka Y, et al, TULIP-2 Trial Investigators. Trial of anifrolu-mab in active systemic lupus erythematosus. N Engl J Med 2020;382(3):211–21.

32. Wallace DJ, Kalunian K, Petri A, et al. Efficacy and safety of epratuzumab in pa-tients with moderate/severe active systemic lupus erythematosus: results from EMBLEM, a phase IIb, randomised, double-blind, placebo-controlled, multi-centre study. Ann Rheum Dis 2014;73:183–90.

33. Clowse MEB, Wallace D, Furie R, et al. Efficacy and safety of epratuzumab in moderately to severely active systemic lupus erythematosus. Arthritis Rheumatol 2017;69:362–75.

34. Albrecht J, Taylor L, Berlin JA, et al. The CLASI (Cutaneous Lupus Erythematosus Disease Area and Severity Index): an outcome instrument for cutaneous lupus er-ythematosus. J Invest Dermatol 2005;125:889–94.

35. Albrecht J, Werth VP. Development of the CLASI as an outcome instrument for cutaneous lupus erythematosus. Dermatol Ther 2007;20:93–101.

36. Ball EM, Bell AL. Lupus arthritis–do we have a clinically useful classification? Rheumatology (Oxford) 2012;51(5):771–9.

37. Wallace DJ, Furie RA, Tanaka Y, et al. Baricitinib for systemic lupus erythemato-sus: a double-blind, randomised, placebo-controlled, phase 2 trial. Lancet 2018; 392(10143):222–31 [Erratum in: Lancet. 2018 Aug 11;392(10146):476].

38. Touma Z, Gladman DD, Urowitz MB. Development validation and reliability of the Systemic Lupus Erythematosus Disease Activity Index 2000 Responder Index-50. Arthritis Res Ther 2012;14(Suppl 3):A55.

39. Prevoo ML, van 't Hof MA, Kuper HH, et al. Modified disease activity scores that include twenty-eight-joint counts. Development and validation in a prospective longitudinal study of patients with rheumatoid arthritis. Arthritis Rheum 1995; 38(1):44–8.

40. Cheng L, Amoura Z, Cheah B, et al. A randomized, double-blind, parallel-group, placebo-controlled, multiple-dose study to evaluate AMG 557 in patients with systemic lupus erythematosus and active lupus arthritis. Arthritis Rheumatol 2018;70:1071–6.

41. Rovin BH, Furie R, Latinis K, et al, for the LUNAR Investigator Group. Efficacy and safety of rituximab in patients with active proliferative lupus nephritis: the Lupus Nephritis Assessment with Rituximab study. Arthritis Rheum 2012;64:1215–26.

42. Appel GB, Contreras G, Dooley MA, et al. Mycophenolate mofetil versus cyclo-phosphamide for induction treatment of lupus nephritis. J Am Soc Nephrol 2009;20:1103–12.
43. Askanase A, Byron M, Keyes-Elstein L, et al. Treatment of lupus nephritis with abatacept: the abatacept and cyclophosphamide combination efficacy and safety study. Arthritis Rheumatol 2014;66:3096–104.
44. Wofsy D, Hillson JL, Diamond B. Abatacept for lupus nephritis. Alternative defini-tions of complete response support conflicting conclusions. Arthritis Rheum 2012;64:3660–5.
45. Fung WA, Su J, Touma Z. Predictors of good long-term renal outcomes in lupus nephritis: results from a single lupus cohort. Biomed Res Int 2017;2017:5312960.
46. Tamirou F, Lauwerys BR, Dall'Era M, et al. A proteinuria cut-off level of 0.7 g/day after 12 months of treatment best predicts long-term renal outcome in lupus nephritis: data from the MAINTAIN Nephritis Trial. Lupus Sci Med 2015;2: e000123. https://doi.org/10.1136/lupus-2015-000123.
47. Touma Z, Urowitz MB, Ibañez D, et al. Time to recovery from proteinuria in pa-tients with lupus nephritis receiving standard treatment. J Rheumatol 2014; 41(4):688–97.
48. Furie R, Rovin BH, Houssiau F, et al. Two-year, randomized, controlled trial of be-limumab in lupus nephritis. N Engl J Med 2020;383(12):1117–28.
49. Golder V, Kandane-Rathnayake R, Huq M, et al. Lupus low disease activity state as a treatment endpoint for systemic lupus erythematosus: a prospective valida-tion study. Lancet Rheumatol 2019;1(2):e95–102.
50. Franklyn K, Lau CS, Navarra SV, et al. Definition and initial validation of a Lupus Low Disease Activity State (LLDAS). Ann Rheum Dis 2016;75:1615–21.
51. Golder V, Kandane-Rathnayake R, Huq M, et al. Evaluation of remission defini-tions for systemic lupus erythematosus: a prospective cohort study. Lancet Rheu-matol 2019;1:E103–10.
52. Morand EF, Trasieva T, Berglind A, et al. Lupus Low Disease Activity State (LLDAS) attainment discriminates responders in a systemic lupus erythematosus trial: post -hoc analysis of the phase IIb MUSE trial of anifrolumab. Ann Rheum Dis 2018;77:706–13.
53. Morand EF, Isenberg D, Wallace DJ, et al. Attainment of treat-to-target endpoints in SLE patients with high disease activity in the atacicept phase 2b ADDRESS II study. Rheumatology 2020;59:2930–8.

Abnormal Mitochondrial Physiology in the Pathogenesis of Systemic Lupus Erythematosus

Chris Wincup, MBBS, MRCP[a,b,]*, Anna Radziszewska, MSc[a,b]

KEYWORDS

- Systemic lupus erythematosus • Mitochondria • Immunometabolism
- Reactive oxygen species • T-cells • Autoimmunity • Mitophagy
- Antimitochondrial antibodies

KEY POINTS

- Activation of immune responses requires a significant increase in cellular energy generation in order to initiate and sustain effector cell functions.
- Aside from their role in energy metabolism, mitochondria are the primary source of endogenous reactive oxygen species and orchestrate apoptosis.
- Both T cells and macrophages from patients with SLE have been shown to demonstrate enhanced cellular energy demands.
- Oxidative stress–induced damage to genomic and mitochondrial DNA can promote the formation of autoantibodies directed against nuclear components.
- Metabolic reprogramming may restore homeostatic immune cell function and thus represents a potentially novel avenue of future drug development in SLE.

INTRODUCTION

Systemic lupus erythematosus (SLE) is a chronic, systemic autoimmune condition characterized by the formation for autoantibodies directed against nuclear components.[1] Over recent years there have been several significant advances in the understanding of the underlying pathologic mechanisms at play in the development of this highly heterogenous disease.[2–4] Abnormalities within both the innate and adaptive immune responses have been demonstrated to play a role in the pathogenesis.[5] These

[a] Department of Rheumatology, Division of Medicine, Rayne Institute, University College London, 5 University Street, London WC1E 6JF, UK; [b] Centre for Adolescent Rheumatology Versus Arthritis at UCL, UCLH, GOSH, London, UK
* Corresponding author.
E-mail address: c.wincup@ucl.ac.uk
Twitter: @chriswincup (C.W.)

Rheum Dis Clin N Am 47 (2021) 427–439
https://doi.org/10.1016/j.rdc.2021.05.001
0889-857X/21/© 2021 Elsevier Inc. All rights reserved.

immune processes require significant changes in cellular activation and proliferation in order to induce antibody and proinflammatory cytokine production. Until recently, however, the way in which these vast and highly active systemic immune responses are initiated and maintained in terms of cellular bioenergetics has been poorly understood. This article reports on the latest understanding with regard to the changes in cellular energy metabolism observed within the immune system and how this these result in SLE pathogenesis. Furthermore, how these advances may be utilized in clinical care as a novel target for future therapeutic options in the management of the disease is considered. In particular, the role of the mitochondria, the intracellular organelle that plays an essential role not only in energy metabolism but also in several other cellular processes that are relevant to the underlying pathogenesis of SLE, is focused on.

THE ROLE OF MITOCHONDRIA IN ENERGY METABOLISM IN HEALTH

All cellular processes require a careful balance between energy generation and energy consumption. Before considering how this is altered in SLE, it is important to understand energy biogenesis in health. A variety of metabolic substrates are required for energy production and predominantly include carbohydrates (such as polysaccharides), lipids (including triglycerides), and proteins (that are broken down into amino acids). Conversion of these substrates to energy in the form of adenosine triphosphate (ATP) can occur through either the breakdown of glucose molecules via glycolysis or through oxidative phosphorylation (OXPHOS) within the mitochondria. Cellular energy metabolism is summarized in **Fig. 1**.

Glycolysis is the primary metabolic pathway and foundation of both aerobic respiration and anaerobic respiration. The process centers on the breakdown of glucose (a 6-membered ring molecule) through a series of reactions. This is a large molecule that enters the cell from the circulation by facilitated diffusion through cell surface glucose transporters. Oxidation of a single glucose molecule results in the generation of 4 ATP molecules; however, 2 ATP molecules are used in this series of reactions, thereby resulting in a net gain of 2 ATP molecules per glucose. Oxidation of glucose results in the release of electrons that in turn results in the generation of intermediate molecules through the reduction of Nicotinamide adenine dinucleotide (NAD^+) to NAD

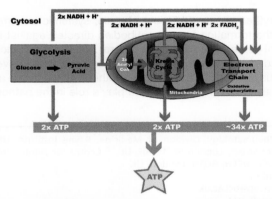

Fig. 1. Cellular energy metabolism consists of a series of enzymatic reactions in which glucose is broken down to pyruvic acid, which forms acetyl-CoA before entering the Krebs cycle. The metabolic products of this process allow for OXPHOS on the inner mitochondrial membrane ETC under aerobic conditions.

dinucleotide ($NADH^+$). Another important product of glycolysis is pyruvic acid, which under anaerobic conditions forms lactic acid. Importantly, if there is sufficient oxygen (O_2), then pyruvic acid enters the mitochondria, where it is converted to acetyl coenzyme A (CoA), which enters the Krebs cycle.

When a sufficient supply of glucose is not available, lipids can be converted into fatty acids by the enzyme lipase, which also is able to be converted to acetyl-CoA. Within the Krebs cycle, acetyl-CoA is converted to citrate and the continued oxidation of the intermediate molecules produced during glycolysis occurs, which in turn results in the production of carbon dioxide. Ultimately, this series of chemical reactions generates energy through the oxidation of acetyl-CoA and the resultant hydrogen-carrying compounds generated from these reactions ($NADH^+$) and flavin adenine dinucleotide ($FADH_2$) then are used to generate ATP through OXPHOS.

The most abundant source of ATP generation is through OXPHOS, which takes place on the inner mitochondrial membrane electron transport chain (ETC). $NADH^+$ and $FADH_2$ generated from the Krebs cycle carry high-energy electrons that are used to generate a proton gradient across the membrane as it allows for hydrogen ions (H^+) to be actively pumped across the membrane from the mitochondrial matrix to the intermembrane space. The ETC is composed of 5 respiratory chain complexes that generate an electric potential within the mitochondrion. This is known as the mitochondrial transmembrane potential ($\Delta\Psi m$), in which the mitochondrial membrane is negatively charged on the outside and positively charged on the inside.[6] Finally, H^+ is able to flux back across the membrane through the fifth respiratory chain complex (ATP synthase), which forms ATP via the phosphorylation of adenosine diphosphate (ADP). The key steps in ATP production via oxidative phosphorylation on the mitochondrial electron transport chain is summarized in **Fig. 2**.

ABNORMAL MITOCHONDRIAL BIOENERGETICS IN SYSTEMIC LUPUS ERYTHEMATOSUS
Oxidative Phosphorylation Versus Glycolysis

Several recent studies have shown evidence of abnormal mitochondrial energy biosynthesis in the immune response in lupus. In health, quiescent T cells have very

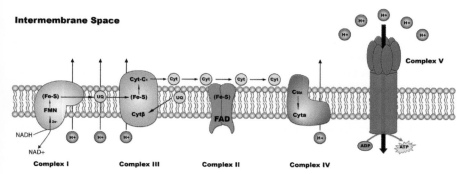

Mitochondrial Matrix

Fig. 2. The ETC is situated on the inner mitochondrial membrane and is the site of ATP generation via OXPHOS. The ETC is composed of 5 respiratory chain complexes that generate a proton gradient across the membrane, which is essential for the conversion of ADP to ATP. CuA, copper ion A; Cyt, cytochrome; Cyta, cytochrome A; Cytβ, cytochrome beta; e⁻, electron; FAD, flavin adenine dinucleotide; Fe-S, iron-sulphur cluster; FMN, flavin mononucleotide; UQ, ubiquinone.

low cellular energy demands and can use a combination of glucose, lipids, and amino acids as substrates for OXPHOS.[7,8] Upon activation of the T-cell receptor, the naïve T cell undergoes a rapid increase in biosynthesis. In order to meet these energy demands, the resultant T effector cell relies on increased ATP production predominantly through glycolysis in order to fuel the inflammatory effector function.[9] Upon conclusion of the immune response, as the cell transitions toward a memory T-cell phenotype, it returns to a more quiescent metabolic state in which fatty acid oxidation is the primary substrate of OXPHOS energy metabolism.[10] These memory T cells display increased mitochondrial mass and spare respiratory capacity, which suggests that they are primed to respond upon repeat activation in the future.[8,11] In the state of chronic T-cell activation, mitochondrial metabolism has been shown to be the predominant source of cellular ATP.[12]

Studies in murine models of SLE have demonstrated that CD4[+] T cells harvested from lupus-prone mice show significantly increased rates of both mitochondrial OXPHOS and glycolysis compared with healthy mice.[13] In the same study, CD4[+] T cells from patients with SLE were analyzed and this too revealed enhanced ATP energy production through increased rates of glycolysis and OXPHOS compared with healthy controls. Further evidence supporting enhanced glycolysis in the autoimmune response comes from mouse models in which overexpression of the key glucose transporter, Glut1, was noted on CD4[+] T cells. The investigators also noted that the T-cell costimulatory molecule CD28 was required to induce maximal glucose uptake by the cell,[14] suggesting that this has a vital role in facilitating energy metabolism required during T-cell proliferation and effector function. Further evidence of the role of altered metabolism is provided by the intracellular effects of complement on mitochondria within T cells.[15] Activation of the complement system is a hallmark of SLE with low C3 and C4 levels suggestive of active disease. Previously it has been suggested that complement can have numerous effects on the metabolic state of immune cells. For example, intracellular complement C1q has been shown to drive OXPHOS protein expression in muscle cells[16] and also has been demonstrated to restrict the adaptive immune response to self-antigens through altering CD8[+] T-cell metabolism.[17] More recently, it has been proposed that this response is predominantly driven by type I interferon (IFN), another key driver of SLE pathogenesis.[18] This represents an interesting area of potential further research exploring the interaction between abnormal T-cell metabolism and complement activation in SLE.

In addition to T-cell energy metabolism, macrophage metabolism has shown to be abnormal in SLE. In the context of inflammation, tissue resident macrophages switch to glycolysis as the primary source of energy production and this is associated with a reduction in OXPHOS derived energy biosynthesis.[19] A study by Jing and colleagues[20] found that IgG immune complexes were capable of inducing glycolysis in macrophages. The investigators also found that in vivo inhibition of glycolytic pathways resulted in reduced macrophage interleukin (IL)-1β production and decreased neutrophil recruitment to kidneys in a murine model of lupus nephritis. This suggests that by directly targeting cellular metabolism, it may be possible to reduce immune-mediated inflammation in SLE in the future.

Mitochondria Transmembrane Potential

There is growing evidence to support that the T-cell $\Delta\Psi m$ is elevated in SLE. A study by Perl and colleagues[21] reported that T cells from patients with SLE had higher $\Delta\Psi m$ and were in a state of persistent mitochondrial hyperpolarization, thus suggesting that, at a bioenergetic level, T-cell mitochondria are primed for a sudden increase in OXPHOS-dependent ATP production. As such, this may drive rapid effector T-cell responses that could be present in active SLE; however, the precise balance between glycolysis and OXPHOS in the chronically activated immune response context of SLE still is poorly understood. The investigators also reported that there was an increase in cytoplasmic alkalinization, more reactive oxygen species (ROS) generation, and reduced intracellular ATP in T cells derived from patients with SLE.

In addition to the activation and proliferation of T cells, mitochondria play an important role in cell death through apoptosis and the clearance of this apoptotic cellular matter has been found defective in the pathogenesis of SLE. It previously has been reported that $\Delta\Psi$m disruption is an essential, irreversible step in the induction of apoptosis.[22] Therefore, altered T-cell mitochondrial bioenergetics not only may play a vital role in the effector immune response in SLE but also may have a secondary role in apoptosis that ultimately may result in the exposure of self-antigens to autoantibodies in the disease. The precise reason for this persistent mitochondrial hyperpolarization in SLE is not clear, although it previously has been shown that several of the central proinflammatory mediators of SLE can induce hyperpolarization.[23]

Abnormalities in the Mitochondrial Electron Transport Chain

As previously outlined, OXPHOS occurs at the site of the ETC on the inner mitochondrial membrane. As shown in **Fig. 2**, the ETC is composed of 5 individual respiratory chain complexes that allow for the sequential transfer of energy and ultimately generates the transmembrane gradient required to convert ADP to ATP. Several studies have sought to investigate the function of the ETC and its components as a possible cause of abnormal immune cell bioenergy synthesis in SLE. A study by Leishangthem and colleagues[24] used spectrophotometry to evaluate the activity of these complexes in peripheral blood mononuclear cells from patients with SLE and in healthy controls. Complex I and complex IV activity was noted to be lower in those with SLE compared with healthy controls. In addition, complex V enzymatic activity was found significantly reduced in SLE, which may have implications for ATP generation, because this complex plays an essential role in the conversion of ADP to ATP.[24] The underlying reason for the reduced enzymatic respiratory chain activity in SLE, however, is not understood. Conversely, a subsequent study evaluated ETC activity using oxygraphy to measure mitochondrial O_2 consumption. Complex I activity was measured through the addition of its inhibitor rotenone. The investigators report that complex I activity was increased in SLE T cells after 24 hours of in vitro stimulation compared with healthy controls. It also was found that complex I is the main source of oxidative stress in SLE.[25]

MITOCHONDRIAL OXIDATIVE STRESS IN THE PATHOGENESIS OF SYSTEMIC LUPUS ERYTHEMATOSUS

Oxidative stress refers to the state of impaired equilibrium in the body's ability to neutralize ROS. This often occurs as a result of excessive production of ROS that cannot sufficiently be counterbalanced by scavenging antioxidant reactions. ROS can include superoxide anions (O_2^-), hydrogen peroxide, and hydroxyl radicals.[26] These radicals are the result of incomplete reduction of O_2 molecules and often may include toxic by-products induced through impaired mitochondrial bioenergetics within the ETC.[25,27,28] The role of oxidative stress in the pathogenesis of SLE has been well described; however, the precise implication of mitochondrial-derived ROS in the disease state is not yet fully understood.[29] It is possible that several environmental factors that have reported to play a role in SLE pathogenesis also may do so through induction of ROS generation,[30] such as UV light,[31] tobacco smoking[32] and silica exposure.[33]

Mitochondrial ROS have been reported to have a direct influence on immune cells. T cells, in particular, are susceptible to oxidative stress, which can alter their activation and induce proinflammatory cytokine release.[6] T cells derived from patients with SLE hve previously have been shown to display significantly higher amounts of ROS, especially in those with active disease.[34] Furthermore, it has been reported that oxidative stress may induce lupus flares through inhibition of the intracellular ERK signaling pathway within T cells.[35] ROS also play a vital role as an induction signal in the initiation of apoptosis, which has been demonstrated to be markedly abnormal in SLE and ultimately results in increased exposure of self-antigens from cellular debris that in turn results in autoantibody formation. In addition, ROS may be generated as a result of increased mitochondrial permeability, which is a terminal event in cell death.[36]

ROS also have been shown to result in oxidative stress through interaction with other metabolites involved in cellular bioenergetics, such as lipids (in which mitochondria play a key role in fatty acid oxidation). This has been demonstrated by Park and colleagues,[37] who investigated how oxidative stress results in changes to oxidation status and susceptibility to oxidation of lipoproteins in patients with SLE. It was found that in spite of similar serum levels of low-density lipoproteins (LDLs) between SLE patients and healthy controls, those derived from patients with SLE were significantly more oxidized. Furthermore, in vitro studies confirmed that LDLs derived from patients with SLE exhibited higher rates of de novo oxidation.[37] The investigators suggest that this may in turn result in vascular inflammation that may prompt premature atherosclerosis, which is a major challenge in the clinical management of SLE.

Another potential role for ROS in the pathogenesis of SLE is through their role in damaging DNA, which is a primary antigenic target of autoantibodies in the disease.[38] This has the potential to induce immunogenicity against self-antigens, in particular to nuclear components, which is a hallmark of SLE pathogenesis. Oxidative stress not only may give rise to damage of genomic DNA but also has the potential to target mitochondrial DNA (mtDNA), which is particularly susceptible to the effects of oxidative stress.[39] This damage may, in turn, result in impaired cellular energy metabolism, given that mtDNA encodes the 13 proteins that give rise to the ETC complexes.[40]

Mitochondria not only are capable of inducing an autoimmune inflammatory response as a result of oxidative stress but also may play a role in the pathogenesis as a result of an abnormal response to impaired repair of damage that they sustain following exposure to ROS.

IMPAIRED MITOCHONDRIAL REPAIR IN SYSTEMIC LUPUS ERYTHEMATOUS
Mitophagy

Within the cell, mitochondria constantly are undergoing a state of fusion and fission. When a mitochondrion is damaged, it is removed by a specialist type of autophagy, known as mitophagy.[41] This process is essential for maintaining mitochondrial homeostasis and keeping the immune system in check. The persistence of dysfunctional mitochondria can have an impact on on ROS generation, which in turn can lead to inflammatory cytokine secretion and immune cell activation.[42] In addition, as discussed previously, the presence of mtDNA from fragmented mitochondria can elicit abnormal immune responses.[42]

It has been shown that lupus T cells are resistant to autophagy and that mitophagy is suppressed in T cells of SLE patients and in lupus-prone mice.[43,44] In T cells from lupus patients, mitochondrial hyperpolarization leads to increased mammalian target of rapamycin (mTOR) activation, which in turn leads to overexpression of HRES-1/RAB4 protein and depletion of Drp1 (a key mediator of mitophagy).[45] Overexpression of RAB4A protein (the mouse equivalent of the human HREs-1/RAB4) in lupus-prone mice results in accumulation of mitochondria, antinuclear antibody (ANA) production, and nephritis.[44] These disease manifestations, however, can be alleviated by RAB4A blockade, indicating that the modulation of mitophagy may serve as a potential therapeutic strategy.[44]

Current evidence also suggests that in SLE monocytes IFN-α signaling induces oxidative stress and affects lysosomal alkalinization through mTOR.[46] The resultant impairment of mitophagy leads to accumulation of mtDNA, which is sensed by stimulator of IFN genes to promote the differentiation of monocytes into autoreactive dendritic cells.[46] Taken together, growing evidence of defects in mitophagy in multiple immune cell lineages in lupus suggests that aberrations in this process may be important in the pathology of the disease and this avenue of research warrants further investigation.

Antimitochondrial Antibody Formation

More recently, there has been increased focus on mitochondria as a possible target for autoantibody formation in SLE. A variety of cell linages, including T cells[47] and neutrophils,[48] are able to extrude their mitochondria outside the cell as a consequence of cell death pathway activation. Mitochondria also may be released from cells during tissue damage and inflammation and mitochondrial components, such as mtDNA, can enter the extracellular milieu during cell death.[49,50] These processes expose mitochondrial antigens, which under normal conditions would be sequestered inside cells, and this may contribute to breaking of tolerance in predisposed individuals.

Antibodies directed at several components of the mitochondrion, including at mtDNA, the inner mitochondrial membrane, and mitochondrial RNA (mtRNA), as well as antibodies to whole mitochondria have been reported in lupus. Anti-mtDNA antibodies are present in a subset of lupus patients,[51] particularly in those with active disease and in lupus nephritis,[52,53] raising the possibility that mtDNA can be a source of antigen for double-stranded DNA (ds-DNA) antibodies common in SLE.[54]

Antibodies targeting inner mitochondrial components also are found in SLE. For instance, antibodies to cardiolipin (a phospholipid found uniquely on the inner mitochondrial membrane) are detectable in some patients with SLE and antiphospholipid syndrome.[53] The presence of these antibodies is clinically associated with increased risk of thrombotic events and thrombocytopenia.[55] HSP60, which is a chaperonin involved in mitochondrial protein transport, is another potential mitochondrial antigen. Antibodies to HSP60 are present in patients with SLE[56] and are associated with vascular events in patients with antiphospholipid antibodies.[57]

A recent study found that antibodies to mtRNA (AmtRNA) also are present in lupus patients.[58] AmtRNA-IgG levels correlated with anti-mtDNA antibody titers and were highest in patients with anti-dsDNA antibodies. Although further studies are needed to confirm these findings, the researchers were able to use AmtRNA-IgG titers to specifically discriminate patients from healthy controls. AmtRNA-IgG titers also were found negatively associated with plaque formation and nephritis, suggesting the potential for using AmtRNA-IgG titers to stratify patients and help predict those at risk of kidney damage.[58]

Finally, patients with SLE also have been reported to have higher levels of antibodies to whole mitochondria.[53,59] In a large study of 204 participants with SLE, levels of anti–whole-mitochondria antibodies were higher in active patients and correlated with levels of anti-dsDNA.[59]

Collectively, these findings suggest that in SLE the adaptive immune system recognizes mitochondrial components. It is as yet unclear, however, whether antimitochondrial antibodies are initiators of the autoimmune response or whether they are the consequence of aberrant immune activation. The suggestion that various clinical disease manifestations of SLE associate with different mitochondrial antibody specificities raises the possibility of using antimitochondrial antibody titers to predict disease activity and to stratify SLE patients in the future.[53]

TARGETING MITOCHONDRIA IN THE TREATMENT OF SYSTEMIC LUPUS ERYTHEMATOSUS

Having highlighted the various ways in which mitochondrial physiology is altered in SLE, in is important to consider how restoring bioenergetic homeostasis may in turn improve symptoms of the disease. Furthermore, these new treatment options potentially may convey additional benefits as metabolic reprogramming could restore normal cellular function without resulting in systemic immunosuppression. Novel metabolic therapeutic targets have shown promise in both in vitro and animal models of SLE.

Evidence for the use of treatment targeting the mitochondria in animal models of SLE recently was reported by Fortner and colleagues,[60] who demonstrated the efficacy of oral MitoQ, a mitochondrial antioxidant, which was found to significantly reduce neutrophil ROS formation in the MRL-*lpr* murine model of SLE. The investigators also noted that in the mice treated with MitoQ also had a significant reduction in serum type I IFN, which is known to play a central role in SLE pathogenesis. This provides interesting evidence to support the role of directly altering mitochondrial function to bring about restoration of immune homeostasis. This also has been considered in a study by Blanco and colleagues,[61] in which the investigators investigated the potential benefits of the mitochondrial coenzyme analog, idebenone, on metabolic and immunologic markers of SLE in the MRL-*lpr* murine model. Mice that received idebenone for 8 weeks were found to have improved survival substantially compared with untreated mice. Furthermore, those receiving idebenone were noted to have less glomerular damage and improved mitochondrial metabolism (with a 30% increase in ATP production observed).[61]

In addition to investigating novel drugs that directly target the mitochondria, several recent studies have looked at the potential role of repurposing drugs that already are used in the treatment of a variety of other disorders in clinical practice that act by restoring cellular bioenergetics. Metformin, which commonly is used in the management of diabetes, has been demonstrated to restore metabolic homeostasis in $CD4^+$ T cells derived from a murine mouse model of SLE. The investigators also evaluated the potential benefit of 2-deoxy-D-glucose, which acts a competitive inhibitor in the production of glucose-6-phosphate from glucose (a rate-limiting step in glycolysis). This was demonstrated to reduce the production of IFN-γ by $CD4^+$ T cells in vitro, thus suggesting that it may be possible to down-regulate generation of this key inflammatory mediator of SLE.[13] In addition to targeting T-cell glycolysis, inhibition of macrophage glycolytic pathways has been shown to reduce disease severity and attenuated proinflammatory cytokine release in animal models of lupus nephritis.[20]

Another potential target for metabolic reprogramming in SLE is mTOR, which can be inhibited through the use of rapamycin. This macrolide compound that has been shown to reduce the activity of T-cells by reducing their sensitivity to IL-2 as an effect of mTOR inhibition.[62] The efficacy of rapamycin previously has been investigated in mouse models of lupus. It was found that mice treated with the drug had significantly reduced levels of anti-dsDNA antibodies, lower proteinuria, and significant increase in survival compared with untreated mice.[63] This also has been translated into human studies by Fernandez and colleagues, who studied the efficacy of rapamycin in patients with refractory SLE, in which previous treatments had not been successful in controlling the disease. Nine patients were given a dose of 2 mg a day for between 6 months and 48 months, whereas 7 patients with refractory SLE receiving standard care were recruited as controls. In those treated with rapamycin, there was a statistically significant reduction in disease activity as measured by both the British Isles Lupus Assessment Group score and Systemic Lupus Erythematosus Disease Activity Index.[64] The investigators also reported how this treatment mechanistically altered T-cell metabolism and noted that although mitochondrial hyperpolarization persisted, T-cell activation was reduced in those taking rapamycin.

In addition, N-acetylcysteine (NAC), which is used more commonly in the management of paracetamol overdose, has demonstrated to be effective in stabilizing mitochondrial metabolism in vitro. A study by Doherty and colleagues[25] found that NAC selective inhibits the activity of complex I on the ETC. The investigators measured mitochondrial respiration as a marker of ETC activity in peripheral blood lymphocytes from patients with SLE and noted increased O_2 consumption following T-cell stimulation. When these cells were treated with NAC, mitochondrial respiration was reduced significantly, thus suggesting that this drug could have an immunomodulatory effect on immune cell metabolism in SLE. Further studies, especially larger clinical trials, however, are required to assess whether these drugs could be effective in long-term management of the disease.

SUMMARY

In summary, there is increasing evidence that abnormal immunometabolism may play a role in the pathogenesis of SLE. In particular, there is a growing understanding of how these changes occur in both T-cell and macrophage bioenergetics and how this plays a role in pathogenesis. Given the wide array of effector cells involved in mediating the autoimmune responses of the disease, however, there still is much to learn (in particular, in relation to the role played by alteration to B-cell metabolism). Future studies are required in order to better translate this understanding into clinical care. It is possible that, in the future, SLE could be stratified by immunometabolic signature and strategies directed at restoring immune homeostasis through metabolic reprogramming could pave the way for newer, more targeted, and better tolerated treatments for this disease.

CLINICS CARE POINTS

- Systemic lupus erythematosus (SLE) is an autoimmune condition presenting with a wide array of both clinical symptoms and immunological abnormalities. There is now growing evidence supporting the role of abnormal immune metabolism in driving pathogenesis in the disease.

- Mitochondria play a key role in cellular energy metabolism, which is essential for activation and proliferation of the immune response seen in SLE.

- Several recent studies in animal models have shown that targetting mitochondrial metabolism may represent a promising, novel future therapeutic option in the management of the disease in the future.

DISCLOSURE

The authors have nothing to disclose.

FUNDING

Dr. Wincup is funded by Versus Arthritis (ref 21992).

REFERENCES

1. Bakshi J, Segura BT, Wincup C, et al. Unmet needs in the pathogenesis and treatment of systemic lupus erythematosus. Clin Rev Allergy Immunol 2018;55(3): 352–67.
2. Bruce IN, O'Keeffe AG, Farewell V, et al. Factors associated with damage accrual in patients with systemic lupus erythematosus: results from the Systemic Lupus International Collaborating Clinics (SLICC) inception cohort. Ann Rheum Dis 2015;74(9):1706–13.
3. Carter EE, Barr SG, Clarke AE. The global burden of SLE: prevalence, health disparities and socioeconomic impact. Nat Rev Rheumatol 2016;12(10):605–20.
4. Murphy G, Isenberg DA. New therapies for systemic lupus erythematosus - past imperfect, future tense. Nat Rev Rheumatol 2019;15(7):403–12.
5. Tsokos GC, Lo MS, Costa Reis P, et al. New insights into the immunopathogenesis of systemic lupus erythematosus. Nat Rev Rheumatol 2016;12(12):716–30.
6. Perl A, Gergely P Jr, Nagy G, et al. Mitochondrial hyperpolarization: a checkpoint of T-cell life, death and autoimmunity. Trends Immunol 2004;25(7):360–7.
7. Fox CJ, Hammerman PS, Thompson CB. Fuel feeds function: energy metabolism and the T-cell response. Nat Rev Immunol 2005;5(11):844–52.
8. Pearce EL, Poffenberger MC, Chang CH, et al. Fueling immunity: insights into metabolism and lymphocyte function. Science 2013;342(6155):1242454.
9. Frauwirth KA, Riley JL, Harris MH, et al. The CD28 signaling pathway regulates glucose metabolism. Immunity 2002;16(6):769–77.
10. MacIver NJ, Michalek RD, Rathmell JC. Metabolic regulation of T lymphocytes. Annu Rev Immunol 2013;31:259–83.
11. Michalek RD, Gerriets VA, Jacobs SR, et al. Cutting edge: distinct glycolytic and lipid oxidative metabolic programs are essential for effector and regulatory CD4+ T cell subsets. J Immunol 2011;186(6):3299–303.
12. Byersdorfer CA, Tkachev V, Opipari AW, et al. Effector T cells require fatty acid metabolism during murine graft-versus-host disease. Blood 2013;122(18): 3230–7.
13. Yin Y, Choi SC, Xu Z, et al. Normalization of CD4+ T cell metabolism reverses lupus. Sci Transl Med 2015;7(274):274ra18.
14. Jacobs SR, Herman CE, Maciver NJ, et al. Glucose uptake is limiting in T cell activation and requires CD28-mediated Akt-dependent and independent pathways. J Immunol 2008;180(7):4476–86.
15. Rahman J, Singh P, Merle NS, et al. Complement's favourite organelle-Mitochondria? Br J Pharmacol 2020;1–16.
16. Feng H, Wang JY, Zheng M, et al. CTRP3 promotes energy production by inducing mitochondrial ROS and up-expression of PGC-1α in vascular smooth muscle cells. Exp Cell Res 2016;341(2):177–86.
17. Ling GS, Crawford G, Buang N, et al. C1q restrains autoimmunity and viral infection by regulating CD8(+) T cell metabolism. Science 2018;360(6388):558–63.

18. Buang N, Tapeng L, Gray V, et al. Type I interferons affect the metabolic fitness of CD8(+) T cells from patients with systemic lupus erythematosus. Nat Commun 2021;12(1):1980.

19. Galván-Peña S, O'Neill LA. Metabolic reprograming in macrophage polarization. Front Immunol 2014;5:420.

20. Jing C, Castro-Dopico T, Richoz N, et al. Macrophage metabolic reprogramming presents a therapeutic target in lupus nephritis. Proc Natl Acad Sci U S A 2020; 117(26):15160–71.

21. Perl A, Hanczko R, Doherty E. Assessment of mitochondrial dysfunction in lymphocytes of patients with systemic lupus erythematosus. Methods Mol Biol 2012;900:61–89.

22. Susin SA, Zamzami N, Castedo M, et al. The central executioner of apoptosis: multiple connections between protease activation and mitochondria in Fas/APO-1/CD95- and ceramide-induced apoptosis. J Exp Med 1997;186(1):25–37.

23. Gergely P, Niland B, Gonchoroff N, et al. Persistent mitochondrial hyperpolarization, increased reactive oxygen intermediate production, and cytoplasmic alkalinization characterize altered IL-10 signaling in patients with systemic lupus erythematosus. J Immunol 2002;169(2):1092–101.

24. Leishangthem BD, Sharma A, Bhatnagar A. Role of altered mitochondria functions in the pathogenesis of systemic lupus erythematosus. Lupus 2016;25(3): 272–81.

25. Doherty E, Oaks Z, Perl A. Increased mitochondrial electron transport chain activity at complex I is regulated by N-acetylcysteine in lymphocytes of patients with systemic lupus erythematosus. Antioxid Redox Signal 2014;21(1):56–65.

26. Nagy G, Koncz A, Fernandez D, et al. Nitric oxide, mitochondrial hyperpolarization, and T cell activation. Free Radic Biol Med 2007;42(11):1625–31.

27. Chen SX, Schopfer P. Hydroxyl-radical production in physiological reactions. A novel function of peroxidase. Eur J Biochem 1999;260(3):726–35.

28. Schopfer P, Plachy C, Frahry G. Release of reactive oxygen intermediates (superoxide radicals, hydrogen peroxide, and hydroxyl radicals) and peroxidase in germinating radish seeds controlled by light, gibberellin, and abscisic acid. Plant Physiol 2001;125(4):1591–602.

29. Shah D, Mahajan N, Sah S, et al. Oxidative stress and its biomarkers in systemic lupus erythematosus. J Biomed Sci 2014;21(1):23.

30. Somers EC, Richardson BC. Environmental exposures, epigenetic changes and the risk of lupus. Lupus 2014;23(6):568–76.

31. Golan TD, Dan S, Haim H, et al. Solar ultraviolet radiation induces enhanced accumulation of oxygen radicals in murine SLE-derived splenocytes in vitro. Lupus 1994;3(2):103–6.

32. Cui J, Raychaudhuri S, Karlson EW, et al. Interactions between genome-wide genetic factors and smoking influencing risk of systemic lupus erythematosus. Arthritis Rheumatol 2020;72(11):1863–71.

33. Morotti A, Sollaku I, Catalani S, et al. Systematic review and meta-analysis of epidemiological studies on the association of occupational exposure to free crystalline silica and systemic lupus erythematosus. Rheumatology (Oxford) 2021; 60(1):81–91.

34. Oates JC, Gilkeson GS. The biology of nitric oxide and other reactive intermediates in systemic lupus erythematosus. Clin Immunol 2006;121(3):243–50.

35. Li Y, Gorelik G, Strickland FM, et al. Oxidative stress, T cell DNA methylation, and lupus. Arthritis Rheumatol 2014;66(6):1574–82.

36. Jabs T. Reactive oxygen intermediates as mediators of programmed cell death in plants and animals. Biochem Pharmacol 1999;57(3):231–45.

37. Park JK, Kim JY, Moon JY, et al. Altered lipoproteins in patients with systemic lupus erythematosus are associated with augmented oxidative stress: a potential role in atherosclerosis. Arthritis Res Ther 2016;18(1):306.

38. Cooke MS, Mistry N, Wood C, et al. Immunogenicity of DNA damaged by reactive oxygen species–implications for anti-DNA antibodies in lupus. Free Radic Biol Med 1997;22(1–2):151–9.

39. Jönsen A, Yu X, Truedsson L, et al. Mitochondrial DNA polymorphisms are associated with susceptibility and phenotype of systemic lupus erythematosus. Lupus 2009;18(4):309–12.

40. Lemarie A, Grimm S. Mitochondrial respiratory chain complexes: apoptosis sensors mutated in cancer? Oncogene 2011;30(38):3985–4003.

41. Palikaras K, Lionaki E, Tavernarakis N. Mechanisms of mitophagy in cellular homeostasis, physiology and pathology. Nat Cell Biol 2018;20(9):1013–22.

42. Xu Y, Shen J, Ran Z. Emerging views of mitophagy in immunity and autoimmune diseases. Autophagy 2020;16(1):3–17.

43. Alessandri C, Barbati C, Vacirca D, et al. T lymphocytes from patients with systemic lupus erythematosus are resistant to induction of autophagy. FASEB J 2012;26(11):4722–32.

44. Caza TN, Fernandez DR, Talaber G, et al. HRES-1/Rab4-mediated depletion of Drp1 impairs mitochondrial homeostasis and represents a target for treatment in SLE. Ann Rheum Dis 2014;73(10):1888–97.

45. Fernandez DR, Telarico T, Bonilla E, et al. Activation of mammalian target of rapamycin controls the loss of TCRζ in Lupus T Cells through HRES-1/Rab4-regulated lysosomal degradation. J Immunol 2009;182(4):2063–73.

46. Gkirtzimanaki K, Kabrani E, Nikoleri D, et al. IFNα Impairs autophagic degradation of mtDNA promoting autoreactivity of SLE monocytes in a STING-dependent fashion. Cell Rep 2018;25(4):921–33.e5.

47. Maeda A, Fadeel B. Mitochondria released by cells undergoing TNF-α-induced necroptosis act as danger signals. Cell Death Dis 2014;5(7):e1312.

48. Lood C, Blanco LP, Purmalek MM, et al. Neutrophil extracellular traps enriched in oxidized mitochondrial DNA are interferogenic and contribute to lupus-like disease. Nat Med 2016;22(2):146–53.

49. McDonald B, Pittman K, Menezes GB, et al. Intravascular danger signals guide neutrophils to sites of sterile inflammation. Science 2010;330(6002):362–6.

50. Oka T, Hikoso S, Yamaguchi O, et al. Mitochondrial DNA that escapes from autophagy causes inflammation and heart failure. Nature 2012;485(7397):251–5.

51. Caielli S, Athale S, Domic B, et al. Oxidized mitochondrial nucleoids released by neutrophils drive type I interferon production in human lupus. J Exp Med 2016; 213(5):697–713.

52. Wang H, Li T, Chen S, et al. Neutrophil extracellular trap mitochondrial DNA and its autoantibody in systemic lupus erythematosus and a proof-of-concept trial of metformin. Arthritis Rheumatol 2015;67(12):3190–200.

53. Becker Y, Loignon R-C, Julien A-S, et al. Anti-mitochondrial autoantibodies in systemic lupus erythematosus and their association with disease manifestations. Sci Rep 2019;9(1):4530.

54. Reimer G, Rubin RL, Kotzin BL, et al. Anti-native DNA antibodies from autoimmune sera also bind to DNA in mitochondria. J Immunol 1984;133(5):2532–6.

55. Hudson M, Herr AL, Rauch J, et al. The presence of multiple prothrombotic risk factors is associated with a higher risk of thrombosis in individuals with anticardiolipin antibodies. J Rheumatol 2003;30(11):2385–91.

56. Dieudé M, Senécal JL, Raymond Y. Induction of endothelial cell apoptosis by heat-shock protein 60-reactive antibodies from anti-endothelial cell autoantibody-positive systemic lupus erythematosus patients. Arthritis Rheum 2004;50(10):3221–31.

57. Dieudé M, Correa JA, Neville C, et al. Association of autoantibodies to heat-shock protein 60 with arterial vascular events in patients with antiphospholipid antibodies. Arthritis Rheum 2011;63(8):2416–24.

58. Becker Y, Marcoux G, Allaeys I, et al. Autoantibodies in systemic lupus erythematosus target mitochondrial RNA. Front Immunol 2019;10:1026.

59. Pisetsky DS, Spencer DM, Mobarrez F, et al. The binding of SLE autoantibodies to mitochondria. Clin Immunol 2020;212:108349.

60. Fortner KA, Blanco LP, Buskiewicz I, et al. Targeting mitochondrial oxidative stress with MitoQ reduces NET formation and kidney disease in lupus-prone MRL-lpr mice. Lupus Sci Med 2020;7(1):e000387.

61. Blanco LP, Pedersen HL, Wang X, et al. Improved mitochondrial metabolism and reduced inflammation following attenuation of murine lupus with coenzyme Q10 analog idebenone. Arthritis Rheumatol 2020;72(3):454–64.

62. Ray JP, Staron MM, Shyer JA, et al. The Interleukin-2-mTORc1 kinase axis defines the signaling, differentiation, and metabolism of T Helper 1 and Follicular B Helper T Cells. Immunity 2015;43(4):690–702.

63. Warner LM, Adams LM, Sehgal SN. Rapamycin prolongs survival and arrests pathophysiologic changes in murine systemic lupus erythematosus. Arthritis Rheum 1994;37(2):289–97.

64. Fernandez D, Bonilla E, Mirza N, et al. Rapamycin reduces disease activity and normalizes T cell activation-induced calcium fluxing in patients with systemic lupus erythematosus. Arthritis Rheum 2006;54(9):2983–8.

Management of Pregnancy in Lupus

Amanda Moyer, MD[a], Eliza F. Chakravarty, MD, MS[b],*

KEYWORDS

- Systemic lupus erythematosus • Pregnancy • Preeclampsia • Disease flare
- Antiphospholipid • Antibody syndrome • Lupus nephritis

KEY POINTS

- Many risk factors for adverse pregnancy outcomes in women with lupus can be modified and optimized prior to conception.
- Factors intrinsic to lupus may confer increases in pregnancy complications, so active monitoring is necessary throughout pregnancy.
- Active use of pregnancy-compatible medications to control SLE and co morbitics can improve pregnancy outcomes.

INTRODUCTION

Less than 100 years ago, a diagnosis of systemic lupus erythematosus (SLE) was considered an absolute contraindication for pregnancy given high rates of maternal and fetal mortality. Fortunately, as medical management of SLE has improved, pregnancy and childrearing has become feasible for women with SLE. Although pregnancy outcomes in women with SLE have improved dramatically over the last 30 years, pregnancy is still associated with increased morbidity and mortality in mother and fetus compared with the general population.[1,2] Increased experience and numerous studies have led to better quantitation of factors contributing to adverse pregnancy outcomes (APOs) in women with SLE, allowing physicians and patients to proactively pursue management strategies to improve outcomes. Open discussions with patients regarding future pregnancy plans help ensure adequate timing of medication changes for continued disease suppression. Outcomes are optimized by preconceptual counseling from rheumatology and obstetrics and comanagement throughout the pregnancy, delivery, and the postpartum period.

[a] Deapartments of Medicine and Pediatrics, University of Oklahoma School of Medicine, Oklahoma City, OK, USA; [b] Arthritis and Clinical Immunology, Oklahoma Medical Research Foundation, Oklahoma City, OK, USA
* Corresponding author.
E-mail address: eliza-chakravarty@omrf.org

Rheum Dis Clin N Am 47 (2021) 441–455
https://doi.org/10.1016/j.rdc.2021.04.008
0889-857X/21/© 2021 Elsevier Inc. All rights reserved.

PERIPARTUM RISK

Despite advancements in SLE management and pregnancy outcomes, multiple studies have shown an increased rate of pregnancy loss, preeclampsia/eclampsia, maternal death (180 vs 12 deaths per 100,000 admissions), and cesarean-section delivery in women with SLE compared with the general population.[1,3] Identification of risk factors, preconception disease control, prompt recognition of flares, and a multidisciplinary approach can meaningfully improve outcomes.

Infertility

Infertility is defined as the failure to conceive after 12 months of regular intercourse and is estimated to affect 10% of couples of childbearing age.[4] Few robust studies have directly examined infertility among women with SLE, but patients with SLE face many factors that can negatively affect conception.[5–8]

Women with SLE have fewer children compared with women without SLE. Clowse and colleagues[9] found that 64% of patients with lupus had fewer children than originally planned, partially because of concerns about the child's health and personal welfare. In addition, a 3-fold higher rate of miscarriage was seen in patients with SLE who had fewer children than planned compared with patients with SLE who had the same number of children as originally desired, suggesting that inability to successfully carry a child may have altered original wishes.[9] SLE can also result in fatigue, pain, and depression, leading to poor self-esteem and loss of libido, which can hinder a couple's ability to conceive.[10]

Decreased ovarian reserve and premature ovarian failure have been described in patients with SLE. Lawrenz and colleagues[11] analyzed the influence of SLE on ovarian reserve in premenopausal patients with SLE without a history cyclophosphamide treatment by measuring antimüllerian hormone (AMH) levels, a well-established biomarker of ovarian reserve. Compared with healthy age-matched controls, AMH values in patients with SLE were significantly lower independent of SLE activity scores (2.15 ng/mL vs 3.17 ng/mL, $P<.05$). A strongly reduced ovarian reserve (AMH<0.4 ng/mL) was found in 15.2% of patients with SLE compared with only 3% of controls.[11]

Chronic inflammation from active disease and autoantibodies likely contributes to decreased fertility in patients with SLE. Autoantibodies directed against the corpus luteum, oocytes, and endometrial antigens have been identified in patients with SLE, and autoimmune oophoritis is well documented.[12] SLE-associated antibodies, specifically antiphospholipid (APL) antibodies, have also been associated infertility (odds ratio [OR], 5.11; confidence interval [CI], 1.2–25.4).[13]

Medication commonly used in SLE can affect conception through a variety of mechanisms (**Table 1**).[6,10,14,15] Careful planning, targeted treatments, and prompt referral can help mitigate infertility risk.

Table 1
Medications used in systemic lupus erythematosus that affect conception

Medication	Mechanism
Nonsteroidal antiinflammatories	Cyclooxygenase inhibition blocks prostaglandin synthesis, which prevents oocyte release and leads to transient infertility
Steroids	Metabolic syndrome, hypothalamic-pituitary-ovarian axis dysfunction, anovulatory cycles
Cyclophosphamide	Gonadotoxin leading to dose-dependent and duration-dependent premature ovarian failure

Pregnancy Loss

Women with SLE experience increased risk of early, late, and recurrent pregnancy loss.[2,3,16] A 2020 meta-analysis reported that those with SLE have an increased risk of stillbirth (relative risk [RR], 16.49; 95% CI, 2.95–92.13; P = .001), fetal loss (RR, 7.55; 95% CI, 4.75–11.99; P = .00001), and abortion (RR, 4.70; 95% CI, 3.02–7.29; P = .00001).[3]

Mechanisms of increased pregnancy loss are likely multifactorial and incompletely understood, but it is hypothesized that abnormal compliment activation and/or the presence of APL antibodies in women with SLE likely contributes to pathologic placental development and increases the risk of miscarriage. This possibility is supported by multiple studies that have associated active SLE and APL antibodies with increased risk of pregnancy loss in women with SLE.[2,8,9,11,13,16–19] APL antibodies, in particular, are associated with recurrent pregnancy loss (OR, 4.8; 95% CI, 1.2–22.2).[4] Recognition of risk factors, disease management, and appropriate support is imperative to prevent and/or manage pregnancy loss in women with SLE.

Disease Flare

Multiple studies show an increased rate of SLE flares during pregnancy compared with nonpregnant women with SLE (HR, 1.59; 95% CI, 1.27–1.96).[20] Active disease before conception or during pregnancy carries a strong association with APOs (see **Box 2**).[2,3,20–30] Overall, the risk of major flare during pregnancy is low if disease is stable at conception. Hydroxychloroquine (HCQ) use further decreases this risk.[20,21,24]

The increased flare propensity during pregnancy may be caused by abnormal immune tolerance mechanisms and increased estrogen exposure. Several observational studies support the potential role of estrogen in development and progression of SLE.[7] Huong and colleagues[31] found that, compared with clomiphene, the use of gonadotropins for ovulation induction increased the rate of SLE flares from 6% to 27%.[7,31] Several risk factors for disease flare during pregnancy have been well described and are listed in **Box 1**.[7,20–24,32]

Disease flares can be challenging to distinguish from physiologic changes of pregnancy or pathologic preeclampsia. Interpretation of complement levels during pregnancy is difficult because levels are affected by increased consumption and estrogen-enhanced synthesis. However, low complement levels early in pregnancy or failure of complement levels to increase as pregnancy progresses may indicate active disease.[19,22,28,32]

Hypertensive Disease of Pregnancy

Preeclampsia/eclampsia is more common in women with SLE (RR, 3.38; 95% CI, 3.25–3.62; P = .00001)[3] and can have devastating effects to mother and

---

Box 1
Risk factors for systemic lupus erythematosus flare during pregnancy

Young maternal age

Low complement levels or failure of levels to increase throughout pregnancy

Active disease at conception or within 6 months prior

History of or active renal disease

APL antibody positivity

Prednisone use (doses ≥10.5 mg daily)

Box 2
Adverse pregnancy outcomes

Spontaneous abortion

Stillbirth

Preterm delivery

Intrauterine growth restriction

Small for gestational age

Low or very low birthweight

Fetal or neonatal death

---

child.[23,29,33,34] Hypertensive disease of pregnancy (HDP) in patients with SLE is associated with a higher incidence of preterm birth (RR, 4.70; 95% CI, 3.02–7.29; $P = .00001$), intrauterine growth restriction (IUGR)/small for gestation age (SGA) (RR, 2.50; 95% CI, 1.41–4.45; $P = .002$), and low birthweight infants (RR, 4.78; 95% CI, 3.65–6.26; $P = .00001$) compared with patients with lupus without HDP.[3] Women with lupus anticoagulant and/or antiphospholipid syndrome (APLS) have a particularly high risk of severe preeclampsia. Risk factors for preeclampsia in women with SLE include active disease, APLS, lupus nephritis (LN), chronic kidney disease, hypertension, declining complements, and thrombocytopenia (**Boxes 2** and **3**).[2,3,16,18,20–30,33]

Furthermore, a prospective observational study of 129 SLE pregnancies that were not complicated by known risk factors (ie, Hispanic race/ethnicity, antihypertensive therapy, active disease, APL/lupus anticoagulant positivity, platelet count <100 × 10^9 cells/L, diabetes mellitus, hypertension, serum creatinine >1.2 mg/dL, prednisone>20 mg daily, or >1000 mg proteinuria) found the rate of APO (composite outcome) to be 7.8% (CI, 3.8%–13.8%). Although this APO rate is significantly lower than other studies that were confounded by known risk factors, it was still significantly higher than of healthy controls participating in the study (3%; CI, 1.1%–6.4%), suggesting that other factors intrinsic to SLE may confer increased risk.[27]

Delivery

Patients with SLE face more complicated delivery courses compared with the general population. In addition to the increased risk of preterm delivery and associated

---

Box 3
Adverse pregnancy outcome risk factors

Maternal flare or active SLE

Hypertension/preeclampsia

Antiphospholipid antibody syndrome

Lupus nephritis

Advanced maternal age

Thrombocytopenia

Minority race

Maternal anti-Ro/anti-La positivity

---

prolonged hospitalization, they face increased risk of cesarean section (RR, 1.85; 95% CI, 1.63–2.10; P = .00001), thromboembolic disease (RR, 11.29; 95% CI, 6.05–21.07; P = .00001), and postpartum infection (RR, 4.35; 95% CI, 2.69–7.03; P = .00001).[2] Delivery complications can negatively affect mother, newborn, and family unit.

FETAL AND NEONATAL COMPLICATIONS

Although rate of APO and fetal death associated with maternal SLE have drastically improved, maternal SLE remains a strong predictor of adverse fetal outcomes.[1,30] Mehta and colleagues[1] observed an overall 2.3 times increased rate of fetal death in infants born to mothers with SLE. Neonates born to mothers with anti-Ro/La antibodies carry the additional risk of developing a neonatal lupus (NL) syndrome, most notably cardiac NL. Maternal risk factors for APOs have been described (see **Box 3**). Maternal health and risk factors contribute significantly to fetal outcomes, with an APO rate of 7.8% in women without baseline risk factors, increasing to 58% in mothers with significant risk factors; additionally, fetal/neonatal mortality increases to 22% in the latter.[22] Maternal use of HCQ, disease optimization, and frequent fetal monitoring, including Doppler ultrasonography and fetal biometry, are important to minimize fetal risk in babies born to mothers with SLE.[20,30]

Preterm Delivery

Prematurity is a major cause of morbidity and mortality in infants born to mothers with SLE. Rates of preterm birth range from 16% to 50% in women with SLE compared with approximately 11% in the general population.[2,19] Premature infants have an increased risk of sepsis, necrotizing enterocolitis, respiratory failure, intraventricular hemorrhage, hypoglycemia, jaundice, and death.[33,34] Newborns of mothers with SLE are more likely to require admission to the neonatal intensive care unit (RR, 2.79; 95% CI, 2.31–3.37; P = .0001), which can lead to additional emotional and financial stress.[3]

Intrauterine Growth Restriction and Low Birthweight

Infants born to mothers with SLE have a significantly increased risk of IUGR, SGA, and low birthweight. Depending on the cohort, risk can be more than quadrupled compared with healthy controls. In a 2019 study, Chen and colleagues[23] reported a 37.8% versus 11.8% rate of IUGR, 62.2% versus 17.2% rate of low birthweight infants, and 37.8% versus 2.7% rate of very low birthweight infants in mothers with SLE compared with health controls. APLS and hypertensive disorders of pregnancy are strongly associated with placental insufficiency and the outcomes discussed earlier.[2,3,19,23,25,33,34]

Neonatal Lupus Syndromes

NL can occur when there is transplacental transfer of maternal anti-Ro/La autoantibodies leading to cardiac, liver, hematologic, and/or skin abnormalities. Anti-Ro/La autoantibodies are immunoglobulin G directed toward intracellular ribosomal nuclear proteins. Starting at ~12 weeks' gestation, these autoantibodies cross the placenta and can damage the developing fetal tissue, producing the spectrum of NL syndromes.[35] Anti-Ro/La antibodies can be found in those with SLE, Sjögren syndrome, or people without diagnosed connective tissue disease. Half of asymptomatic mothers who have a child affected by NL develop symptoms of autoimmune disease after a median of 3 years and should be assessed and monitored for an underlying connective tissue disease.[36,37] In general, NL manifestations resolve as maternal autoantibodies clear from the neonatal circulation. However, the cardiac manifestations are irreversible and carry significant morbidity and mortality.[29,36]

Cardiac neonatal lupus (Congenital heart block)

Fetal cardiac disease, manifesting as atrioventricular (AV) block, dilated cardiomyopathy, and/or endocardial fibroelastosis, has been linked to maternal anti-Ro (less commonly anti-La) antibodies. Increased maternal anti-Ro levels, not disease activity, correlate with risk of cardiac complications in the fetus. Jaeggi and colleagues[38] found that antibody-related cardiac complications occurred exclusively when a fetus was exposed to anti-Ro antibody levels greater than or equal to 50 U/mL, independent of anti-La titers. Cardiac NL accounts for more than 80% of severe AV blocks in newborns with structurally normal hearts.[36,39] Cardiac NL occurs in approximately 1% to 2% of fetuses exposed to anti-Ro antibodies and carries a 15% to 18% mortality, primarily driven by hydrops, prematurity, and dilated cardiomyopathy (**Box 4**).[39–42] Occurrence of fetal cardiac disease in subsequent pregnancies is increased to approximately 18%.[43,44]

Izmirly and colleagues[39] found the probability of survival at 10 years for a child diagnosed with cardiac NL and born alive to be 86%. However, they also found a significantly higher case fatality rate in minority infants compared with white children with cardiac NL who died after birth, but not for fetuses who died in utero, suggesting that racial disparities play a role in mortality.[39] Screening for fetal cardiac NL in women with anti-Ro/La antibodies is recommended beginning at 16 weeks and continuing weekly or biweekly until 28 weeks of gestation in coordination with maternal fetal medicine and pediatric cardiology.[30,39,45]

Few therapies have proved effective in the prevention of cardiac NL. Maternal HCQ use in pregnancy has been found to decrease the incidence of cardiac NL, possibly because of inhibition of toll-like receptor, thus reducing cardiac inflammation and scarring.[36,43,46,47] Use of steroids, intravenous immunoglobulin, and β-agonists (ie, terbutaline) to increase fetal heart rate, and plasmapheresis remains inconclusive and poorly studied.[42,46,48–50]

A third-degree AV block from cardiac NL is irreversible and carries a mortality of approximately 17%.[29,39,46] Infants with AV block who survive usually require a permanent pacemaker placement (70%–90% by 10 years of age).[36,39]

Noncardiac neonatal lupus

Liver, skin, or hematologic abnormalities can be seen in infants of mothers with SLE. Several studies suggest that infants exposed to anti-La antibodies are more likely to

---

Box 4
Fetal echocardiogram findings associated with increased mortality in fetuses exposed to anti-Ro antibodies

Hydrops

Dilated cardiomyopathy

Endocardial fibroelastosis

Valvar dysfunction

Early gestation age at diagnosis

Ventricular dysfunction

Lower ventricular nadir rate

have noncardiac NL and that the rate of recurrence in subsequent pregnancies nearly doubles.[38,51]

Cutaneous NL has been reported to occur in up to 16% of infants born to women with anti-La, less commonly anti-Ro, antibodies.[40,51] Affected infants develop a rash resembling subacute cutaneous lupus lesions, which can be exacerbated by ultraviolet light. Lesions are usually not apparent at birth but develop before the first month of life. The rash is often misdiagnosed, leading to unnecessary investigations. Biopsy is not required to make the diagnosis. The rash is often transient, resolving by 6 to 9 months of age without residual dyspigmentation or scarring.[36] Maternal use of HCQ is associated with a reduced risk of cutaneous NL. Barsalou and colleagues[51] also showed a trend toward decreased rates of cutaneous NL in patients whose mothers were treated with nonfluorinated steroids plus or minus azathioprine, suggesting that general disease control is likely important in decreasing rates of NL.

Findings of hepatic or hematologic NL have been associated with increased morbidity in affected infants.[39] Transient anemia, thrombocytopenia, or neutropenia are the most common manifestations.[35] Hematological and hepatobiliary involvement often occurs in conjunction with cardiac and/or cutaneous NL. Symptoms resolve as maternal antibodies are cleared from fetal circulation, usually without specific intervention.[36]

MANAGEMENT AND RISK FACTOR MITIGATION

Most patients with SLE can have successful and safe pregnancies. Fertility preservation, prepregnancy disease optimization, appropriate medications, and frequent maternal and fetal monitoring via a multidisciplinary team are essential. Active maternal disease has been consistently found to be a strong predictor of APO and significantly increases the risk of hypertensive disease in the mother and thus IUGR, stillbirth, and preterm delivery in the fetus. The odds for preeclampsia have been shown to be increased in mothers with active disease, but not inactive disease, underscoring the importance of disease control before conception and throughout pregnancy.[33]

Counseling

Given the increased risk of infertility and premature ovarian failure in patients with SLE, family planning and fertility preservation options should be routinely discussed with patients, especially during times of disease quiescence or before cytotoxic therapy. However, cyclophosphamide is only used in cases of severe lupus, often semiemergently, leaving little time to implement fertility preservation strategies. However, gonadotropin-releasing hormone analogues can offer benefit if used before or concomitantly with alkylating agents.[30] Induction therapy for LN and other organ-threatening manifestations that minimize or eliminate cytotoxic therapy are increasingly being studied and used. Referral to a fertility specialist should be considered early in the family planning course for patients with lupus.

Medication Management

Judicious use of medication before and throughout pregnancy is critical for suppression of SLE disease activity and management of comorbid conditions that can lead to APOs. If a woman with SLE is considering pregnancy or discovers she is pregnant, her medications should be promptly reviewed. Potential teratogenic medication should be discontinued at least 4 to 6 weeks before conception or immediately on discovery of pregnancy. Fortunately, there are only a few medications commonly used in the treatment of SLE that are known teratogens (**Table 2**).[30,52–54]

It is important to remember that such medications are often necessary for optimal health in women with SLE when not pregnant. Therefore, teratogenic medications must be discontinued and replaced with effective medications compatible with pregnancy. It is key to switch from a teratogenic medication to a compatible substitute 6 to 12 months before conception, not for issues of teratogenicity, but in order to ensure that the underlying disease can be managed with the new medication regimen. In general, 4 to 6 weeks is enough time to remove the teratogenic medication from the maternal circulation. Leflunomide is the exception and requires an intensive cholestyramine washout protocol for elimination.[55]

Fortunately, many therapeutics for the management of SLE are compatible with pregnancy and their use is supported by numerous observational studies without evidence of increased risk of congenital anomalies.[53] Expert consensus and guidelines strongly recommend that use of these medications to control disease is critical to minimizing APO because active disease in the periconception pregnancy period is strongly associated with adverse outcomes in both mother and fetus.[30,54] Many outstanding review articles are available that discuss individual immunosuppressive agents for use during pregnancy.[56–58] Teratogenic immunosuppressants can be replaced by medications compatible with pregnancy, including azathioprine, calcineurin inhibitors, and sulfasalazine. In cases of organ-threatening or life-threatening SLE manifestations, rituximab is a reasonable alternative to cyclophosphamide.[30,53,54]

Table 2
Medications contraindicated in pregnancy

Medication	Mechanism	Adverse Effects	Clinical Pearls
Mycophenolate mofetil	Purine synthesis inhibitor	• Increased first-trimester miscarriage • Teratogenic	Stop at least 6 wk before attempting pregnancy
Cyclophosphamide	Alkylating agent	• Premature ovarian insufficiency • Teratogenic	Use of gonadotropin-releasing hormone analogues can reduce premature ovarian failure
Methotrexate	Antimetabolite	• Teratogen • Abortion	Likely has dose-dependent effects
Leflunomide	Pyrimidine synthesis inhibitor	• Teratogenic in animal studies • Limited human data during pregnancy	Washout procedure recommended in the case of unintentional pregnancy
Angiotensin-converting enzyme inhibitors	—	• Teratogenic early in pregnancy • Fetal renal abnormalities • Oligohydramnios later in pregnancy	Maternal proteinuria may increase secondary to discontinuation
Warfarin	—	• Teratogen • Hemorrhagic complications in fetus and mother	May be used in second trimester after organogenesis if benefits outweigh risks

For ancillary medications, including warfarin and angiotensin-converting enzyme (ACE) inhibitors, the switch can be made closer to pregnancy. Warfarin needs to be replaced by low molecular weight or unfractionated heparin. ACE inhibitors should be replaced by labetalol or other antihypertensives compatible with pregnancy. Alternatives to ACE inhibitors are unlikely to have the same effects on proteinuria; increased proteinuria alone during pregnancy does not necessarily reflect an increase in inflammatory glomerulonephritis.[30,54]

Several medications used in SLE deserve special attention. There is ample evidence that use of HCQ before conception and throughout pregnancy and lactation is associated with significantly improved pregnancy outcomes in women with SLE irrespective of disease activity. Not only do quality indicators for the treatment of SLE recommend initiation and continuation of HCQ at SLE diagnosis, it is also strongly recommended to initiate HCQ in women with SLE who are considering pregnancy or are pregnant if they are not taking it already. Benefits of HCQ during pregnancy include reduction of risk of disease flare, preeclampsia, and NL syndromes. Furthermore, HCQ is not immunosuppressive, so there is no theoretic concern for increased risk of maternal or neonatal infection.[20,24,30,47,51,54]

The use of corticosteroids during pregnancy in women with SLE is an additional point for discussion. Nonfluorinated corticosteroids are inactivated by the placental enzyme 11 β-dehydrogenase type 2; doses less than 20 mg daily do not reach fetal circulation. In contrast, fluorinated corticosteroids are used when treatment of the fetus is the goal, such as in cases of enhanced fetal lung maturation in settings of impending premature delivery. Because low-dose fluorinated corticosteroids are compatible with pregnancy, women who have stable disease on chronic low doses should not necessarily be tapered or discontinued in anticipation or discovery of pregnancy because they can safely continue on their baseline dose and avoid the increased risk of flare if tapered.[48] The addition of low-dose or an increase of baseline steroids in a woman with otherwise stable disease in the setting of pregnancy is not recommended. There is no benefit to supposedly prophylactic steroid use for flare reduction during pregnancy.[59,60] If signs and symptoms of flare develop during pregnancy, steroids have the shortest onset of action and should be considered for immediate treatment while changes in steroid-sparing agents are considered. Often, doses higher than 20 mg daily are required for moderate to severe flares during pregnancy. Disease control is paramount, but, as in the nonpregnant situation, the lowest dose of steroids should be used for the shortest period of time to treat SLE flare and maintain disease quiescence.

Management of Specific Situations

Antiphospholipid syndrome

APS in women with SLE greatly increases risk of severe complications including preeclampsia, prematurity, and pregnancy loss. Diagnosis of APLS requires positive serologies (lupus anticoagulant, antibodies against phospholipids, cardiolipins, and/or β2 glycoprotein I) on 2 occasions at least 12 weeks apart as well as evidence of a thrombotic event. For women who have had a non–obstetric-related thrombotic event before pregnancy, treatment of the syndrome during pregnancy is therapeutic doses of low molecular weight or unfractionated heparin plus low-dose aspirin (LDA) throughout pregnancy and at least 6 to 12 weeks postpartum.[30,54,61]

Obstetric APLS is defined as positive serologies in addition to (1) greater than or equal to 3 consecutive early pregnancy losses (<10 weeks' gestation); or (2) any late pregnancy complication (pregnancy loss, preeclampsia, or severe prematurity) associated with placental insufficiency and without other known cause. For women who have a diagnosis of obstetric APLS, treatment consists of prophylactic doses of heparin in addition to LDA.[30,54,61]

Less is known regarding the optimal treatment of women with positive serologies for APLS without a prior thrombotic event, particularly in women who have never been pregnant. In these cases, LDA alone can be considered (along with HCQ), but the addition of heparin is not currently recommended because the absolute risk of pregnancy complications in the setting of positive serologies alone is low and not quantifiable.[60] Primigravid patients with known triple-positive serologies (positive lupus anticoagulant, high titers of both antiphospholipid antibodies and β2 glycoprotein 1) may benefit from shared decision making regarding the risks and benefits of adding prophylactic doses of heparin to their regimens.[28,30,54,61]

Renal disease

Renal disease is the most common organ-threatening manifestation of SLE, with LN occurring in up to 30% of patients with SLE.[62] Active LN, uncontrolled hypertension, and renal insufficiency are relative contraindications to pregnancy and all attempts to achieve control should be undertaken before conception. Women who are currently receiving induction treatment of LN should defer conception until remission has been achieved and maintained on azathioprine and/or calcineurin inhibitors. In addition, ACE inhibitors should be discontinued, and alternative antihypertensive medications substituted before pregnancy whenever possible so that changes in proteinuria can be understood before conception.[63]

It is common for LN to flare or manifest during pregnancy. This situation can be challenging for multiple reasons. During the second half of pregnancy, LN may be indistinguishable from preeclampsia, a pregnancy-related medical emergency. All pregnant women with SLE, irrespective of past manifestations, should be routinely monitored for changes in blood pressure and proteinuria. If significant increases are detected, then it is important to look for other signs of active SLE that may increase overall SLE disease activity and suggest LN. Aggressive BP control should be initiated as well as presumptive treatment of LN, including increases in nonfluorinated corticosteroid levels. If the pregnancy is close to term, indicated delivery may be considered to resolve potential preeclampsia and allow for renal biopsy and induction therapy in case of LN. In the previable weeks of gestation, treatment of presumed LN is reasonable with careful monitoring for progressive symptoms of preeclampsia, which may necessitate delivery to prevent eclampsia and/or fetal demise.[16,30,54,63]

Pulmonary hypertension

Pulmonary arterial hypertension (PAH) is an uncommon, but highly morbid, manifestation of SLE that is one of the most significant contraindications to pregnancy given the inability of the pulmonary vasculature to accommodate the excess blood plasma volume of pregnancy. Women with known PAH should be strongly counseled against pregnancy and those who become pregnant should be counseled regarding the high risk of fetal and maternal morbidity and mortality. In cases where women with PAH wish to continue with pregnancy, endothelin receptor inhibitors should be discontinued because they are teratogenic. Calcium channel blockers, sildenafil, and prostanoids are compatible with pregnancy and should be used instead. The highest-risk period of pregnancy for women with moderate to severe PAH is during delivery and immediately postpartum, when dramatic shifts in fluids can maximally strain the pulmonary arteries.[64,65]

Contraindications to Pregnancy

Many known risk factors for pregnancy complications in women with SLE are amenable to modification, such as active underlying disease, uncontrolled hypertension, diabetes mellitus, and use of teratogenic medications. Other risk factors can be managed during pregnancy to reduce the chance of adverse outcomes, including use of HCQ, congenital heart block (CHB) screening in fetuses of mothers affected by SSA/Ro, and use of LDA and heparin in the setting of obstetric or thrombotic APLS. In contrast, several risk factors may be present that are not readily modifiable, including past pregnancy complications, race/ethnicity, end-organ damage, and genetics.

Rather than framing issues of pregnancy risks as contraindications, it may be more helpful to discuss risk stratification with patients considering pregnancy in order to allow for discussion and nonjudgmental shared decision making. Even in settings of extremely high risk, including severe active internal-organ SLE or PAH, many pregnancies are strongly desired and women elect to proceed despite risks. Honest and nonjudgmental discussions with affected women should include frank assessment of risk, recommendations for management, and nonjudgmental respect for and support of each woman's individual decisions in order to facilitate open communication and rapid assessment of change in health status.

SUMMARY

Although pregnancy in patients with SLE carries increased risk to mother and fetus, significant improvements have been made. Compared with the general population, patients with SLE have witnessed a marked improvement in in-hospital maternal mortality, decreasing from a rate of 34 times higher in 1998 to 2000 to less than 5 times higher in 2013 to 2015.[1] Most patients with SLE are able to become pregnant and deliver a healthy infant. However, as with many other chronic conditions, careful planning before conception is essential to maximize the mother's health and ensure disease quiescence on medications compatible with pregnancy. It is just as important to ensure that women with childbearing potential use reliable contraception to ensure that any pregnancies can be timed appropriately. Known risk factors associated with higher incidence of APOs include active disease within 6 months of conception, APLS, uncontrolled hypertension, renal insufficiency, use of teratogenic medications, nonuse of HCQ, and abrupt discontinuations of disease-suppressing medications.

Recent advances in special situations related to SLE pregnancies include the use of HCQ to significantly reduce the risk of NL in SSA/Ro-positive mothers as well as the use of combination of LDA with heparin in cases of obstetric and thrombotic APLS.

Shared decision making, open communication, and a multidisciplinary approach are essential to maximize the experience and health for mother and infant. With few exceptions, pregnancy and childbirth is achievable for most women with SLE.

CLINICS CARE POINTS

- Successful pregnancy is achievable for most women with lupus provided that underlying disease is well controlled 6 to 12 months before conception through the delivery and postpartum period.
- Pregnancy-compatible medications are available for most manifestations of lupus that arise before or during pregnancy.

- Use of HCQ throughout pregnancy may increase healthy maternal and fetal outcomes for SLE pregnancies, including a significant reduction in the incidence of SSA/Ro-associated CHB.
- Risk stratification, support, open communication, and shared decision making between patient and providers further enhance the pregnancy experience and safety for mothers with SLE and their offspring.

DISCLOSURE

The author has nothing to disclose.

REFERENCES

1. Mehta B, Luo Y, Xu J, et al. Trends in maternal and fetal outcomes among pregnant women with systemic lupus erythematosus in the United States: a cross-sectional analysis. Ann Intern Med 2019;171:164–71.
2. Bundhun PK, Soogund MZ, Huang F. Impact of systemic lupus erythematosus on maternal and fetal outcomes following pregnancy: a meta-analysis of studies published between years 2001-2016. J Autoimmun 2017;79:17–27.
3. He WR, Wei H. Maternal and fetal complications associated with systemic lupus erythematosus: An updated meta-analysis of the most recent studies (2017-2019). Medicine (Baltimore) 2020;99:e19797.
4. Carp HJ, Selmi C, Shoenfeld Y. The autoimmune bases of infertility and pregnancy loss. J Autoimmun 2012;38:J266–74.
5. Grossmann B, Saur S, Rall K, et al. Prevalence of autoimmune disease in women with premature ovarian failure. Eur J Contracept Reprod Health Care 2020; 25:72–5.
6. Ebrahimi M, Akbari Asbagh F. The role of autoimmunity in premature ovarian failure. Iran J Reprod Med 2015;13:461–72.
7. Oktem O, Yagmur H, Bengisu H, et al. Reproductive aspects of systemic lupus erythematosus. J Reprod Immunol 2016;117:57–65.
8. Angley M, Lim SS, Spencer JB, et al. Infertility among African American women with systemic lupus erythematosus compared to healthy women: a pilot study. Arthritis Care Res (Hoboken) 2020;72:1275–81.
9. Clowse ME, Chakravarty E, Costenbader KH, et al. Effects of infertility, pregnancy loss, and patient concerns on family size of women with rheumatoid arthritis and systemic lupus erythematosus. Arthritis Care Res (Hoboken) 2012;64:668–74.
10. Hickman RA, Gordon C. Causes and management of infertility in systemic lupus erythematosus. Rheumatology (Oxford) 2011;50:1551–8.
11. Lawrenz B, Henes J, Henes M, et al. Impact of systemic lupus erythematosus on ovarian reserve in premenopausal women: evaluation by using anti-Muellerian hormone. Lupus 2011;20:1193–7.
12. Moncayo R, Moncayo HE. A new endocrinological and immunological syndrome in SLE: elevation of human chorionic gonadotropin and of antibodies directed against ovary and endometrium antigens. Lupus 1995;4:39–45.
13. Shoenfeld Y, Carp HJ, Molina V, et al. Autoantibodies and prediction of reproductive failure. Am J Reprod Immunol 2006;56:337–44.
14. Micu MC, Micu R, Ostensen M. Luteinized unruptured follicle syndrome increased by inactive disease and selective cyclooxygenase 2 inhibitors in women with inflammatory arthropathies. Arthritis Care Res (Hoboken) 2011;63: 1334–8.

15. Khizroeva J, Nalli C, Bitsadze V, et al. Infertility in women with systemic autoimmune diseases. Best Pract Res Clin Endocrinol Metab 2019;33:101369.
16. Smyth A, Oliveira GH, Lahr BD, et al. A systematic review and meta-analysis of pregnancy outcomes in patients with systemic lupus erythematosus and lupus nephritis. Clin J Am Soc Nephrol 2010;5:2060–8.
17. Hardy CJ, Palmer BP, Morton SJ, et al. Pregnancy outcome and family size in systemic lupus erythematosus: a case-control study. Rheumatology (Oxford) 1999; 38:559–63.
18. Rajaei E, Shahbazian N, Rezaeeyan H, et al. The effect of lupus disease on the pregnant women and embryos: a retrospective study from 2010 to 2014. Clin Rheumatol 2019;38:3211–5.
19. Kim JW, Jung JY, Kim HA, et al. Lupus low disease activity state achievement is important for reducing adverse outcomes in pregnant patients with systemic lupus erythematosus. J Rheumatol 2021;48(5):707–16.
20. Eudy AM, Siega-Riz AM, Engel SM, et al. Effect of pregnancy on disease flares in patients with systemic lupus erythematosus. Ann Rheum Dis 2018;77:855–60.
21. Davis-Porada J, Kim MY, Guerra MM, et al. Low frequency of flares during pregnancy and post-partum in stable lupus patients. Arthritis Res Ther 2020;22:52.
22. Buyon JP, Kim MY, Guerra MM, et al. Kidney outcomes and risk factors for nephritis (flare/de novo) in a multiethnic cohort of pregnant patients with lupus. Clin J Am Soc Nephrol 2017;12:940–6.
23. Chen D, Yuan S, Lao M, et al. Umbilical arterial Doppler ultrasonography predicts late pregnancy outcomes in patients with lupus nephritis: a multicenter study from Southern China. Lupus 2019;28:1312–9.
24. Janardana R, Haridas V, Priya V, et al. Maternal and fetal outcomes of lupus pregnancies: a collective effort by Karnataka rheumatologists. Lupus 2020;29: 1397–403.
25. Palma Dos Reis CR, Cardoso G, Carvalho C, et al. Prediction of adverse pregnancy outcomes in women with systemic lupus erythematosus. Clin Rev Allergy Immunol 2020;59:287–94.
26. Phansenee S, Sekararithi R, Jatavan P, et al. Pregnancy outcomes among women with systemic lupus erythematosus: a retrospective cohort study from Thailand. Lupus 2018;27:158–64.
27. Buyon JP, Kim MY, Guerra MM, et al. Predictors of pregnancy outcomes in patients with lupus: a cohort study. Ann Intern Med 2015;163:153–63.
28. Kim MY, Guerra MM, Kaplowitz E, et al. Complement activation predicts adverse pregnancy outcome in patients with systemic lupus erythematosus and/or antiphospholipid antibodies. Ann Rheum Dis 2018;77:549–55.
29. Limaye MA, Buyon JP, Cuneo BF, et al. A review of fetal and neonatal consequences of maternal systemic lupus erythematosus. Prenat Diagn 2020;40(9): 1066–76.
30. Andreoli L, Bertsias GK, Agmon-Levin N, et al. EULAR recommendations for women's health and the management of family planning, assisted reproduction, pregnancy and menopause in patients with systemic lupus erythematosus and/ or antiphospholipid syndrome. Ann Rheum Dis 2017;76:476–85.
31. Huong DL, Wechsler B, Vauthier-Brouzes D, et al. Importance of planning ovulation induction therapy in systemic lupus erythematosus and antiphospholipid syndrome: a single center retrospective study of 21 cases and 114 cycles. Semin Arthritis Rheum 2002;32:174–88.
32. Ueda A, Chigusa Y, Mogami H, et al. Predictive factors for flares of established stable systemic lupus erythematosus without anti-phospholipid antibodies during

pregnancy. J Matern Fetal Neonatal Med 2020;1–6. https://doi.org/10.1080/14767058.2020.1843626.

33. Skorpen CG, Lydersen S, Gilboe IM, et al. Influence of disease activity and medications on offspring birth weight, pre-eclampsia and preterm birth in systemic lupus erythematosus: a population-based study. Ann Rheum Dis 2018;77:264–9.

34. Chen YJ, Chang JC, Lai EL, et al. Maternal and perinatal outcomes of pregnancies in systemic lupus erythematosus: a nationwide population-based study. Semin Arthritis Rheum 2020;50:451–7.

35. Zuppa AA, Riccardi R, Frezza S, et al. Neonatal lupus: follow-up in infants with anti-SSA/Ro antibodies and review of the literature. Autoimmun Rev 2017;16:427–32.

36. Vanoni F, Lava SAG, Fossali EF, et al. Neonatal systemic lupus erythematosus syndrome: a comprehensive review. Clin Rev Allergy Immunol 2017;53:469–76.

37. Rivera TL, Izmirly PM, Birnbaum BK, et al. Disease progression in mothers of children enrolled in the research registry for neonatal lupus. Ann Rheum Dis 2009;68:828–35.

38. Jaeggi E, Laskin C, Hamilton R, et al. The importance of the level of maternal anti-Ro/SSA antibodies as a prognostic marker of the development of cardiac neonatal lupus erythematosus a prospective study of 186 antibody-exposed fetuses and infants. J Am Coll Cardiol 2010;55:2778–84.

39. Izmirly PM, Saxena A, Kim MY, et al. Maternal and fetal factors associated with mortality and morbidity in a multi-racial/ethnic registry of anti-SSA/Ro-associated cardiac neonatal lupus. Circulation 2011;124:1927–35.

40. Cimaz R, Spence DL, Hornberger L, et al. Incidence and spectrum of neonatal lupus erythematosus: a prospective study of infants born to mothers with anti-Ro autoantibodies. J Pediatr 2003;142:678–83.

41. Levesque K, Morel N, Maltret A, et al. Description of 214 cases of autoimmune congenital heart block: results of the French neonatal lupus syndrome. Autoimmun Rev 2015;14:1154–60.

42. Eliasson H, Sonesson SE, Sharland G, et al. Isolated atrioventricular block in the fetus: a retrospective, multinational, multicenter study of 175 patients. Circulation 2011;124:1919–26.

43. Izmirly PM, Kim MY, Llanos C, et al. Evaluation of the risk of anti-SSA/Ro-SSB/La antibody-associated cardiac manifestations of neonatal lupus in fetuses of mothers with systemic lupus erythematosus exposed to hydroxychloroquine. Ann Rheum Dis 2010;69:1827–30.

44. Llanos C, Izmirly PM, Katholi M, et al. Recurrence rates of cardiac manifestations associated with neonatal lupus and maternal/fetal risk factors. Arthritis Rheum 2009;60:3091–7.

45. Sonesson SE, Ambrosi A, Wahren-Herlenius M. Benefits of fetal echocardiographic surveillance in pregnancies at risk of congenital heart block: single-center study of 212 anti-Ro52-positive pregnancies. Ultrasound Obstet Gynecol 2019;54:87–95.

46. Izmirly P, Saxena A, Buyon JP. Progress in the pathogenesis and treatment of cardiac manifestations of neonatal lupus. Curr Opin Rheumatol 2017;29:467–72.

47. Barsalou J, Jaeggi E, Laskin CA, et al. Prenatal exposure to antimalarials decreases the risk of cardiac but not non-cardiac neonatal lupus: a single-centre cohort study. Rheumatology (Oxford) 2017;56:1552–9.

48. Saxena A, Izmirly PM, Mendez B, et al. Prevention and treatment in utero of autoimmune-associated congenital heart block. Cardiol Rev 2014;22:263–7.

49. Izmirly P, Kim M, Friedman DM, et al. Hydroxychloroquine to prevent recurrent congenital heart block in fetuses of anti-SSA/Ro-positive mothers. J Am Coll Cardiol 2020;76:292–302.
50. Izmirly PM, Saxena A, Sahl SK, et al. Assessment of fluorinated steroids to avert progression and mortality in anti-SSA/Ro-associated cardiac injury limited to the fetal conduction system. Ann Rheum Dis 2016;75:1161–5.
51. Barsalou J, Costedoat-Chalumeau N, Berhanu A, et al. Effect of in utero hydroxychloroquine exposure on the development of cutaneous neonatal lupus erythematosus. Ann Rheum Dis 2018;77:1742–9.
52. Singh AG, Chowdhary VR. Pregnancy-related issues in women with systemic lupus erythematosus. Int J Rheum Dis 2015;18:172–81.
53. Ostensen M, Forger F. How safe are anti-rheumatic drugs during pregnancy? Curr Opin Pharmacol 2013;13:470–5.
54. Fanouriakis A, Kostopoulou M, Alunno A, et al. 2019 update of the EULAR recommendations for the management of systemic lupus erythematosus. Ann Rheum Dis 2019;78:736–45.
55. Cassina M, Johnson DL, Robinson LK, et al. Pregnancy outcome in women exposed to leflunomide before or during pregnancy. Arthritis Rheum 2012;64:2085–94.
56. Tosounidou S, Gordon C. Medications in pregnancy and breastfeeding. Best Pract Res Clin Obstet Gynaecol 2020;64:68–76.
57. Lateef A, Petri M. Systemic lupus erythematosus and pregnancy. Rheum Dis Clin North Am 2017;43:215–26.
58. Maynard S, Guerrier G, Duffy M. Pregnancy in women with systemic lupus and lupus nephritis. Adv Chronic Kidney Dis 2019;26:330–7.
59. Bandoli G, Palmsten K, Forbess Smith CJ, et al. A review of systemic corticosteroid use in pregnancy and the risk of select pregnancy and birth outcomes. Rheum Dis Clin North Am 2017;43:489–502.
60. Sammaritano LR, Bermas BL, Chakravarty EE, et al. 2020 American College of Rheumatology Guideline for the Management of Reproductive Health in Rheumatic and Musculoskeletal Diseases. Arthritis Rheumatol 2020;72:461–88.
61. Tektonidou MG, Andreoli L, Limper M, et al. EULAR recommendations for the management of antiphospholipid syndrome in adults. Ann Rheum Dis 2019;78:1296–304.
62. Hiraki LT, Feldman CH, Liu J, et al. Prevalence, incidence, and demographics of systemic lupus erythematosus and lupus nephritis from 2000 to 2004 among children in the US Medicaid beneficiary population. Arthritis Rheum 2012;64:2669–76.
63. Attia DH, Mokbel A, Haggag HM, et al. Pregnancy outcome in women with active and inactive lupus nephritis: a prospective cohort study. Lupus 2019;28:806–17.
64. de Raaf MA, Beekhuijzen M, Guignabert C, et al. Endothelin-1 receptor antagonists in fetal development and pulmonary arterial hypertension. Reprod Toxicol 2015;56:45–51.
65. Galie N, Humbert M, Vachiery JL, et al. 2015 ESC/ERS Guidelines for the diagnosis and treatment of pulmonary hypertension: The Joint Task Force for the Diagnosis and Treatment of Pulmonary Hypertension of the European Society of Cardiology (ESC) and the European Respiratory Society (ERS): Endorsed by: Association for European Paediatric and Congenital Cardiology (AEPC), International Society for Heart and Lung Transplantation (ISHLT). Eur Heart J 2016;37:67–119.

Lupus Cohorts

Christopher Redmond, MD, Omer Pamuk, MD,
Sarfaraz A. Hasni, MD, MSc*

KEYWORDS

• Lupus • Cohort • Registry • Database

KEY POINTS

- Studies based on data from systemic lupus erythematosus (SLE)cohorts have made significant contributions, such as new SLE classification criteria, premature cardiovascular events as a major cause of mortality, and validation of disease activity and damage indices.
- Long-term follow-up based on prospective cohort studies allows measurement of outcomes and evaluation of prognostic factors that may change over time.
- Cohort studies provide valuable information to analyze differences between treatment modalities in SLE when used in real-life scenarios.
- Limitations of cohort-based studies include selection bias, presence of unmeasured confounders, and missing data.

Systemic lupus erythematosus (SLE) is a chronic heterogenous autoimmune disease involving multiple organ systems and resulting in significant morbidity, mortality at a younger age, and a poor quality of life.[1] There is a lack of therapeutic advancement in SLE because of the heterogeneity of clinical manifestations, and racial/ethnic differences in disease severity and response to treatment.[2] To this end, large lupus cohorts with diverse ethnic and racial backgrounds, especially those possessing varied clinical features, have been instrumental in understanding the pathogenesis and natural history of lupus as well as the therapeutic response to candidate medications.[3] A strength of the cohort study design is that study subjects do not have the outcome of interest at enrollment. Because they are enrolled based on an exposure of interest, such a design ultimately provides the opportunity to assess relative risk. Shortcomings of cohort study design include the need for consistent high-quality follow-up and vulnerability to study subject attrition. Although a cohort study design may be optimal for rare diseases, it may be inefficient in the situation of rare outcomes of interest.

National Institute of Arthritis and Musculoskeletal and Skin Diseases, National Institutes of Health, Bethesda, MD 20892, USA
* Corresponding author. National Institute of Arthritis and Musculoskeletal and Skin Diseases, National Institutes of Health, 9000 Rockville Pike, Bldg 10, Room 3-2340, Bethesda, MD 20892, USA.
E-mail address: sarfaraz.hasni@nih.gov

Rheum Dis Clin N Am 47 (2021) 457–479
https://doi.org/10.1016/j.rdc.2021.04.009
0889-857X/21/Published by Elsevier Inc.
rheumatic.theclinics.com

A cohort is defined as "any group of individuals affected by common diseases, environmental or temporal influences, treatments, or other traits whose progress is assessed in a research study."[4] According to the World Health Organization (WHO), a registry is "a file of documents containing uniform information about individual persons, collected in a systematic and comprehensive way, to serve a predetermined purpose."[5] In addition, "database" is used as an alternative term for registry and cohort. Although these 3 terms (cohort, registry, and database) are not exactly interchangeable, they have been used reciprocally in research and publications.

TYPES OF COHORTS

Lupus cohorts or registries are designed in many ways (**Box 1**). Initially, lupus registries were mostly cross-sectional and included only basic clinical or prognostic characteristics.[6] In recent years, electronic medical record systems have provided the tools required for continuous and repeated monitoring of longitudinal data collection, which has resulted in a mushrooming of lupus cohorts worldwide.[7]

The primary difference between cohort studies and randomized clinical trials (RCTs) is the lack of randomization. In cohort studies, exposure status is determined by chance (eg, genetic factors, antibody positivity), environment (eg, smoking, sun exposure), or clinical judgment (eg, therapy selection).[8] In prospective cohort studies, exposure is assessed at the baseline and the study follows patients over time for prespecified outcomes, such as end-stage renal disease (ESRD) or mortality. In retrospective cohorts, the study tries to assess the potential exposures that may predict a predefined event.[8] In the evidence hierarchy, prospective studies are generally of higher quality owing to more systematic and robust data collection.[9]

Cohorts may be based in a network that is single center, multicenter, national, or international. The size of a cohort is typically determined by the aim and specific objectives. For instance, some cohorts may include all patients with SLE, whereas others may focus on a subset of patients with SLE, such as lupus nephritis or pediatric patients with lupus. The outcomes of interest in lupus cohorts often include disease activity, prognosis, drug response, toxicity, end-organ damage, and patient-reported outcomes.

Role of Cohorts in Studying Systemic Lupus Erythematosus

RCTs are considered the gold standard for determining the efficacy of a new treatment modality.[10] However, RCTs have narrow inclusion criteria and necessarily include a

---

Box 1
Types of cohorts

- Administrative cohorts
- Cross-sectional cohorts
- Longitudinal retrospective cohorts
- Longitudinal prospective cohorts
- Single-center cohorts
- Multicenter or international cohorts
- Cohorts including all patients
- Cohorts for special patient subgroups (specific ethnic group or treatment groups, and so forth)

smaller number of patients for a short duration, all ultimately limiting the ability to generalize the results.[8]

In contrast, observational cohort studies may yield real-life data about the natural course of disease and therapeutic response, which can be particularly valuable for a heterogenous multisystem disease such as SLE. For example, an RCT of rituximab (RTX) in SLE failed to achieve the primary efficacy outcomes, whereas multiple lupus cohort studies showed efficacy of RTX in the situations of immune cytopenias,[11] cutaneous lupus,[12] recalcitrant lupus, and even lupus nephritis.[13]

Cohort studies can also capture information about patient populations underrepresented in RCTs, and that may be limited because of restrictive inclusion criteria.[14] In addition, the dichotomous nature of RCTs sometimes means they are not feasible because of ethical or logistical issues with adjusting or withholding care. For example, when evaluating the efficacy of treatment of lupus nephritis, either withholding care or using a placebo-based RCT could have significant consequences for patient morbidity and mortality. In these instances, cohort studies are ideal for studying treatment effect.[15] For cohort-based studies to have a meaningful impact on clinical practice, they similarly need to be well defined in terms of scope, population, inclusion criteria, and rigorous definition of case ascertainment, as well as characterized by regular follow-up and extensive data collection.[16,17] Single-center cohorts usually have higher-quality and more uniform data compared with multicenter cohorts, but because they are usually located in large tertiary care centers, the ability to generalize from their data may be a significant limitation.

Existing Lupus Cohorts

Some of the well-established SLE cohorts that have contributed to the understanding of SLE natural history, prognosis, and treatment response are discussed here. This enumeration is by no means a comprehensive list of SLE cohorts, but is a description of cohorts that allows us to highlight different aims, outcomes, geographic regions, and patient populations. Some of the cohorts described as national cohorts may also contribute data to the international cohorts, but, for the sake of simplicity, are handled individually (**Table 1**).

INTERNATIONAL COHORTS
Systemic Lupus Erythematosus International Collaborating Clinics Cohort

The Systemic Lupus Erythematosus International Collaborating Clinics (SLICC) cohort was founded in 1991, serving as a collaboration between providers from Canada, the United Kingdom, Switzerland, and the United States in order to achieve better understanding of the natural history of SLE, SLE disease activity, and SLE-related damage.[18–20] The group subsequently expanded to 42 full-time members deriving from various parts of the world. More than 1300 patients with SLE were included in the cohort. In 1998, the SLICC group established a longitudinal cohort of newly diagnosed patients with lupus (SLICC Inception Cohort) aiming to better understand risk factors for atherosclerosis and metabolic syndrome, and also to better characterize nervous system involvement.[21] Some of the seminal contributions of this cohort have been the development of the SLICC/American College of Rheumatology (ACR) Damage Index for SLE, the SLICC SLE Classification Criteria, and formalizing a definition of disease flare. In addition, ancillary studies based on the SLICC cohort have made significant contributions to the understanding of fertility and pregnancy in patients with SLE. The large, prospective nature of the SLICC cohort has allowed it to

Table 1
Various international, national, single-center, and pediatric lupus cohorts and their major features

Cohort	Centers	Year Established	Design	Patients	Ethnicity	Published Articles[a]	Objectives
International/Multicenter Cohorts							
SLICC	Worldwide	1991	Prospective, longitudinal	>1300	Multiethnic	>60	Classification, severity, and outcomes
Euro-Lupus Cohort	Multicenter, Europe	1991	Prospective, longitudinal	>1000	White	>19	Epidemiology, treatment, outcomes
LUMINA Cohort	Alabama, Texas, Puerto Rico	1994	Prospective, longitudinal	>700	Hispanic, African American, white	92	Disease course in minority
GLADEL Cohort	9 Latin American countries	1997	Prospective, longitudinal	>1500	Mestizo, white, African, Latin American	29	Epidemiology and outcomes in Latin America
PROFILE	Multicenter, United States, Puerto Rico	1998	Longitudinal, prospective	>2322	African American, Hispanic, white	6	Genetic and clinical outcome of patients
APLC	Asia Pacific	2013	Prospective, longitudinal	>2160	Multiethnic	9	Outcome and clinical features
National Cohorts							
Centers for Disease Control and Prevention	California, Georgia, Michigan, New York, Indian American/Alaska Native communities	2002	Longitudinal	200–1000/site	Multiethnic	19	Epidemiology and outcomes

							Clinical phenotype
Hong Kong Cohort	Tuen Mun Hospital, Hong Kong	1997	Retrospective	>1000	Southern China	110	Disease outcome, epidemiology
Portugal	Rheumatology departments throughout Portugal	1976	Retrospective Prospective (2012 onward)	>1200	Multiethnic	24	Disease outcome, epidemiology
Spain (RELESSER)	Rheumatology departments throughout Spain	2011	Prospective	>4000	White	23	Epidemiology and outcomes
Egypt	Single center	1980	Retrospective	>1100	Egyptian	2	Disease outcome, epidemiology
China (CSTAR)	Multicenter	2009	Prospective	>2000	Chinese	11	Disease outcome, epidemiology
1000 Canadian Faces of Lupus	Multicenter, Canada	2005	Cross-sectional	>1000	White, Asian, Afro-Caribbean, Native Canadians	13	Clinical features of adult and pediatric SLE
INSPIRE India	Multicenter, India	2018	Prospective	>1000	Asian Indian	1	Epidemiology
Carolina Lupus Study	Multicenter, United States	1995	Prospective	265	White, African American	20	Disease outcome, epidemiology
Institutional/Single-center Cohorts							
Johns Hopkins Lupus Cohort	Maryland	1985	Prospective	>1500	White, African American	215	Epidemiology, outcome, genetics
Toronto Lupus Database	Toronto, Canada	1970	Prospective	>1500	White	151	Epidemiology and outcomes
Birmingham Lupus Cohort	Birmingham, United Kingdom	1989	Prospective	>380	Multiethnic	26	Disease outcome, epidemiology
University College London Hospitals Lupus Cohort	London, United Kingdom	1975	Prospective	>636	Multiethnic	211	Outcome and clinical features

(continued on next page)

Table 1
(continued)

Cohort	Centers	Year Established	Design	Patients	Ethnicity	Published Articles[a]	Objectives
NIAMS, NIH Lupus cohort	Maryland	1994	Prospective	>1000	Multiethnic	150	Natural history and pathogenesis
UCSF Cohort	California	2002	Prospective	>2000	Multiethnic	15	Genetic association and outcome
Renji Hospital Lupus Database	Shanghai, China	1992	Prospective	>4000	Chinese	32	Clinical phenotype, genetic
Lupus Database of University of Santo Tomas	Manila, Philippines	2000	Retrospective	>350	Filipino	12	Clinical phenotype, outcome
SLEIGH	South Carolina	2003	Retrospective	>700	Gullah/Geechee population in South Carolina	19	Clinical phenotype
Mexico City Cohort	Mexico City, Mexico,	2009	Prospective	>350	Latin American	16	Outcome in pregnant patients with lupus
Lupus Family Registry and Repository	United States	1992	Prospective,	>3500	Multiethnic	>124	Discovery of genetic associations
Pittsburgh Lupus Databank	Pittsburgh, Pennsylvania	1980	Prospective	>1000	Multiethnic	70	Genetics and outcome
CSMC Lupus Cohort	California	1988	Prospective	>2000	Multiethnic	65	Epidemiology, outcomes, and genetics
UNC Glomerular Disease Collaborative Network	North Carolina	1985	Prospective	>2600	Multiethnic	15	Outcomes

Tock Seng Hospital SLE Study Group	Singapore	2002	Prospective	>500	Asian	19	Epidemiology and outcomes
Pediatric Cohorts							
Brazilian childhood-onset SLE group	Multicenter, Brazil	2020	Retrospective	>1500	Brazilian	15	Epidemiology and outcomes
CARRA	Multicenter, North America, Italy, Brazil	2017	Prospective	>1200	Multiethnic	80	Epidemiology and outcomes

Abbreviations: APLC, Asia Pacific Lupus Collaboration; CARRA, Childhood Arthritis and Rheumatology Research Alliance; CSMC, Cedar-Saini Medical Center; CSTAR, Chinese SLE Treatment and Research; GLADEL, Grupo Latinoamericano de Estudia del Lupus; INSPIRE, Indian SLE Inception Cohort for Research; LUMINA, Lupus in Minorities: Nature vs Nurture; NIAMS, National Institute for Arthritis and Musculoskeletal Disease and Skin; NIH, National Institutes of Health; RELESSER, SLE Registry of the Spanish Society of Rheumatology; SLEIGH, SLE in Gullah Health; SLICC, SLE International Collaborating Clinics; UCSF, University of California, San Francisco; UNC, University of North Carolina.

[a] Tabulating cohort publications: the primary investigators were identified for each cohort through review of cohort publications. All publications from these primary investigators were then reviewed through PubMed, and those publications using the cohort for demographic, clinical, or laboratory data were included in the publication count. Studies where cohort data were used as part of a multicenter cohort were only counted toward the multicenter cohort. In cohorts with multiple primary investigators, such as the SLICC cohort and Lupus Family Registry and Repository, multiple searches were completed to identify a minimum number of publications, identified as greater than x=1, x being the number of publications.

make invaluable contributions to the understanding of lupus as a whole. However, as with any large cohort, the ability to make broad general comments may come at the cost of identifying unique features of lupus limited to particular regions, races, or ethnicities.

Euro-Lupus Project Cohort

The prospective study of the epidemiology, natural history, and long-term evaluation of SLE in the European population, also known as the Euro-Lupus Project cohort, was established in 1991. The project included 12 university centers from Spain, United Kingdom, Italy, Poland, Turkey, Norway, and Belgium.[22] Initial data from 1000 patients with SLE showed similarities to other cohorts such as a significant female predominance and an average age of onset at 31 years old.[22] In addition, the data from this cohort revealed that symptoms such as malar rash, renal disease, and arthritis were more prevalent in childhood-onset SLE but that this prevalence decreased with age. It also confirmed that different extractable nuclear antigen antibodies were associated with unique clinical profiles.[23]

The large size and prospective nature of this cohort allowed researchers to study multiple variables, including treatment comparisons via nested RCTs. Most notably, the Euro-Lupus nephritis trial of induction therapy randomly assigned 90 patients with class III, IV, or VI lupus nephritis to receive either high-dose monthly intravenous cyclophosphamide over 6 months or low-dose intravenous cyclophosphamide every 2 weeks over 3 months. No difference in primary treatment failure (the primary end point), glucocorticoid reduction, kidney remission, or renal failure was seen.[24] In addition, 10-year follow-up after patients were put on azathioprine for purposes of maintenance therapy showed encouraging outcomes compared with low-dose intravenous cyclophosphamide.[25] In short, the Euro-Lupus Project is an example of a large prospective cohort capitalizing on the breadth of data and flexibility for additional studies that may be found in such a study design.

Lupus in Minorities: Nature Versus Nurture Cohort

The Lupus in Minorities: Nature Versus Nurture (LUMINA) cohort was a prospective cohort established in 1994 specifically to study the effects of genetics, social demographics, and behavior on racial and ethnic minority patients with SLE in the United States.[26] Patients with early onset SLE (defined as diagnosis <5 years before enrollment) were recruited from the southern continental United States, particularly Alabama and Texas, along with Puerto Rico. Genetic analysis showed that human leukocyte antigen alleles associated with higher SLE disease activity seen in black patients were also more prevalent in Hispanic patients from Texas as opposed to those from Puerto Rico. However, being a Hispanic patient from Texas was itself also an independent risk factor for increased disease activity, cyclophosphamide use, and higher daily dose of corticosteroids.[27] Taken together, this suggests that, for Hispanic patients in the United States, both genetics and disparities in access to care likely contribute to worse SLE outcomes. The LUMINA cohort is an example of how the balance of racial and ethnic diversity can be used to determine the impact of multiple variables on disease outcomes. Going 1 step further, other cohorts have subdivided those patients identified as Hispanic into more specific categories based on their ancestry, in order to better elucidate the genetic component to SLE in this population.

Grupo Latinoamericano de Estudia del Lupus Cohort

In 1991, rheumatology providers from Argentina, Brazil, Columbia, Cuba, Chile, Guatemala, Mexico, Peru, and Venezuela created a cohort of patients meeting the

ACR SLE classification criteria. Demographic, socioeconomic, clinical, and laboratory data for more than 1000 patients were collected from 34 referral clinics throughout the countries mentioned earlier.[28] Patients from the cohort were divided into white (European ancestry), Mestizo (Amerindian and white ancestry), African–Latin American (Latin and African ancestry), and Amerindian. The data from the Grupo Latinoamericano de Estudia del Lupus (GLADEL) cohort showed both nonwhite groups and those with lower education had higher mortality, incidence of renal disease, and damage accrual.[28] Although previous groups have evaluated Latin American patients with SLE as a single group, results from GLADEL cohort established for the first time that there is significant heterogeneity among patients with SLE from this region. GLADEL shows that, although it is not possible to make generalized statements regarding SLE, regional cohorts play an important role in identifying the heterogeneity that exists within the SLE population.

Asia Pacific Lupus Collaboration Cohort

The Asia Pacific Lupus Collaboration (APLC) was formed in 2012 and comprises 23 sites in 13 countries.[29] It constitutes 2160 patients with lupus with greater than 12,000 visits. Data are collected using a standardized case report form. One of the major contributions from this cohort is the development and validation of lupus low disease activity state (LLDAS) criteria and their association with health-related quality of life. Although a relatively new cohort with few longitudinal data, further long-term observations from this cohort are expected to provide prospective evaluation of LLDAS and its association with damage accrual.

NATIONAL COHORTS
Centers for Disease Control and Prevention Lupus Registries

In order to accurately monitor SLE disease in diverse geographic regions of United States, the Centers for Disease Control and Prevention (CDC) funded 5 regional lupus registries for SLE and primary cutaneous lupus.[30] The primary focus of these registries was to determine ethnic and racial differences in incidence, prevalence, and severity of SLE in their respective regions. The 5 registries were established in specific regions of California, Georgia, Michigan, New York, and the Indian Health Service. Cases were identified using hospital databases, physician office records, laboratory data, and population databases situated in these regions.

The California Lupus Surveillance Project (CLSP) studied 724 patients with SLE residing in San Francisco County, California, from 2007 to 2009. This cohort was unique in its significant representation of Asian/Pacific Islander patients with SLE living in the United States. In the CLSP cohort, African Americans, Asian/Pacific Islanders, and Hispanic patients had increased prevalence of lupus nephritis, and the African American patients manifested increased neurologic and hematologic complications.[31]

The Georgians Organized Against Lupus (GOAL) was a cohort of more than 1000 mostly African American patients with SLE and chronic cutaneous lupus from the Fulton and DeKalb counties, Georgia. Research from the GOAL cohort showed that African Americans with SLE are at an increased risk of depression, poor medication adherence, and increased mortality.[32] Patient surveys further showed that up to 80% of the African American patients with SLE in the GOAL cohort reported experiencing racism, which itself was associated with greater lupus disease activity.[33] The data from the GOAL cohort provided powerful insights into the impact of social determinants on lupus.[34]

The Michigan Lupus Epidemiology and Surveillance (MILES) cohort consists of 2278 patients with SLE residing in Wayne or Washtenaw Counties and observed from 2002 to 2004.[30] Research from this cohort showed a higher prevalence of SLE in black patients in general (2.3-fold higher than white) and a prevalence of 1 in 537 among black women, specifically. The study further established racial disparity in the burden of SLE. Black patients experience earlier age of diagnosis and increased proportions of renal disease and progression to ESRD compared with white patients.[35] The studies from this cohort also identified that diets high in omega-3 fatty acids are protective against self-reported lupus activity, that a high rate of cost-related medication nonadherence may be found in patients with lupus, and that laboratory patterns may help differentiate flare versus infection.[36–38]

The Manhattan Lupus Surveillance Program (MLSP) was a registry of 1854 patients with lupus living in New York County, New York, from 2007 to 2009.[39] The data from MLSP again revealed that the incidence and prevalence of lupus were highest among black women, followed by Hispanic and Asian patients.[39,40] Data on primary discoid lupus also showed a higher prevalence in black and Hispanic women compared with other racial and ethnic groups.[41] The Indian Health Service (IHS) Lupus Registry comprised 304 individuals with SLE residing in 1 of the 3 IHS active clinical catchments from 2007 to 2009. The age-adjusted prevalence and incidence of SLE was 178 per 100,000 person-years and 7.4 per 100,000 person-years.[42] The prevalence was highest in women aged 50 to 59 years and in patients from the Phoenix Area IHS. The age-adjusted prevalence of SLE in American Indian/Alaska Native women (271 per 100,000) from the IHS Lupus Registry was similar or higher than that in black women.[42] The IHS Lupus Registry for the first time revealed interesting insights into the clinical phenotype of the indigenous North American people. Specifically, the 3 most common ACR classification criteria met by the cases in this registry were antinuclear antibody positivity (98.2%), hematologic disorder (89.8%), and arthritis (80.4%). Discoid rash and neurologic disorders were the least common criteria met. Similar to black patients with SLE, renal disorder was present in close to 40% of patients. Furthermore, the American Indian and Alaskan Native patients with SLE were more likely to be diagnosed and managed by their primary care providers, highlighting the need for enhanced access to specialist care in these communities.[43]

By using 5 different cohorts throughout the United States, the CDC was able to identify general trends and variations in symptoms of the different racial and ethnic groups that encompass the US SLE population. Although these cohorts did have short study times, they have inspired many retrospective and further prospective cohort studies of SLE in the United States.

Hong Kong Lupus Cohort

The Hong Kong Lupus cohort was established in 1995 and includes more than 1000 patients with lupus. Data from this cohort showed that patients with SLE had a significantly reduced life expectancy, increased risk of depression, and increased incidence of disability compared with the general population.[44] More recent data from the cohort showed that patients diagnosed with lupus between 2005 and 2018 had significantly improved 5-year and 10-year cumulative survival rates compared with patients diagnosed between 1995 and 2004, in part because of lower organ damage accrual.[45] Although reliance on provider-reported outcomes and diagnostic codes can affect the quality of cohort data, the relatively all-inclusive nature of this cohort provided an excellent depiction of SLE in Hong Kong over several decades.

Portugal Lupus Cohort

In 2012, the Portuguese Society of Rheumatology started a longitudinal registry to understand the natural history of SLE in Portugal. A total of 1296 mostly female patients between the ages of 20 and 40 years were enrolled over a period of 1 year.[46] Although the short inclusion period may have limited the cohort's ability to comment on the changing characteristics of SLE, it also limited confounding from changes in community standard of care over time. The most frequent clinical features of SLE of this mostly white cohort were musculoskeletal (91%), cutaneous and mucous membrane (90%), and hematological (58%). Myositis was more common in black patients and renal disease and serositis occurred more often in men in this cohort.[47]

Spanish Society of Rheumatology Systemic Lupus Erythematosus Registry

The Spanish Society of Rheumatology SLE Registry (RELESSER) is a multicenter, hospital-based registry of patients with SLE. The registry included more than 4000 patients from 45 centers and consists of 2 phases: a transversal phase (RELESSER-T) to describe sociodemographic, clinical, and laboratory characteristics of patients with SLE and incomplete SLE; and a longitudinal prospective study on a selected sample of patients included in the initial cohort (RELESSER-PROS) to answer different research questions.[48] The data from RELESSER-T suggest that patients with incomplete SLE (meeting <4 ACR classification criteria) have stable, mild disease.[49] As the largest registry of European patients with lupus, the RELESSER cohort is able to use subsets of its patients to answer multiple questions regarding SLE. RELESSER continues to be a source of robust data about differences between various subsets of patients with lupus.[50,51]

Egyptian Lupus Cohorts

Although some nations use a large, centralized cohort to describe their patients with lupus, multiple lupus cohorts have been used to describe patients in Egypt. One of the largest cohorts concerns 1109 patients with SLE who presented to an outpatient clinic over 35 years. Data from this cohort revealed that arthritis (76.7%) and malar rash (48.5%) were the most common clinical manifestations, followed by renal involvement (33.1%).[52] Another single-center study out of Egypt showed patients with juvenile-onset SLE with higher disease activity and a more aggressive disease course compared with their adult counterparts.[53] A recent study of a cohort of 569 patients with SLE from 3 centers in Egypt highlighted clinical characteristics and damage accrual.[54] This cohort reported alopecia as the most common clinical manifestation (76.1%), along with a notably higher rate of nephritis (65.7%).

Chinese Systemic Lupus Erythematosus Treatment and Research Group Registry

Founded in 2009, the Chinese SLE Treatment and Research (CSTAR) cohort consists of 104 rheumatology centers in 30 provinces in China with 2104 patients with SLE. All CSTAR centers used the same methods to collect demographic data, clinical features, laboratory examination, and disease activity indices. Furthermore, patient samples, including DNA samples and serum, are stored in a biobank for future studies. The data from the CSTAR cohort identify some clinical features unique to Chinese patients with lupus, such as higher incidence of hematologic (56.1%) and renal involvement (47.4%) and lower incidence of neurologic manifestations (4.8%) compared with similar-sized European cohorts.[55] Initial quality-control issues with providers incorporating disease activity indices have improved over time, and the data from CSTAR registry continue to provide significant insights into prevalence of various clinical manifestations of lupus as well as the effect of gender on the phenotypes of Chinese patients with SLE.[56–58]

INSTITUTIONAL
Johns Hopkins Lupus Cohort

Established in 1987, the Hopkins Lupus Cohort started with 185 patients with SLE receiving care at Johns Hopkins University in Baltimore, Maryland. Over the past 3 decades, the Hopkins Lupus Cohort has grown to more than 2000 participants. It comprises 56% white and 36% African American patients.[59] Data from this cohort showed that advanced age, lower income, lower education, hypertension, and positive lupus anticoagulant were all associated with higher SLE Damage Index (SDI) scores.[60] Studies from the Hopkins Cohort have also highlighted disparities in disease trajectories by showing that African American patients take longer to achieve low disease activity.[61] Other studies from this institution have validated disease activity measures such as the SLE Disease Activity Index for assessing end-organ damage and mortality in patients with SLE.[62]

The large size and consistency of follow-up for the patient population in the Johns Hopkins Lupus Cohort has made it an invaluable source of information for determinants of long-term patient outcomes. However, the lack of significant Hispanic or Asian patients within the Hopkins Lupus Cohort may lead to limitations for purposes of the ability to generalize their data.[59]

University of Toronto Lupus Clinic Cohort

The University of Toronto Lupus Clinic Cohort is one of the oldest databases of patients with lupus in the world, following patients prospectively, and according to a standard protocol, since 1970.[63] The cohort started with 110 patients and has grown to more than 1700 patients. The coordinators of the Toronto Lupus Clinic Cohort have noted that the observational nature of this cohort renders it vulnerable to confounding variables and associations.[63] In spite of these obstacles, this cohort has made several seminal observations, including the bimodal mortality pattern of SLE, the recognition that patients with SLE are at risk for accelerated atherosclerosis, and the description of a subset of patients with serologically active but clinically quiescent lupus. Data from this cohort have shown that increased SLEDAI, steroid use, and immunosuppressants use at the time of enrollment are associated with greater organ damage.[64] Other studies from this cohort have identified risk factors (poor medication compliance, thrombotic microangiopathy, and concentric anti-Glomerular Basement Membrane nephropathy) for rapid-onset ESRD and that menopause is not associated with significant improvement in symptoms.[65–67]

Birmingham Systemic Lupus Erythematosus Cohort

Established in 1989, there are more than 380 patients in The Birmingham Lupus Cohort followed regularly with prospective data collection concerning the British Isles Lupus Assessment Group index, treatment, and damage (as measured by the SDI). The data from this cohort showed that patients with SLE had an increased mortality, with the most common cause of death being infection, followed by cardiovascular disease and malignancy. The damage accrual rate was lower than for the Hopkins Lupus Cohort, and exposure to cyclophosphamide and glucocorticoids was associated with damage accrual. Interestingly, ethnicity in this cohort was not predictive of damage accrual. This finding is perhaps caused by the national health care system, which provides equal access to everyone.[68]

University College London Lupus Cohort

The study cohort consists of patients attending the Lupus Clinic of University College Hospital London, with follow-up extending up to 40 years. The data from this cohort provide significant insights into predictors of damage accrual, mortality, longitudinal outcomes in lupus nephritis, the impact of thrombocytopenia on SLE outcomes, and immune phenotypes in juvenile SLE.[69–72] Similar to other cohorts, data from this cohort also showed that use of high-dose steroids and immunosuppressives early in the disease course is associated with poorer outcomes. Surprisingly, the use of hydroxychloroquine was not found to be protective against disease damage.

National Institute of Arthritis and Musculoskeletal and Skin Disease Lupus Cohort

The National Institute of Arthritis and Musculoskeletal and Skin Disease (NIAMS) lupus cohort at the National Institutes of Health (NIH) in Bethesda, Maryland, was formally established in 1994 as part of a pathogenesis and natural history of SLE protocol. There are more than 1000 patients in this cohort, who are followed longitudinally and at regular intervals. Data regarding disease manifestations, medications, comorbidities, and laboratory test results are routinely collected. Disease activity and damage indices are calculated, and patient-reported outcomes and research samples for biobank are collected. The strength of the cohort is the well-phenotyped data that are longitudinal and linked to a stored biospecimen repository, and all codified within a research database. The cohort is ethnically diverse, with more than 25% African American and 18% Hispanic patients. One weakness of this cohort is that the patients typically have more severe disease or have failed initial treatment.

Discoveries made through this cohort resulted in several early-phase proof-of-concept clinical trials. More than 150 publications have resulted from this effort. An offshoot of this protocol has been an ongoing thrust to understand premature vascular atherosclerosis in these patients by virtue of longitudinal multimodal vascular assessment. An outcome of this project has been an appreciation of the role of low-density granulocyte and neutrophil extracellular traps in vascular inflammation and coronary atherosclerosis.[73] In addition, with an aim to determine genetic factors for early onset and for severe SLE, another subset of patients in this cohort is undergoing whole-exome sequencing.

PEDIATRIC LUPUS COHORTS

Childhood-onset lupus represents less than 10% of the total lupus population. Pediatric patients with SLE have clinical and biological features that differ from adult patients, which underscores the need for dedicated pediatric SLE cohorts.

Brazilian Childhood-Onset Systemic Lupus Erythematosus Group Cohort

This multicenter observational cohort of 27 pediatric rheumatology university centers in Brazil includes 1519 patients with childhood SLE.[74,75] This cohort showed that patients diagnosed with SLE before the age of 6 years had more organ system involvement, higher disease activity indices, and higher mortality.[74] Later studies showed that patients with positive double stranded DNA, low C3 level, and proteinuria were all associated with early-onset lupus nephritis, worse morbidity, and higher mortality.[76] Another study from this cohort showed that childhood-onset SLE-related antiphospholipid syndrome is a rare condition, present in only 4% of patients; however, when present, it is associated with a high damage accrual.[75] By virtue of being one of the largest cohorts of pediatric patients with lupus, this cohort has provided unique insights into the characteristics of pediatric SLE. In contrast, the data from this cohort are from a single nation. Hence, the ability to generalize may be limited.

Childhood Arthritis and Rheumatology Research Alliance

The Childhood Arthritis and Rheumatology Research Alliance (CARRA) was founded in 2002 as an investigator-led collaborative research network seeking to pool resources and create meaningful contributions to research on rare pediatric rheumatic diseases. CARRA has continued to grow, and now includes 72 different registry sites, predominantly in North America but with 1 site in Italy and another in Israel. CARRA began collecting information on SLE in March 2017. The registry has collected observational data regarding clinical manifestations, treatments, and outcomes in pediatric SLE, in addition to the collection of biospecimens. To date, the CARRA group members have more than 80 publications on SLE, including consensus treatment plans for lupus nephritis, predictors of disability in pediatric SLE, and randomized placebo-controlled trials on the use of atorvastatin.[77–79] As with most cohorts, the CARRA registry is vulnerable to selection bias. Nevertheless, it is a good example of the breadth of data and projects that are attainable when providers work together to enhance the understanding of rare rheumatic conditions.

Social Media and Lupus Cohorts

Social media platforms have hundreds of millions of subscribers and provide an easily accessible way to reach a larger population of individuals with rare diseases such as SLE. For example, online surveys have been used to study SLE in the United Kingdom to assess the impact of SLE on patients and their caretakers.[80] In another example, online surveys from the Lupus Foundation identified patients on supratherapeutic doses of hydroxychloroquine.[81] At the same time, there are multiple lupus apps available for download to portable devices, mostly focused on helping patients better manage their symptoms and with a few focused on collecting patient-reported outcomes and enrolling patients in lupus clinical research.[82,83] These studies have shown that social media are able to reach a large number of patients, allow open-ended answers, require a minimal time commitment, and allow anonymity, which may make patients more forthcoming. However, these studies also highlight some of the downsides of social media, including reliance on unverifiable patient-provided information, lack of longitudinal follow-up, self-selected study populations, and various reporter biases, such as those based on a priori perceptions about disease and/or the topic under study.

Coronavirus Disease 2019 Global Rheumatology Alliance Registry

Health care providers worldwide have responded to the severe acute respiratory syndrome coronavirus-2 (SARS-CoV2) pandemic by joining forces to deliver fast and effective means of monitoring, treating, and preventing coronavirus disease 2019 (COVID-19) infection. The rheumatology community responded in kind, creating the COVID-19 Global Rheumatology Alliance (GRA). The GRA is unique among rheumatology registries or cohorts in both the manner and time frame in which it was established. The initial impetus for GRA, which was started on social media and communication platforms, was to spotlight the lack of data regarding COVID-19 in rheumatology patients. It is on these platforms that providers proposed a deidentified survey for the purpose of data collection. Within 2 months, the registry parameters were established, the protocol was approved by more than 300 international organizations, and enrollment commenced after more than 30 sites obtained ethical approval for data submission.[84] The GRA collects online data from the providers and patients regarding their experiences with SARS-CoV2 and rheumatic disease. As of December 1, 2020, there are data entered for 788 (20%) patients with SLE with COVID-19 in the registry. Data from the GRA have highlighted the use of 10 mg/d or more of prednisone, with higher rates of hospitalization and tumor necrosis factor inhibitor use associated with a decreased risk of hospitalization in patients with rheumatic disease.[85] Although this is not an SLE-specific cohort, per se, it exemplifies how the global rheumatology community can amass valuable data in a short period of time.

Steps to Establish a Systemic Lupus Erythematosus Cohort

The cohorts discussed earlier show the diversity of data that may be obtained through various types of cohort study design.

For researchers interested in establishing a cohort, the differences in approach to establishing a cohort may make starting such a project seem daunting. However, there are some underlying common principles that may help guide the development of such a project (**Fig. 1**). For more detailed information on planning a registry or cohort, the authors suggest the guide developed by US Agency for Healthcare Research and Quality.[86,87]

1. The initial step in establishing a cohort or patient registry is to articulate a specific aim or purpose. In some cases, the purpose of a cohort may be a specific research hypothesis, but often the purpose of a cohort is broad; namely, to understand the natural history of disease by capturing data about prognosis, quality of life, and patient outcomes.[87] Cohorts designed with a specific research question in mind may have a short duration, such as months to years, whereas those focused on natural history or prognosis may take decades to achieve their aims.[77]
2. The next steps are to identify key stakeholders, build a registry team, and establish an oversight plan. It is important to identify the key stakeholders at an early stage so as to incorporate their input into the type and scope of data to be collected. The registry team requires a variety of individuals with different kinds of knowledge and skills, such as project management, subject matter experts, database management, biostatistics, patient privacy, and quality assurance. Establishment of an oversight plan helps with financial and legal concerns, data access, and publications.
3. The final steps in establishing a cohort are defining the core datasets, identifying the target population, and developing a study plan or protocol. The information set needed to address the specific aim of the registry defines the core dataset variables to be collected through the registry. However, it is also useful to add noncore variables to answer any future research questions. Defining the target population is the foundation for planning the registry because they will be affected by the results. The inclusion criteria for a cohort are usually broad so as to enable generalization of results to a larger population. The study plan or protocol should include the objectives of the registry, outcomes of interest, eligibility criteria, data collection procedures, and plans for ethical obligations, especially patient privacy.
4. Often overlooked in the development and planning is a marketing strategy for securing patient enrollees, community trust building in order to remove cultural barriers to research participation, addressing financial and technological barriers to participation, and giving back to the study group participants.
5. When designing a cohort study, it is essential to consider issues such as the expected rate of study attrition (and strategies to preserve study subject engagement), handling of incomplete data, and identifying confounding variables.

Strength and Limitations of Cohort Studies

The most important strength of prospective cohort studies is the accuracy of their data concerning exposures, confounders, and outcomes (**Table 2**). This type of design is

Initial steps

- Description of the purpose of the cohort
- Is a cohort study the right method for this objective (ie, to evaluate whether a cohort is a convenient way to achieve the scientific objectives)?
- Identification of primary and secondary stakeholders
- Evaluation of the feasibility of a cohort,

Next steps

- Establish a registry team
- Define decision-making system, concept, execution, and reporting of results
- Scope of data and scientific rigor

Final steps

- Description of core dataset, outcomes, and study population
- Writing a research plan or study protocol
- End of the cohort and study closeout (if necessary)

Fig. 1. Steps for establishing a cohort.

expensive and time consuming owing to long follow-up.[15] Another positive aspect of the cohort study design is the ability to investigate multiple exposures and outcomes. Cohort studies are also positioned to observe rare clinical events and to follow groups with rare diseases longitudinally. Compared with RCTs, the cohort-based studies generally have less strict inclusion and exclusion criteria and thus are able to represent a broad patient population, often representative of patients who are seen in routine clinical practice. Therefore, they may provide more generalizable knowledge and may be more applicable to real-life scenarios.[3]

Table 2
Strength and weakness of cohorts

Strength	Weakness
• Shows a full spectrum of the disease, and real-life experience • Shows response to new therapies, may identify the most cost-effective treatment • Includes large number and diverse patient population • Longer follow-up • Enables real-time safety and effectiveness data • May determine very rare subtypes, events, or complications • Study design may be quick and inexpensive • Many outcomes may be studied concomitantly	• Expensive to design and maintain • Uniformity of data, especially in multicenter cohorts • Nonrandomized groups with possibility of selection bias and unmeasured confounders • Real-life dose adjustment may be a problem for comparison • Incomplete data collection at certain time intervals • Nonrandom loss to follow-up can significantly affect outcomes • Lack of uniform therapeutic and diagnostic approaches between centers in multicenter studies

Perhaps, the most important advantage of cohort studies is their longitudinal follow-up and data collection.[88] By following patients at regular intervals, this allows measurement of outcomes and evaluation of prognostic factors that may change over time. Cohort studies provide valuable information to analyze differences between treatment modalities in SLE in the long term and are useful for the development of diagnostic and prognostic biomarkers.[15] Studies based on various lupus cohorts have revealed that patients with SLE develop premature cardiovascular disease. Cohorts also help determine the effects of comorbidities on lupus outcomes. In addition, the importance of patient-reported outcome, quality of life, cognitive dysfunction, and the role of psychological and social factors in SLE have been better recognized in recent years all because of data from observational cohorts.[15]

Some of the limitations of cohort studies derive from susceptibility to selection bias as well as the potential for unmeasured confounders that in turn may overwhelm treatment effects because of lack of randomization.[8] The results of cohort studies carry risk of bias caused by inhomogeneous treatment groups because treatment decision is based on clinical judgment rather than predefined criteria. Another problem in cohort design is the potential for censored data caused by lost-to-follow-up patients, which may not be random.[8] This situation may necessitate the use of statistical methods to handle truncated or censored data in longitudinal datasets. Data quality is another potential problem in cohorts, and the long-term maintenance of high-quality data collection and recording is labor intensive and complex.[6] Another potential weakness of cohorts is heterogeneity of diagnostic and therapeutic approaches, especially in multicenter cohorts.[89] A recent consortium (MASTERPLANS) focused on data harmonization and integration of different SLE cohorts. They published their experiences tackling large, heterogenous datasets.[90]

In conclusion, real-life experience, greater power for the detection of rare events, the ability to simultaneously study many research questions, and the ability to generate observations of multiple outcomes are strengths of cohort studies. Together, these assets of the cohort design promise an enriched perspective of a complex disease.[14,91] A well-planned and organized cohort can be a valuable source of knowledge to understand and improve outcomes in chronic diseases such as SLE.

CLINICS CARE POINTS

- Lupus Cohorts provide a full spectrum of disease in a real-life clinical setting.
- Includes a large diverse population with long term follow-up.
- Several outcomes can be studied simultaneously.
- Cohorts are expensive, time consuming to establish and maintain.
- Incomplete data collection, selection bias, and unmeasured confounders may make it difficult to interpret the data.

DISCLOSURE

This research was supported by the Intramural Research Program of the National Institute of Arthritis and Musculoskeletal and Skin Diseases of the NIH.

REFERENCES

1. Dorner T, Furie R. Novel paradigms in systemic lupus erythematosus. Lancet 2019;393(10188):2344–58.
2. Gordon C, Amissah-Arthur MB, Gayed M, et al. The British Society for Rheumatology guideline for the management of systemic lupus erythematosus in adults. Rheumatology (Oxford) 2018;57(1):e1–45.
3. Villa-Blanco I, Calvo-Alen J. Utilizing registries in systemic lupus erythematosus clinical research. Expert Rev Clin Immunol 2012;8(4):353–60.
4. Patient cohort. Secondary patient cohort. 2009. Available at: https://medical-dictionary.thefreedictionary.com/patient+cohort. Accessed January 7, 2021.
5. Brooke EM, World Health O. The current and future use of registers in health information systems/Eileen M. Brooke. Geneva (Switzerland): World Health Organization; 1974.
6. Camm AJ, Fox KAA. Strengths and weaknesses of 'real-world' studies involving non-vitamin K antagonist oral anticoagulants. Open Heart 2018;5(1):e000788.
7. Brown ML, Gersh BJ, Holmes DR, et al. From randomized trials to registry studies: translating data into clinical information. Nat Clin Pract Cardiovasc Med 2008;5(10):613–20.
8. Euser AM, Zoccali C, Jager KJ, et al. Cohort studies: prospective versus retrospective. Nephron Clin Pract 2009;113(3):c214–7.
9. Vandenbroucke JP. Observational research, randomised trials, and two views of medical science. PLoS Med 2008;5(3):e67.
10. Garrison LP Jr, Neumann PJ, Erickson P, et al. Using real-world data for coverage and payment decisions: the ISPOR Real-World Data Task Force report. Value Health 2007;10(5):326–35.
11. Serris A, Amoura Z, Canoui-Poitrine F, et al. Efficacy and safety of rituximab for systemic lupus erythematosus-associated immune cytopenias: a multicenter retrospective cohort study of 71 adults. Am J Hematol 2018;93(3):424–9.
12. Quelhas da Costa R, Aguirre-Alastuey ME, Isenberg DA, et al. Assessment of response to B-cell depletion using rituximab in cutaneous lupus erythematosus. JAMA Dermatol 2018;154(12):1432–40.
13. Kronbichler A, Brezina B, Gauckler P, et al. Refractory lupus nephritis: when, why and how to treat. Autoimmun Rev 2019;18(5):510–8.

14. Pombo-Suarez M, Gomez-Reino J. The role of registries in the treatment of rheumatoid arthritis with biologic disease-modifying anti-rheumatic drugs. Pharmacol Res 2019;148:104410.

15. Lu LJ, Wallace DJ, Navarra SV, et al. Lupus registries: evolution and challenges. Semin Arthritis Rheum 2010;39(4):224-45.

16. Urowitz MB, Gladman DD. Contributions of observational cohort studies in systemic lupus erythematosus: the university of toronto lupus clinic experience. Rheum Dis Clin North Am 2005;31(2):211-21, v.

17. Petri M. Lupus in Baltimore: evidence-based 'clinical pearls' from the Hopkins Lupus Cohort. Lupus 2005;14(12):970-3.

18. Petri M, Orbai AM, Alarcon GS, et al. Derivation and validation of the Systemic Lupus International Collaborating Clinics classification criteria for systemic lupus erythematosus. Arthritis Rheum 2012;64(8):2677-86.

19. Ehrenstein MR, Conroy SE, Heath J, et al. The occurrence, nature and distribution of flares in a cohort of patients with systemic lupus erythematosus: a rheumatological view. Br J Rheumatol 1995;34(3):257-60.

20. Gladman D, Ginzler E, Goldsmith C, et al. The development and initial validation of the Systemic Lupus International Collaborating Clinics/American College of Rheumatology damage index for systemic lupus erythematosus. Arthritis Rheum 1996;39(3):363-9.

21. Ines L, Rodrigues M, Jesus D, et al. Risk of damage and mortality in SLE patients fulfilling the ACR or only the SLICC classification criteria. A 10-year, inception cohort study. Lupus 2018;27(4):556-63.

22. Cervera R, Khamashta MA, Font J, et al. Systemic lupus erythematosus: clinical and immunologic patterns of disease expression in a cohort of 1,000 patients. The European Working Party on Systemic Lupus Erythematosus. Medicine (Baltimore) 1993;72(2):113-24.

23. Cervera R, Khamashta MA, Hughes GR. The Euro-lupus project: epidemiology of systemic lupus erythematosus in Europe. Lupus 2009;18(10):869-74.

24. Houssiau FA, Vasconcelos C, D'Cruz D, et al. Immunosuppressive therapy in lupus nephritis: the Euro-Lupus Nephritis Trial, a randomized trial of low-dose versus high-dose intravenous cyclophosphamide. Arthritis Rheum 2002;46(8):2121-31.

25. Houssiau FA, Vasconcelos C, D'Cruz D, et al. The 10-year follow-up data of the Euro-Lupus Nephritis Trial comparing low-dose and high-dose intravenous cyclophosphamide. Ann Rheum Dis 2010;69(1):61-4.

26. Reveille JD, Moulds JM, Ahn C, et al. Systemic lupus erythematosus in three ethnic groups: I. The effects of HLA class II, C4, and CR1 alleles, socioeconomic factors, and ethnicity at disease onset. LUMINA Study Group. Lupus in minority populations, nature versus nurture. Arthritis Rheum 1998;41(7):1161-72.

27. Uribe AG, McGwin G Jr, Reveille JD, et al. What have we learned from a 10-year experience with the LUMINA (Lupus in Minorities; Nature vs. nurture) cohort? Where are we heading? Autoimmun Rev 2004;3(4):321-9.

28. Pons-Estel BA, Catoggio LJ, Cardiel MH, et al. The GLADEL multinational Latin American prospective inception cohort of 1,214 patients with systemic lupus erythematosus: ethnic and disease heterogeneity among "Hispanics". Medicine (Baltimore) 2004;83(1):1-17.

29. Kandane-Rathnayake R, Golder V, Louthrenoo W, et al. Development of the Asia Pacific Lupus Collaboration cohort. Int J Rheum Dis 2019;22(3):425-33.

30. Drenkard C, Lim SS. Update on lupus epidemiology: advancing health disparities research through the study of minority populations. Curr Opin Rheumatol 2019; 31(6):689–96.

31. Maningding E, Dall'Era M, Trupin L, et al. Racial and ethnic differences in the prevalence and time to onset of manifestations of systemic lupus erythematosus: the California Lupus Surveillance Project. Arthritis Care Res (Hoboken) 2020; 72(5):622–9.

32. Heiman E, Lim SS, Bao G, et al. Depressive symptoms are associated with low treatment adherence in African American individuals with systemic lupus erythematosus. J Clin Rheumatol 2018;24(7):368–74.

33. Martz CD, Allen AM, Fuller-Rowell TE, et al. Vicarious racism stress and disease activity: the Black Women's Experiences Living with Lupus (BeWELL) study. J Racial Ethn Health Disparities 2019;6(5):1044–51.

34. Lim SS, Drenkard C. Understanding lupus disparities through a social determinants of health framework: the georgians organized against lupus research cohort. Rheum Dis Clin North Am 2020;46(4):613–21.

35. Somers EC, Marder W, Cagnoli P, et al. Population-based incidence and prevalence of systemic lupus erythematosus: the Michigan Lupus Epidemiology and Surveillance program. Arthritis Rheumatol 2014;66(2):369–78.

36. Charoenwoodhipong P, Harlow SD, Marder W, et al. Dietary omega polyunsaturated fatty acid intake and patient-reported outcomes in systemic lupus erythematosus: The Michigan Lupus Epidemiology and Surveillance Program. Arthritis Care Res (Hoboken) 2020;72(7):874–81.

37. Minhas D, Marder W, Harlow S, et al. Access and cost-related non-adherence to prescription medications among lupus cases and controls: the Michigan Lupus Epidemiology & Surveillance (MILES) Program. Arthritis Care Res (Hoboken) 2020. https://doi.org/10.1002/acr.24397.

38. Littlejohn E, Marder W, Lewis E, et al. The ratio of erythrocyte sedimentation rate to C-reactive protein is useful in distinguishing infection from flare in systemic lupus erythematosus patients presenting with fever. Lupus 2018;27(7):1123–9.

39. Izmirly PM, Wan I, Sahl S, et al. The incidence and prevalence of systemic lupus erythematosus in New York County (Manhattan), New York: The Manhattan Lupus Surveillance Program. Arthritis Rheumatol 2017;69(10):2006–17.

40. Izmirly PM, Buyon JP, Wan I, et al. The incidence and prevalence of adult primary Sjogren's Syndrome in New York County. Arthritis Care Res (Hoboken) 2019; 71(7):949–60.

41. Izmirly P, Buyon J, Belmont HM, et al. Population-based prevalence and incidence estimates of primary discoid lupus erythematosus from the Manhattan Lupus Surveillance Program. Lupus Sci Med 2019;6(1):e000344.

42. Ferucci ED, Johnston JM, Gaddy JR, et al. Prevalence and incidence of systemic lupus erythematosus in a population-based registry of American Indian and Alaska Native people, 2007-2009. Arthritis Rheumatol 2014;66(9):2494–502.

43. McDougall JA, Helmick CG, Lim SS, et al. Differences in the diagnosis and management of systemic lupus erythematosus by primary care and specialist providers in the American Indian/Alaska Native population. Lupus 2018;27(7): 1169–76.

44. Mok CC. Epidemiology and survival of systemic lupus erythematosus in Hong Kong Chinese. Lupus 2011;20(7):767–71.

45. Mok CC, Ho LY, Chan KL, et al. Trend of survival of a cohort of chinese patients with systemic lupus erythematosus over 25 years. Front Med (Lausanne) 2020; 7:552.

46. Sousa S, Goncalves MJ, Ines LS, et al. Clinical features and long-term outcomes of systemic lupus erythematosus: comparative data of childhood, adult and late-onset disease in a national register. Rheumatol Int 2016;36(7):955–60.

47. Santos MJ, Capela S, Figueira R, et al. [Characterization of a Portuguese population with systemic lupus erytematosus]. Acta Reumatol Port 2007;32(2):153–61.

48. Rua-Figueroa I, Lopez-Longo FJ, Calvo-Alen J, et al. National registry of patients with systemic lupus erythematosus of the Spanish Society of Rheumatology: objectives and methodology. Reumatol Clin 2014;10(1):17–24.

49. Rua-Figueroa I, Richi P, Lopez-Longo FJ, et al. Comprehensive description of clinical characteristics of a large systemic lupus erythematosus cohort from the Spanish Rheumatology Society Lupus Registry (RELESSER) with emphasis on complete versus incomplete lupus differences. Medicine (Baltimore) 2015; 94(1):e267.

50. Torrente-Segarra V, Salman Monte TC, Rua-Figueroa I, et al. Juvenile- and adult-onset systemic lupus erythematosus: a comparative study in a large cohort from the Spanish Society of Rheumatology Lupus Registry (RELESSER). Clin Exp Rheumatol 2017;35(6):1047–55.

51. Riveros Frutos A, Casas I, Rua-Figueroa I, et al. Systemic lupus erythematosus in Spanish males: a study of the Spanish Rheumatology Society Lupus Registry (RELESSER) cohort. Lupus 2017;26(7):698–706.

52. El Hadidi KT, Medhat BM, Abdel Baki NM, et al. Characteristics of systemic lupus erythematosus in a sample of the Egyptian population: a retrospective cohort of 1109 patients from a single center. Lupus 2018;27(6):1030–8.

53. Abdel-Nabi HH, Abdel-Noor RA. Comparison between disease onset patterns of Egyptian juvenile and adult systemic lupus erythematosus (single centre experience). Lupus 2018;27(6):1039–44.

54. Afifi N, El Bakry SA, Mohannad N, et al. Clinical features and disease damage risk factors in an Egyptian SLE cohort: a Multicenter study. Curr Rheumatol Rev 2020. https://doi.org/10.2174/1573397116666201126161244.

55. Li M, Zhang W, Leng X, et al. Chinese SLE Treatment and Research group (CSTAR) registry: I. Major clinical characteristics of Chinese patients with systemic lupus erythematosus. Lupus 2013;22(11):1192–9.

56. Zhang S, Su J, Li X, et al. Chinese SLE Treatment and Research group (CSTAR) registry: V. gender impact on Chinese patients with systemic lupus erythematosus. Lupus 2015;24(12):1267–75.

57. Zhao J, Bai W, Zhu P, et al. Chinese SLE Treatment and Research group (CSTAR) registry VII: prevalence and clinical significance of serositis in Chinese patients with systemic lupus erythematosus. Lupus 2016;25(6):652–7.

58. Jiang N, Li M, Zhang M, et al. Chinese SLE Treatment and Research group (CSTAR) registry: clinical significance of thrombocytopenia in Chinese patients with systemic lupus erythematosus. PLoS One 2019;14(11):e0225516.

59. Fangtham M, Petri M. 2013 update: Hopkins lupus cohort. Curr Rheumatol Rep 2013;15(9):360.

60. Petri M, Purvey S, Fang H, et al. Predictors of organ damage in systemic lupus erythematosus: the Hopkins Lupus Cohort. Arthritis Rheum 2012;64(12):4021–8.

61. Babaoglu H, Li J, Goldman D, et al. Time to lupus low disease activity state in the Hopkins Lupus Cohort: Role of African American Ethnicity. Arthritis Care Res (Hoboken) 2020;72(2):225–32.

62. Watson P, Brennan A, Birch H, et al. An integrated extrapolation of long-term outcomes in systemic lupus erythematosus: analysis and simulation of the Hopkins lupus cohort. Rheumatology (Oxford) 2015;54(4):623–32.

63. Gladman DD, Urowitz MB. University of Toronto Lupus Clinic turns 40. J Rheumatol 2012;39(5):1074–7.

64. Urowitz MB, Gladman DD, Ibanez D, et al. Effect of disease activity on organ damage progression in systemic lupus erythematosus: University of Toronto Lupus Clinic Cohort. J Rheumatol 2020. https://doi.org/10.3899/jrheum.190259.

65. Tselios K, Gladman DD, Taheri C, et al. Factors associated with rapid progression to end stage kidney disease in lupus nephritis. J Rheumatol 2020. https://doi.org/10.3899/jrheum.200161.

66. Urowitz MB, Ibanez D, Jerome D, et al. The effect of menopause on disease activity in systemic lupus erythematosus. J Rheumatol 2006;33(11):2192–8.

67. Gladman DD, Hirani N, Ibanez D, et al. Clinically active serologically quiescent systemic lupus erythematosus. J Rheumatol 2003;30(9):1960–2.

68. Yee CS, Su L, Toescu V, et al. Birmingham SLE cohort: outcomes of a large inception cohort followed for up to 21 years. Rheumatology (Oxford) 2015;54(5):836–43.

69. Gisca E, Duarte L, Farinha F, et al. Assessing outcomes in a lupus nephritis cohort over a 40-year period. Rheumatology (Oxford) 2020. https://doi.org/10.1093/rheumatology/keaa491.

70. Costa Pires T, Caparros-Ruiz R, Gaspar P, et al. Prevalence and outcome of thrombocytopenia in systemic lupus erythematous: single-centre cohort analysis. Clin Exp Rheumatol 2020. PMID: 32896257.

71. Robinson GA, Peng J, Donnes P, et al. Disease-associated and patient-specific immune cell signatures in juvenile-onset systemic lupus erythematosus: patient stratification using a machine-learning approach. Lancet Rheumatol 2020;2(8):e485–96.

72. Segura BT, Bernstein BS, McDonnell T, et al. Damage accrual and mortality over long-term follow-up in 300 patients with systemic lupus erythematosus in a multi-ethnic British cohort. Rheumatology (Oxford) 2020;59(3):698.

73. Carlucci PM, Purmalek MM, Dey AK, et al. Neutrophil subsets and their gene signature associate with vascular inflammation and coronary atherosclerosis in lupus. JCI Insight 2018;3(8). https://doi.org/10.1172/jci.insight.99276.

74. Lopes SRM, Gormezano NWS, Gomes RC, et al. Outcomes of 847 childhood-onset systemic lupus erythematosus patients in three age groups. Lupus 2017;26(9):996–1001.

75. Islabao AG, Mota LMH, Ribeiro MCM, et al. Childhood-onset systemic lupus erythematosus-related antiphospholipid syndrome: a multicenter study with 1519 patients. Autoimmun Rev 2020;19(12):102693.

76. Miguel DF, Terreri MT, Pereira RMR, et al. Comparison of urinary parameters, biomarkers, and outcome of childhood systemic lupus erythematosus early onset-lupus nephritis. Adv Rheumatol 2020;60(1):10.

77. Mina R, von Scheven E, Ardoin SP, et al. Consensus treatment plans for induction therapy of newly diagnosed proliferative lupus nephritis in juvenile systemic lupus erythematosus. Arthritis Care Res (Hoboken) 2012;64(3):375–83.

78. Hersh AO, Case SM, Son MB, et al. Predictors of disability in a childhood-onset systemic lupus erythematosus cohort: results from the CARRA Legacy Registry. Lupus 2018;27(3):494–500.

79. Schanberg LE, Sandborg C, Barnhart HX, et al. Use of atorvastatin in systemic lupus erythematosus in children and adolescents. Arthritis Rheum 2012;64(1):285–96.

80. Kent T, Davidson A, Newman D, et al. Burden of illness in systemic lupus erythematosus: results from a UK patient and carer online survey. Lupus 2017;26(10): 1095–100.
81. Wallace DJ, Tse K, Hanrahan L, et al. Hydroxychloroquine usage in US patients, their experiences of tolerability and adherence, and implications for treatment: survey results from 3127 patients with SLE conducted by the Lupus Foundation of America. Lupus Sci Med 2019;6(1):e000317.
82. Schumacher KR, Stringer KA, Donohue JE, et al. Social media methods for studying rare diseases. Pediatrics 2014;133(5):e1345–53.
83. Davies W. Insights into rare diseases from social media surveys. Orphanet J Rare Dis 2016;11(1):151.
84. Liew JW, Bhana S, Costello W, et al. The COVID-19 Global Rheumatology Alliance: evaluating the rapid design and implementation of an international registry against best practice. Rheumatology (Oxford) 2020. https://doi.org/10.1093/rheumatology/keaa483.
85. Gianfrancesco M, Hyrich KL, Al-Adely S, et al. Characteristics associated with hospitalisation for COVID-19 in people with rheumatic disease: data from the COVID-19 Global Rheumatology Alliance physician-reported registry. Ann Rheum Dis 2020;79(7):859–66.
86. Gliklich R, Dreyer N, Leavy M, eds. Registries for Evaluating Patient Outcomes: A User's Guide. Rockville, MD:Agency for Healthcare Research and Quality. April 2014.
87. Gliklich RE, Leavy MB, Dreyer NA (sr eds). Registries for Evaluating Patient Outcomes: A User's Guide. 4th ed. Rockville, MD: Agency for Healthcare Research and Quality; September 2020.
88. Lim LSH, Feldman BM. Using registry data to understand disease evolution in inflammatory myositis and other rheumatic diseases. Curr Rheumatol Rep 2019; 22(1):2.
89. Urschel S. Apples, oranges, and statistical magic: limitations of registry studies and need for collaborative studies. J Heart Lung Transplant 2015;34(9):1136–8.
90. Le Sueur H, Bruce IN, Geifman N, et al. The challenges in data integration - heterogeneity and complexity in clinical trials and patient registries of Systemic Lupus Erythematosus. BMC Med Res Methodol 2020;20(1):164.
91. Nikiphorou E, Buch MH, Hyrich KL. Biologics registers in RA: methodological aspects, current role and future applications. Nat Rev Rheumatol 2017;13(8): 503–10.

Innovative Trials and New Opportunities in SLE

Yashaar Chaichian, MD[a],*, Daniel J. Wallace, MD, FACP, MACR[b,1]

KEYWORDS

- Systemic lupus erythematosus • Treatment • Innovation • Clinical trials
- Preclinical studies

KEY POINTS

- Anifrolumab data from the second of 2 parallel phase 3 randomized controlled trials (RCTs) combined with those from the phase 2 study indicate that type 1 interferon (IFN) blockade through IFNAR inhibition is effective and safe, and will hopefully expand the treatment armamentarium in systemic lupus erythematosus (SLE).
- Voclosporin and belimumab each demonstrated efficacy and safety in recent phase 3 RCTs in lupus nephritis (as did obinutuzumab in phase 2). Accordingly, belimumab and voclosoprin were both recently approved by the Food and Drug Administration (FDA) for use in lupus nephritis, each in combination with standard therapy.
- Results of other clinical trials targeting diverse pathways, including inhibition of Janus kinase/signal transducer and activator of transcription, plasmacytoid dendritic cells, and mammalian target of rapamycin, along with cerebron modulation and treatment with low-dose interleukin-2, provide hope for additional therapeutic options down the line in SLE.
- Recent insights provide greater clarity regarding the subsets of patients who may respond more favorably toward rituximab in severe refractory SLE, as well as how to safely withdraw glucocorticoids and maintenance immunosuppression in patients with stable SLE.
- Last, preclinical data targeting several novel immunologic approaches demonstrate potential avenues worth consideration for future clinical trials in SLE.

INTRODUCTION

Although progress has been made in the treatment of systemic lupus erythematosus (SLE), remission rates remain disappointingly low.[1] This is in stark contrast to several other autoimmune-driven diseases, including psoriasis, inflammatory bowel disease, and rheumatoid arthritis. In addition, the significant burden of disease is reinforced by

[a] Division of Immunology and Rheumatology, Stanford University, 1000 Welch Road, Suite 203, Palo Alto, CA 94304, USA; [b] Division of Rheumatology, Cedars-Sinai Medical Center, David Geffen School of Medicine, UCLA, Los Angeles, CA, USA, 8750 Wilshire Boulevard Suite 350, Beverly Hills, CA 90211
[1] Present address: 8750 Wilshire Boulevard Suite 350, Beverly Hills, CA 90211.
* Corresponding author.
E-mail address: ychaich@stanford.edu

Rheum Dis Clin N Am 47 (2021) 481–499
https://doi.org/10.1016/j.rdc.2021.04.010
0889-857X/21/© 2021 Elsevier Inc. All rights reserved.

rheumatic.theclinics.com

low health-related quality of life measures among many patients with SLE.[2] The paucity of successful SLE clinical trials, stemming from issues related to both study design and significant disease heterogeneity, is a painful reminder that we still have a long way to go. Nevertheless, there are clear signs of hope amidst the disappointment, including several recent positive phase III clinical trials, and Food and Drug Administration (FDA) approval of two additional treatment options for lupus nephritis. In this article, we highlight results from clinical and preclinical studies of novel therapeutic strategies based on emerging insights into our understanding of SLE disease mechanisms. We also highlight several studies that inform optimal use of existing treatments in ways that improve efficacy and/or limit toxicity. Together, these developments suggest we may yet unlock the key toward more satisfactory treatment outcomes in SLE.

DISCUSSION
Inhibition of Type 1 Interferon: Anifrolumab

With the recognition that interferon-alpha (IFN-α) represents the main type I IFN important in the pathogenesis of SLE,[3] therapeutic blockade of this subtype has been explored in multiple studies. The most successful have been with anifrolumab, a fully human, immunoglobulin (Ig)G1kappa monoclonal antibody (mAb) that binds to the type I IFN receptor (IFNAR), inhibiting all type I IFNs from mediating downstream effects. In the phase 2 randomized controlled trial (RCT), the primary endpoint of an SRI-4 response at week 24 plus sustained reduction in oral glucocorticoids (GC) from week 12 to 24 was met for anifrolumab compared with placebo (PBO), although there was no dose response.[4] Apart from a higher incidence of herpes zoster and influenza, the rate of adverse events was similar to PBO.

TULIP-1 and TULIP-2 were the 2 parallel phase 3 RCTs of anifrolumab in patients with moderate-to-severely active SLE. In TULIP-1, the primary efficacy endpoint of an SRI-4 response at week 52 was not met.[5] Nevertheless, several secondary endpoints including British Isles Lupus Assessment Group (BILAG)-Based Composite Lupus Assessment (BICLA) responses at week 52 suggested clinical benefit of anifrolumab. The negative results from TULIP-1 prompted a mid-trial switch in the primary endpoint in TULIP-2 from an SRI-4 at week 52 to the BICLA response at that time point.[6] Anifrolumab met this new primary endpoint, along with several key secondary endpoints. In a subsequent analysis, anifrolumab-treated patients in both TULIP-1 and TULIP-2 had decreases in total number of flares and annualized flare rates, as well as a prolonged time to first flare when compared with PBO.[7]

Aspects of the design and reporting of the 2 phase 3 anifrolumab RCTs have been criticized. These include (1) the change in the TULIP-2 primary endpoint (although this was done before unblinding), and (2) publishing the negative TULIP-1 trial results in a journal not indexed in PubMed.[8] These factors notwithstanding, we still believe that the results from TULIP-2 are noteworthy and demonstrate the therapeutic benefit in SLE of type I IFN blockade through IFNAR inhibition. Ongoing studies of anifrolumab in SLE include a phase 3 long-term extension study,[9] as well as a phase 2 RCT in active proliferative lupus nephritis (LN).[10]

Calcineurin Inhibitors in Lupus Nephritis: Tacrolimus and Voclosporin

Calcineurin inhibitors (CNIs) suppress T-cell activation and are a cornerstone of treatment to prevent allograft rejection among patients undergoing kidney transplantation.[11] Tacrolimus has been widely used for LN, especially in Asia. RCT data for induction therapy of LN suggests tacrolimus in combination with steroids is noninferior to cyclophosphamide (CYC)[12] or mycophenolate mofetil (MMF)[13] at 6 months. Similar long-term renal outcomes have been observed for patients treated with tacrolimus or MMF for induction therapy of LN.[14] The 2019 Update of the Joint EULAR/ERA-EDTA recommendations for the management of LN added tacrolimus to their treatment algorithm for selected cases: induction failure to standard therapy in either proliferative or pure class V nephritis, or following failure of standard maintenance therapy for pure class V nephritis, either alone or in combination.[15]

Indeed, suboptimal response rates in LN with standard of care treatment has led to interest in combining a CNI with MMF and GCs, that is, multitarget therapy. In the largest such multicenter randomized trial conducted in China, at week 24, complete remission was achieved by more patients in the multitarget group that included tacrolimus (45.9%) compared with the IV CYC group (25.6%) (*P*<.001).[16] Incidence of adverse events were similar between groups. However, the open-label design and short duration of follow-up are notable limitations of this study.

As a novel agent, voclosporin may be preferable to traditional CNIs currently in use. It is more potent than cyclosporine, has a more favorable glucose profile compared to tacrolimus, and has predictable pharmacokinetics and pharmacodynamics without need for therapeutic drug monitoring.[17,18] Voclosporin, in combination with MMF (2 g/d) and a quick taper of low-dose oral GCs, was studied in a phase 2, multicenter, randomized, double-blind, PBO-controlled trial (AURA-LV) for induction of remission in LN.[19] Significantly greater complete renal response (CRR) at week 24 was achieved among patients receiving either low or high-dose voclosporin compared with PBO, although CRR was higher in the low-dose group, indicating a lack of a dose response.

Results from the recently completed phase 3 AURORA 1 study confirm the efficacy findings of voclosporin in AURA-LV.[20] The primary endpoint of RR at 52 weeks was met, without unexpected safety signals. The results of the phase 3 AURORA trial indicate promise for voclosporin plus MMF as a treatment option in LN, and accordingly, voclosporin was granted FDA approval for this indication in January 2021. A long-term phase 3 continuation study (AURORA 2) will assess the safety and tolerability of continuing voclosporin for an additional 24 months among those who completed 52 weeks in the AURORA 1 study.[21]

Belimumab in Lupus Nephritis

Belimumab is a fully human IgG1-gamma mAb that selectively inhibits soluble B lymphocyte stimulator (BLyS), also known as B-cell activating factor (BAFF).[22] Based on the positive findings from the large BLISS-52 and BLISS-76 multicenter RCTs,[23,24] the FDA approved belimumab in 2011 as the first new agent for the treatment of SLE in more than 50 years.[25] Despite its approval for the treatment of seropositive patients with SLE with an inadequate response to standard of care (SOC) therapy, the role of belimumab in patients with severe active LN remained unclear, as these patients were excluded from both BLISS-52 and BLISS-76. Nevertheless, approximately 15% of patients in these studies had LN of lesser activity, and a post hoc analysis indicated belimumab was helpful in decreasing proteinuria and renal flares.[26]

Recently published results from the BLISS-LN study provide the most comprehensive picture to date regarding the safety and efficacy of belimumab for the induction management of LN. BLISS-LN was a phase 3 double-blind RCT in which 448 patients with SLE with biopsy-proven, active LN (class III, IV, and/or V) were randomized to monthly belimumab infusions or matching PBO, in addition to SOC therapy (MMF or cyclophosphamide-azathioprine).[27] The primary endpoint, a primary efficacy RR at week 104, was met by significantly more patients in the belimumab group (43%) than in the PBO group (32%) (*P* = .03). A similar pattern was observed for the major secondary end point of CRR (30% vs 20%, respectively; $P = .02$). Belimumab-treated patients had a lower risk of a renal-related event or death compared with those who received PBO (hazard ratio, 0.51; 95% confidence interval, 0.34–0.77; $P = .001$). The safety profile of belimumab was similar to that observed in prior trials of this medication.

It must be noted that the initial primary efficacy endpoint, the original ordinal renal response (complete, partial, or no response) at week 104, was altered midway through the trial. In addition, most patients had an estimated glomerular filtration rate $\geq$60 mL/min per 1.73 m^2. As such, whether belimumab is effective in patients with active LN who have moderate to significant renal insufficiency remains unsettled. Furthermore, the separation between treatment and PBO groups with respect to the primary efficacy endpoint, while clearly significant, only emerged at week 24.

Therefore, in our view, data from BLISS-LN suggest that belimumab appears to be most appropriate for the subset of patients with normal or only mildly abnormal renal function, with stable chronic active LN despite SOC induction therapy. Nevertheless, the BLISS-LN findings are significant and have contributed to an expansion of the treatment armamentarium in LN, as belimumab was granted FDA approval for this indication in December 2020.

Combination Therapy with Rituximab and Belimumab

There has been increasing interest in studying the combination of rituximab and belimumab due to complementary effects on B cells. Rituximab therapy followed by belimumab is based on the observation that B-cell depletion leads to elevated BAFF levels, and an ensuing increase in autoreactive B cells.[28] Positive clinical and immunologic responses were noted in a small phase 2A, open-label, single-arm proof-of-concept study with rituximab followed by belimumab administered to patients with severe, refractory SLE.[29] This approach was subsequently studied in patients with recurrent or refractory LN in a small open-label, randomized, phase 2 trial (CALIBRATE).[30] Patients (n = 43) received rituximab, CYC, and GCs followed by weekly belimumab infusions until week 48 (RCB group), or rituximab and CYC without subsequent belimumab (RC group). Designed to assess safety, the number of adverse events between groups were similar. Although CALIBRATE was not powered to fully assess efficacy, the addition of belimumab following rituximab did not lead to improved clinical outcomes at week 48: complete or partial RR was achieved in 51% of the RCB group and 41% of the RC group ($P = .452$).

Two larger studies are under way to further assess combination B-cell therapy in nonrenal SLE. BEAT Lupus is a double-blind, PBO-controlled, 52-week phase 2 RCT in which patients receiving rituximab will be randomized to belimumab or PBO, 4 to 8 weeks following the first rituximab infusion.[31] BLISS-BELIEVE, a double-blind, PBO-controlled phase 3 RCT, will investigate rituximab *following* belimumab therapy.[32] The rationale is that this sequence may lead to greater B-cell depletion than rituximab monotherapy by targeting the rise in B memory cells following belimumab.

Humanized Anti-CD20 Monoclonal Antibody: Obinutuzumab

The use of anti-CD20 therapy with rituximab has led to the development of humanized anti-CD20 mAbs for study in autoimmune disorders.[33] Obinutuzumab, already approved for follicular lymphoma and chronic lymphocytic leukemia,[34] is the one humanized anti-CD20 mAb that has shown promise in SLE thus far. As a result of its type II binding conformation, obinutuzumab results in enhanced B-cell depletion, greater direct cell death, reduced CD20 internalization, and lower complement-dependent cytotoxicity compared with rituximab.[35] In a phase 2 trial in LN, patients (n = 125) with active, biopsy-proven class III or IV LN were randomized to obinutuzumab or PBO in addition to MMF and GCs.[36] The primary endpoint, CRR at week 52, was met in 35% receiving obinutuzumab compared with 23% receiving PBO (P = .115, prespecified alpha level was 0.2). Overall renal response (complete or partial RR) at week 52 was 56% compared with 36% receiving PBO (P = .025). Obinutuzumab was overall safe and well-tolerated, and has been given fast-track designation by the FDA. Follow-up analyses indicated sustained patterns of CRR with obinutuzumab over PBO at week 76 (40% vs 18%, P = .007) and week 104 (41% vs 23%, P = .026).[37] However, they also confirmed significant increases in serum BAFF following treatment, as is seen with rituximab.[28,38] A phase 3 RCT is under way to further assess the efficacy and safety of obinutuzumab in LN.[39]

Janus Kinase/Signal Transducer and Activator of Transcription Pathway Inhibitors

Janus kinase (JAK)/signal transducer and activator of transcription (STAT) inhibitors stimulate intracellular signaling and proinflammatory gene transcription on activation by receptor-ligand interaction.[40] JAK inhibition is already an effective treatment strategy in several rheumatic diseases, including rheumatoid arthritis (RA), psoriatic arthritis, and psoriasis.[41] Inhibition of this pathway represents a biologically plausible therapeutic target in SLE as signal transduction from the activated IFN receptor to the nucleus requires JAK/STAT activation.[42,43]

Baricitinib is an orally administered reversible inhibitor of JAK1 and JAK2 that is approved for use in RA at a dose of 2 mg daily.[44] In a double-blind, randomized, PBO-controlled phase 2 trial (n = 314), the 4-mg but not the 2-mg dose met the primary endpoint of significantly improved SLEDAI-2K arthritis or rash at week 24.[45] Safety findings were similar to prior trials with baricitinib. In a subsequent analysis, baricitinib led to a dose-dependent decrease in the IFN signature.[46] Treatment response was observed regardless of the change in IFN gene signature, indicating some baricitinib effects on cytokine signaling were not IFN-mediated. There are 2 ongoing phase 3 RCTs[47,48] and a long-term extension study[49] that will provide further data on its potential role in the treatment of SLE.

Tofacitinib is a JAK1/JAK3 inhibitor (and to a lesser degree an inhibitor of JAK2), and is approved for RA, psoriasis, and inflammatory bowel disease.[44] In a murine lupus model, it was shown to modify innate and adaptive immune responses, and improve disease activity as well as associated vascular dysfunction and NET formation.[50] In a phase 1b/2a trial in SLE (n = 30), tofacitinib was well-tolerated, safe, and led to improvement in innate and adaptive immune dysregulation as well as lipoprotein phenotype and function.[51] Two additional trials are ongoing: an open-label phase 2 pilot study in adult patients with discoid lupus with or without concurrent SLE,[52] and an open-label RCT in young adults who have moderate to severe cutaneous lupus erythematosus (CLE).[53]

Upadacitinib, a selective JAK1 inhibitor (ABBV-494), is approved for RA.[44] It is currently being investigated as monotherapy and in conjunction with a Bruton tyrosine kinase (BTK) inhibitor, ABBV-105, as ABBV-599, in a phase 2 SLE RCT.[54] Filgotinib, another selective JAK1 inhibitor, was evaluated in comparison with lanraplenib (a Syk kinase inhibitor) or PBO in a phase 2 RCT in CLE that did not meet its primary endpoint for either treatment arm.[55] It was also studied in a multicenter phase 2 RCT in class V LN that was hampered by recruitment difficulties.[56] Although the small number of patients treated with filgotinib had reduced proteinuria, no benefit was seen with lanraplenib (author disclosure: YC served as a principal investigator for this study).

Nonreceptor tyrosine kinase 2 (TYK2), a member of the JAK family, along with JAK1 is constitutively associated with IFNAR.[57] Brepocitinib, a TYK2/JAK1 inhibitor, is currently being evaluated in several autoimmune diseases, including in a phase 2b RCT in SLE.[58] A phase 2 study of BMS-986165, a TYK2 inhibitor, is also under way.[59]

Targeting Plasmacytoid Dendritic Cells

Plasmacytoid dendritic cells (pDC) serve as the main producer of type I IFN,[60] and as such pDC inhibition is an attractive treatment approach in SLE. BIIB059 is a humanized mAb that binds the BDCA-2 receptor on pDCs, inhibiting TLR7/9 signaling and downstream type I IFN production.[61,62] The therapeutic potential of BIIB059 was recently demonstrated in a 2-part phase 2 RCT in patients with SLE with active CLE and joint involvement (part A), as well as in those with CLE with or without systemic manifestations (part B). In part A, the primary endpoint of change in total active joint count from baseline to week 24 was met in BIIB059-treated patients compared with PBO, as was the secondary endpoint of the proportion of patients at week 24 achieving an SRI-4 response.[63] In part B, the primary endpoint defined by percentage change in CLASI-A scores from baseline to week 16 demonstrated a dose response, with a statistically significant difference in CLASI-A score changes compared with PBO.[64] However, results for the phase 2 RCT according to patients' baseline IFN expression have not yet been published.

Inhibition of Mammalian Target of Rapamycin: Sirolimus, N-Acetylcysteine

Metabolic stress in SLE is in part due to activation of mammalian target of rapamycin (mTOR), which skews the immune system toward a proinflammatory lineage.[65,66] The depletion of glutathione underlies the activation of the mechanistic target of rapamycin and T cells. Sirolimus, the medication developed from rapamycin, was evaluated in a single-arm, open-label, phase 1/2 trial of patients with active SLE unresponsive to, or intolerant of, SOC medications.[67] At 12 months, there were reductions in mean SLEDAI and total BILAG index scores, mean GC dose, and proinflammatory T-cell lineage specification. Sirolimus had an overall acceptable safety profile. The open-label nature of this study and recruitment of patients from only a single center are limitations. A phase 2, double-blind RCT will further assess the safety and efficacy of this treatment approach in patients with active SLE despite SOC therapy.[68]

N-acetylcysteine (NAC) is an amino acid precursor of glutathione and improves the outcome of murine lupus.[69] This over-the-counter mucolytic has been available for decades, is safe, and leads to reversal of glutathione depletion and mTOR activation.[70,71] A double-blind, PBO-controlled pilot study in SLE (n = 32) showed improvements in SLEDAI and BILAG scores, as well as the Fatigue Assessment Scale.[72] A recently approved National Institutes of Health grant will study NAC in greater detail.[73]

Cerebron Modulation: Iberdomide

Thalidomide and lenalidomide bind to the protein cereblon, directing a ligase toward transcription factors Ikaros and Aiolos to cause their ubiquitination and degradation.[74] A cerebron modulator (CC-220, iberdomide) has higher affinity and has been studied for myeloma and CLE.[74] An ascending-dose, safety and pharmacokinetics study of 42 subjects with CLE suggested safety and efficacy.[75] A phase 2 study of 288 patients with SLE has been completed and significantly met the SRI-4 primary endpoint at week 24 among patients in the 0.45 mg group (54%) versus PBO (35%) ($P = .011$).[76] Iberdomide also decreased B cells and plasmacytoid dendritic cells, and was well-tolerated.[76,77] Although CLASI-50 skin scores were not improved in the overall population, they were reduced among patients with subacute and chronic CLE. Enhanced effects were observed in 2 biomarker-defined populations (Aiolos-high, type 1 IFN-high),[77] providing an additional rationale for further clinical trials of this novel therapeutic option in SLE.

Low-Dose Interleukin-2 Therapy

Low-dose, but not higher dose interleukin-2 (IL-2), expands regulatory T cells, decreases inflammation, and has demonstrated clinical benefits in type 1 diabetes and graft-versus-host reactions.[78] Furthermore, acquired IL-2 deficiency and related aberrant regulatory T-cell homeostasis are implicated in SLE pathogenesis.[79] Based on these data, and the attractive prospect of potentially identifying a nonimmunosuppressive approach toward lupus treatment, approximately 5 pharmaceutical companies are examining the role of low-dose IL-2 in SLE with a variety of preparations. Preliminary evidence from the small available trials has suggested variable improvements and no safety signals.[80–83] In a PBO-controlled, double-blind phase 2 RCT (n = 60 patients), the primary endpoint of an SRI-4 response at week 12 for low-dose IL-2 (55.2%) compared with PBO (30.0%) ($P = .052$) did not achieve statistical significance.[83] However, the trend in SRI-4 response at week 12 favoring the low-dose IL-2 arm was confirmed at week 24 ($P = .027$). Two additional studies,[84,85] one phase 1, another phase 2, will investigate novel low-dose IL-2 agents in SLE and are currently recruiting participants (disclosure: YC is planning to serve as a principal investigator for the phase 2 RCT).

A summary of SLE treatments discussed previously and their therapeutic targets are presented in **Table 1**.

Rituximab Responders in Severe Refractory Systemic Lupus Erythematosus

Rituximab notably failed to meet its primary endpoints in 2 large RCTs: (1) EXPLORER, which assessed rituximab in patients with moderate to severe nonrenal SLE, and (2) LUNAR, which evaluated rituximab in patients with active proliferative (class III or IV) LN.[86,87] Issues with background GC therapy and selection of primary endpoints have been cited as potential reasons why these were "negative" studies.[88] Nevertheless, significant anecdotal data and results from multiple open-label studies[89–92] have led to rituximab use in severe renal and nonrenal SLE that is refractory to first-line therapy. Divergent factors predictive of rituximab response have previously been reported. In one study, severe disease, lack of hematologic involvement, or prior treatment with high-dose GCs were associated with a favorable response.[93] In another study, younger age and B-cell depletion 6 weeks following rituximab were associated with a good response.[94]

Two recent studies shed further light on specific subsets of patients with SLE who may respond best to rituximab. Cassia and colleagues[95] reviewed the treatment experience of 147 patients with SLE at 4 European centers who received rituximab as induction therapy, focusing on the 80 patients who received maintenance rituximab to prevent relapses. Factors reducing the risk of treatment failure in multivariate analysis were a low number of prior immunosuppressive agents tried and low C4 levels. Freitas and colleagues[96] assessed the treatment course of patients with SLE up to 6 months after treatment with rituximab, identifying those (n = 144) with active disease after 6 months. Patients with renal disease were less likely to fail rituximab, and these patients had elevated anti–double-stranded DNA levels and greater disease activity.

Despite the failure of rituximab in RCTs, significant nonrandomized data and clinical experience support its use in patients with severe renal and nonrenal SLE who fail to

Table 1
Summary of systemic lupus erythematosus clinical trials reviewed

Mechanism (Drug)	Study Population	Highest Phase Study Completed	Primary Endpoint(s) Met	Further Studies Ongoing
Type 1 IFN inhibition (anifrolumab)	SLE	Phase 3	No for TULIP-1 Yes for TULIP-2	Yes
Calcineurin inhibition (tacrolimus, voclosporin)	LN	Phase 3	Yes	Yes
BAFF inhibition (belimumab)	LN	Phase 3	Yes	TBD
Anti-CD20 plus BAFF inhibition (rituximab plus belimumab)	SLE, LN	Phase 2	Yes (safety endpoint)	Yes
Humanized anti-CD20 (obinutuzumab)	LN	Phase 2	Yes	Yes
JAK/STAT inhibition (baricitinib, tofacitinib, upadacitinib, filgotinib, brepocitinib, BMS-986165)	SLE, LN	Phase 2 (baricitinib, filgotinib)	Yes for baricitinib No for filgotinib	Yes
BDCA-2 receptor inhibition on pDCs (BIIB059)	CLE, SLE	Phase 2	Yes	TBD
mTOR inhibition (sirolimus, N-acetylcysteine)	SLE	Phase 2	Yes	Yes
Cerebron modulation (iberdomide)	SLE	Phase 2	Yes	TBD
Low-dose IL-2	SLE	Phase 2b	No	Yes

Abbreviations: BAFF, B-cell activating factor; CLE, cutaneous lupus erythematosus; IL, interleukin; JAK, Janus kinase; LN, lupus nephritis; mTOR, mammalian target of rapamycin; pDC, plasmacytoid dendritic cell; SLE, systemic lupus erythematosus; STAT, signal transducer and activator of transcription; TBD, to be determined.

respond to first-line treatment options. The studies presented here provide greater insights regarding the specific subsets of patients who may be more responsive to rituximab therapy.

Timing of Safe Withdrawal of Glucocorticoids

When to safely withdraw GCs in patients with stable SLE without inducing a disease flare remains a challenging question. The approach in real-world settings has been more empiric than evidence based. However, 2 recent studies[97,98] provide further insights into when GC withdrawal can be safely considered in patients with stable SLE (**Box 1**). Based on these studies, successful GC withdrawal is a realistic goal in many with SLE, particularly patients in long-term remission or lupus low disease activity state, and on immunosuppressive therapy at baseline. Given the side effects and toxicity associated with long-term GC exposure, these data will hopefully contribute to more judicious GC use in the management of SLE going forward.

Timing of Safe Withdrawal of Maintenance Immunosuppression

Another area of clinical interest is when to safely withdraw maintenance immunosuppression in patients with stable SLE. For LN, the 2019 Update of the Joint EULAR/ERA-EDTA recommendations suggest consideration of gradual withdrawal of treatment (GCs followed by immunosuppressive drugs) after at least 3 to 5 years of complete clinical response on therapy.[15] In nonrenal SLE, there is less guidance on appropriate timing of GC withdrawal. Two recent studies[99,100] add to our knowledge of how and when to safely consider withdrawing maintenance immunosuppression in either setting (**Box 2**).

Box 1
Glucocorticoid withdrawal in systemic lupus erythematosus

Tani C et al, 2019[97]:

- prospectively collected data from a monocentric longitudinal cohort of patients (n = 148) with systemic lupus erythematosus (SLE) over a 6-year follow-up period
- patients who were glucocorticoid (GC)-free at last visit were identified, compared with patients on GC at last visit
- most who succeeded in stopping GC were in either complete remission (54%) or clinical remission (37%)
- Lupus low disease activity state was achieved in 97% of these patients
- GC withdrawal was not associated with a trend toward higher risk of disease flare, though these results were not statistically significant

Tselios K et al, 2020[98]:

- long-term longitudinal cohort of patients (n = 270) with 2 consecutive years of clinically quiescent disease
- compared rates of clinical flare and damage accrual among those either maintained on low-dose prednisone (5 mg/d) or undergoing gradual GC withdrawal
- patients in the GC withdrawal group developed significantly less clinical flares at 24 months
- damage accrual at 24 months was reduced in the GC withdrawal group
- immunosuppressive therapy at baseline was associated with a reduced risk of clinical flare (P = .024)

Box 2
Immunosuppressive withdrawal in renal and nonrenal SLE

Zen M et al, 2020[99]:

- patients (n = 206) with biopsy-proven lupus nephritis (LN) ever treated with immunosuppressives (IS) and currently in follow-up

- IS discontinuation was defined as the complete withdrawal of any IS drug in patients in remission

- among patients who underwent IS discontinuation (n = 83), 23% subsequently flared, mostly with extrarenal flares

- longer remission before IS discontinuation and subsequent continuation of antimalarials predicted persistent IS-free remission

Chakravarty E et al, 2020[100]:

- patients (n = 102) with Safety of Estrogens in Lupus Erythematosus National Assessment SLE Disease Activity Index (SELENA-SLEDAI) without serologies <4 taking mycophenolate mofetil (MMF) for ≥2 years (for nephritis) or ≥1 year (for non-nephritis)

- randomized to unblinded MMF or to a 12-week taper off MMF and followed through week 60

- all were receiving stable hydroxychloroquine (HCQ) doses and on ≤10 mg prednisone equivalent

- serious flares were infrequent in both groups

- no significant differences in time to flare between groups

Other Novel Approaches

A number of additional novel therapeutic strategies are being evaluated in SLE clinical trials. Several are briefly mentioned here. KZR-616, a first-in-class selective immuno-proteasome inhibitor was recently evaluated in a phase 1b open-label dose-escalation study of patients (n = 41) with active SLE or LN despite stable background therapy.[101] KZR-616 was well-tolerated and safe at 13 weeks, and early signals of efficacy were observed in multiple disease activity and serologic markers. An open-label phase 2 study in active proliferative LN is planned.[102] Itolizumab, a first-in-class mAb that selectively inhibits the immune checkpoint receptor CD6, is being evaluated in a phase 1b study in patients with SLE with or without active LN.[103] Mesenchymal stem cell therapy has also been investigated in the setting of refractory SLE as well as LN, although studies to date have been small.[104] A phase 2 study is underway to assess this treatment strategy more definitively.[105]

Targeting Mitochondrial Dysfunction

The importance of mitochondrial dysfunction in SLE pathogenesis has gained greater recognition, with mitochondrial DNA damage, mitophagy, oxidate stress, and aberrant mitochondrial biogenesis and energy metabolism all implicated.[106] In addition, increased synthesis of mitochondrial reactive oxygen species by lupus neutrophil subsets correlates with increased formation of NETs in oxidized mitochondrial DNA, leading to type I IFN responses.[107,108] Idebenone is an antioxidant as well as a coenzyme Q10 synthetic quinone analog that has been used in the treatment of Leber hereditary optic neuropathy.[109] Blanco and colleagues[110] evaluated idebenone in a murine model of lupus (MRL/lpr mice) administered over 8 weeks. Idebenone led to significant reductions in disease features, including improved renal function, and also reduced mortality. It also inhibited NET formation in neutrophils and improved mitochondrial metabolism, with similar results seen in NZM2328 mice. Further exploration of treatment strategies that may counteract the mitochondrial dysfunction present in SLE are warranted.

SLAMF1 Inhibition

Aberrant T-cell–B-cell interactions are important facilitators of immune dysregulation in SLE. Signaling lymphocytic activation molecule family members 1 to 9 (SLAMF1-9) are type I transmembrane glycoprotein cell surface receptors expressed on hematopoietic cells.[111] SLAMF1 is expressed on both T and B cells (along with dendritic cells), and homophilic interactions induce immunoglobulin production and cross-talk between T cells/B cells. Karampetsou and colleagues[111] demonstrated that SLAMF1 mAb decreased conjugate formation, IL-6 production by B cells, IL-21 and IL-17A production by T cells, and Ig and autoantibody production in both healthy controls and patients with SLE. As SLAMF1 expression on T-cell and B-cell surfaces in peripheral blood is upregulated in SLE,[112,113] this justifies further studies targeting SLAMF1 to determine if inhibiting abnormal T-cell–B-cell interactions through this mechanism can be a successful therapeutic approach.

Chimeric Antigen Receptor T-Cell–Based Therapy

Cytotoxic T cells express transduced genes for anti-CD19 surface receptors and lead to death of targeted cells once bound.[114,115] CD8+ T cells that express CD19-targeted chimeric antigen receptors (CARs) are a successful therapeutic option for the treatment of multiple B-cell malignancies, often leading to sustained remission.[116] CAR-T-cell–based treatment leads to more complete and prolonged B-cell depletion than rituximab, using a cell-based rather than antibody approach. Additional advantages of CAR-T cells include only needing a single dose, and their ability to evolve into both effector and memory cell populations.[117] These unique characteristics have generated interest in studying CAR-T therapy in SLE.

Kansal and colleagues[117] recently demonstrated that sustained CD19+ B-cell depletion via CAR-T cells can be effective in 2 murine models of lupus: (NZB × NZW) F1 and MRL fas/fas. In this study, CAR-T based treatment led to (1) persistent depletion of CD19+ B cells, (2) prevented autoantibody production, (3) reversed disease manifestations in target organs, and (4) prolonged life spans. Whether CAR-T based therapy is safe and effective in patients with SLE is currently unknown but is worth pursuing.

SUMMARY

The SLE treatment landscape continues to feature a paucity of approved therapeutic options, amidst a backdrop of numerous prior failed clinical trials. Nevertheless, as highlighted in this article, a number of exciting preclinical and clinical breakthroughs have emerged in the past few years, targeting specific and novel immunologic pathways. These developments, particularly the encouraging results from several phase 3 RCTs in both renal and nonrenal SLE, provide reason for optimism that patients will have access to more effective treatments in the not-too-distant future. Indeed, in recent months two new FDA-approved options for the management of lupus nephritis have become available. Lastly, better understanding of the factors associated with both treatment response and safe withdrawal of existing therapies in SLE will hopefully contribute to limiting medication-related toxicity in our patients.

CLINICS CARE POINTS

- Anifrolumab data from the second of 2 parallel phase 3 RCTs combined with those from the phase 2 study indicate that type 1 IFN blockade through IFNAR inhibition is effective and safe, and will hopefully expand the treatment armamentarium in SLE.

- Voclosporin and belimumab each demonstrated efficacy and safety in recent phase 3 RCTs in LN, and were granted FDA approval for this indication in combination with standard therapy. Favorable results for obinutuzumab in phase 2 suggest a potential role in LN for humanized type 2 anti-CD20 mAb therapy, alongside novel calcineurin inhibition and BAFF blockade.

- Combination therapy with rituximab and belimumab has been shown to be safe in limited studies to date, which were not powered for efficacy. Several planned RCTs will further address whether this complementary B-cell targeted approach is efficacious in SLE.

- Results of other clinical trials targeting diverse pathways (inhibition of JAK/STAT, pDCs, and mTOR, along with cerebron modulation and treatment with low-dose IL-2) provide hope for additional therapeutic options down the line in SLE.

- Despite its failure in 2 RCTs, rituximab remains an option for severe refractory SLE, and several studies indicate specific subsets of patients who may have a more favorable response.

- Recent insights into the safe withdrawal of glucocorticoids in SLE as well as maintenance immunosuppression in both renal and nonrenal SLE provide guidance toward limiting excess treatment-related toxicity, which is a major goal.

- Last, preclinical data targeting several novel immunologic approaches demonstrate potential avenues worth consideration for future clinical trials in SLE.

DISCLOSURE

Y. Chaichian has received support from Amgen Inc., AMPEL BioSolutions, Gilead Sciences, Eli Lilly and Company, the Lupus Research Alliance, and Pfizer Inc., to conduct clinical research, and has served in an advisory board role for GlaxoSmithKline plc,. D.J. Wallace has consulted for Amgen Inc., Aurinia, Eli Lilly and Company, EMD Serono, GlaxoSmithKline plc, Janssen Pharmaceuticals, and Merck & Co.

REFERENCES

1. Wilhelm TR, Magder LS, Petri M. Remission in systemic lupus erythematosus: durable remission is rare. Ann Rheum Dis 2017;76(3):547–53.
2. Yazdany J, Yelin E. Health-related quality of life and employment among persons with systemic lupus erythematosus. Rheum Dis Clin North Am 2010; 36(1):15–32, vii.
3. Ronnblom L, Pascual V. The innate immune system in SLE: type I interferons and dendritic cells. Lupus 2008;17(5):394–9.
4. Furie R, Khamashta M, Merrill JT, et al. Anifrolumab, an anti-interferon-α receptor monoclonal antibody, in moderate-to-severe systemic lupus erythematosus. Arthritis Rheumatol 2017;69(2):376–86.
5. Furie RA, Morand EF, Bruce IN, et al. Type I interferon inhibitor anifrolumab in active systemic lupus erythematosus (TULIP-1): a randomised, controlled, phase 3 trial. Lancet Rheumatol 2019;1(4):e208–19.
6. Morand EF, Furie R, Tanaka Y, et al. Trial of anifrolumab in active systemic lupus erythematosus. N Engl J Med 2020;382(3):211–21.

7. Furie R, Morand EF, Askanase A, et al. SAT0174 Flare assessments in patients with active systemic lupus erythematosus treated with anifrolumab in 2 phase 3 trials [abstract]. Ann Rheum Dis 2020;79(Suppl 1).

8. Wofsy D. A tale of two trials. Arthritis Rheumatol 2020;72(8):1256–7.

9. Long term safety of anifrolumab in adult subjects with active systemic lupus erythematosus. Clinicaltrials.gov Identifier: NCT02794285. Available at: https://clinicaltrials.gov/ct2/show/NCT02794285. Accessed December 12, 2020.

10. Safety and efficacy of two doses of anifrolumab compared to placebo in adult subjects with active proliferative lupus nephritis. Clinicaltrials.gov Identifier: NCT02547922. Available at: https://clinicaltrials.gov/ct2/show/NCT02547922. Accessed December 12, 2020.

11. Azzi JR, Sayegh MH, Mallat SG. Calcineurin inhibitors: 40 years later, can't live without. J Immunol 2013;191(12):5785–91.

12. Chen W, Tang X, Liu Q, et al. Short-term outcomes of induction therapy with tacrolimus versus cyclophosphamide for active lupus nephritis: a multicenter randomized clinical trial. Am J Kidney Dis 2011;57(2):235–44.

13. Mok CC, Ying KY, Yim CW, et al. Tacrolimus versus mycophenolate mofetil for induction therapy of lupus nephritis: a randomised controlled trial and long-term follow-up. Ann Rheum Dis 2016;75(1):30–6.

14. Mok CC, Ho LY, Ying SKY, et al. Long-term outcome of a randomised controlled trial comparing tacrolimus with mycophenolate mofetil as induction therapy for active lupus nephritis. Ann Rheum Dis 2020;79(8):1070–6.

15. Fanouriakis A, Kostopoulou M, Cheema K, et al. 2019 Update of the Joint European League Against Rheumatism and European Renal Association–European Dialysis and Transplant Association (EULAR/ERA–EDTA) recommendations for the management of lupus nephritis. Ann Rheum Dis 2020;79:713–23.

16. Liu Z, Zhan H, Liu Z, et al. Multitarget therapy for induction treatment of lupus nephritis: a randomized trial. Ann Intern Med 2015;162(1):18–26.

17. Mayo PR, Ling SY, Huizinga RB, et al. Population PKPD of voclosporin in renal allograft patients. J Clin Pharmacol 2014;54(5):537–45.

18. Kolic J, Beet L, Overby P, et al. Differential effects of voclosporin and tacrolimus on insulin secretion from human islets. Endocrinology 2020;161(11):bqaa162.

19. Rovin BH, Solomons N, Pendergraft WF 3rd, et al. A randomized, controlled double-blind study comparing the efficacy and safety of dose-ranging voclosporin with placebo in achieving remission in patients with active lupus nephritis. Kidney Int 2019;95(1):219–31.

20. Arriens C, Polyakova S, Adzerikho I, et al. OP0277 AURORA phase 3 study demonstrates voclosporin statistical superiority over standard of care in lupus nephritis (LN) [abstract]. Ann Rheum Dis 2020;79(Suppl 1).

21. Aurinia renal assessments 2: Aurinia renal response in lupus with voclosporin (AURORA2). ClinicalTrials.gov Identifier: NCT03597464. Available at: https://clinicaltrials.gov/ct2/show/NCT03597464. Accessed December 12, 2020.

22. Stohl W, Hilbert DM. The discovery and development of belimumab: the anti-BLyS–lupus connection. Nat Biotechnol 2012;30(1):69–77.

23. Navarra SV, Guzman RM, Gallacher AE, et al. Efficacy and safety of belimumab in patients with active systemic lupus erythematosus: a randomised, placebo-controlled, phase 3 trial. Lancet 2011;377(9767):721–31.

24. Furie R, Petri M, Zamani O, et al. A phase III, randomized, placebo-controlled study of belimumab, a monoclonal antibody that inhibits B lymphocyte stimulator, in patients with systemic lupus erythematosus. Arthritis Rheum 2011;63(12):3918–30.

25. Horowitz DL, Furie R. Belimumab is approved by the FDA: what more do we need to know to optimize decision making? Curr Rheumatol Rep 2012;14(4): 318–23.

26. Dooley MA, Houssiau F, Aranow C, et al. Effect of belimumab treatment on renal outcomes: results from the phase 3 belimumab clinical trials in patients with SLE. Lupus 2013;22(1):63–72.

27. Furie R, Rovin BH, Houssiau F, et al. Two-year, randomized, controlled trial of belimumab in lupus nephritis. N Engl J Med 2020;383(12):1117–28.

28. Ehrenstein MR, Wing C. The BAFFling effects of rituximab in lupus: danger ahead? Nat Rev Rheumatol 2016;12(6):367–72.

29. Kraaij T, Kamerling SWA, de Rooij ENM, et al. The NET-effect of combining rituximab with belimumab in severe systemic lupus erythematosus. J Autoimmun 2018;91:45–54.

30. Atisha-Fregoso Y, Malkiel S, Harris KM, et al. CALIBRATE: a phase 2 randomized trial of rituximab plus cyclophosphamide followed by belimumab for the treatment of lupus nephritis. Arthritis Rheumatol 2020. https://doi.org/10.1002/art.41466.

31. Jones A, Muller P, Dore CJ, et al. Belimumab after B cell depletion therapy in patients with systemic lupus erythematosus (BEAT Lupus) protocol: a prospective multicentre, double-blind, randomised, placebo-controlled, 52-week phase II clinical trial. BMJ Open 2019;9(12):e032569.

32. Teng YKO, Bruce IN, Diamond B, et al. Phase III, multicentre, randomised, double-blind, placebo-controlled, 104-week study of subcutaneous belimumab administered in combination with rituximab in adults with systemic lupus erythematosus (SLE): BLISS-BELIEVE study protocol. BMJ Open 2019;9(3):e025687.

33. Du FH, Mills EA, Mao-Draayer Y. Next-generation anti-CD20 monoclonal antibodies in autoimmune disease treatment. Auto Immun Highlights 2017;8(1):12.

34. Chung C. Current targeted therapies in lymphomas. Am J Health Syst Pharm 2019;76(22):1825–34.

35. Reddy V, Klein C, Isenberg DA, et al. Obinutuzumab outperforms rituximab at inducing B-cell cytotoxicity in vitro through Fc-mediated effector mechanisms in rheumatoid arthritis and systemic lupus erythematosus [abstract]. Arthritis Rheumatol 2015;67(suppl 10).

36. Furie R, Aroca G, Alvarez A, et al. A phase II randomized, double-blind, placebo-controlled study to evaluate the efficacy and safety of obinutuzumab or placebo in combination with mycophenolate mofetil in patients with active class III or IV lupus nephritis [abstract]. Arthritis Rheumatol 2019;71(suppl 10).

37. Furie R, Aroca G, Alvarez A, et al. Two-year results from a randomized, controlled study of obinutuzumab for proliferative lupus nephritis [abstract]. Arthritis Rheumatol 2020;72(suppl 10).

38. Vital E, Remy P, Quintana Porras L, et al. Biomarkers of B-cell depletion and response in a randomized, controlled trial of obinutuzumab for proliferative lupus nephritis [abstract]. Arthritis Rheumatol 2020;72(suppl 10).

39. A study to evaluate the efficacy and safety of obinutuzumab in patients with ISN/RPS 2003 class III or IV lupus nephritis (REGENCY). Clinicaltrials.gov Identifier: NCT04221477. Available at: https://clinicaltrials.gov/ct2/show/NCT04221477. Accessed December 12, 2020.

40. Gadina M, Johnson C, Schwartz D, et al. Translational and clinical advances in JAK-STAT biology: the present and future of jakinibs. J Leukoc Biol 2018;104(3): 499–514.

41. Jamilloux Y, El Jammal T, Vuitton L, et al. JAK inhibitors for the treatment of auto-immune and inflammatory diseases. Autoimmun Rev 2019;18(11):102390.

42. Mok CC. The Jakinibs in systemic lupus erythematosus: progress and pros-pects. Expert Opin Investig Drugs 2019;28:85–92.

43. Dong J, Wang QX, Zhou CY, et al. Activation of the STAT1 signalling pathway in lupus nephritis in MRL/lpr mice. Lupus 2007;16:101–9.

44. Damsky W, Peterson D, Ramseier J, et al. The emerging role of Janus kinase in-hibitors in the treatment of autoimmune and inflammatory diseases. J Allergy Clin Immunol 2021;147(3):814–26.

45. Wallace DJ, Furie RA, Tanaka Y, et al. Baricitinib for systemic lupus erythemato-sus: a double-blind, randomised, placebo-controlled, phase 2 trial. Lancet 2018;392(10143):222–31.

46. Dörner T, Tanaka Y, Petri M, et al. Baricitinib-associated changes in type I inter-feron gene signature during a 24-week phase-2 clinical SLE trial [abstract]. Arthritis Rheumatol 2018;70(suppl 10).

47. A study of baricitinib (LY3009104) in participants with systemic lupus erythema-tosus (BRAVE I). ClinicalTrials.gov Identifier: NCT03616912. Available at: https://clinicaltrials.gov/ct2/show/NCT03616912. Accessed December 12, 2020.

48. A study of baricitinib in participants with systemic lupus erythematosus (BRAVE II). ClinicalTrials.gov Identifier: NCT03616964. Accessed December 12, 2020.

49. A study of baricitinib in participants with systemic lupus erythematosus (SLE) (SLE- BRAVE-X). ClinicalTrials.gov Identifier: NCT03843125. Available at: https://clinicaltrials.gov/ct2/show/NCT03843125. Accessed December 12, 2020.

50. Furumoto Y, Smith CK, Blanco L, et al. Tofacitinib ameliorates murine lupus and its associated vascular dysfunction. Arthritis Rheumatol 2017;69(1):148–60.

51. Hasni S, Gupta S, Davis M, et al. A phase 1b/2a trial of tofacitinib, an oral janus kinase inhibitor, in systemic lupus erythematosus [abstract]. Arthritis Rheumatol 2019;71(suppl 10).

52. Oral tofacitinib in adult subjects with discoid lupus erythematosus (DLE) and systemic lupus erythematosus (SLE). Clinicaltrials.gov Identifier: NCT03159936. Available at: https://clinicaltrials.gov/ct2/show/NCT03159936. Accessed December 12, 2020.

53. Open-label study of tofacitinib for moderate to severe skin involvement in young adults with lupus. Clinicaltrials.gov Identifier: NCT03288324. Available at: https://clinicaltrials.gov/ct2/show/NCT03288324. Accessed December 12, 2020.

54. A study to investigate the safety and efficacy of ABBV-105 and upadacitinib given alone or in combination in participants with moderately to severely active systemic lupus erythematosus. Clinicaltrials.gov Identifier: NCT03978520. Avail-able at: https://clinicaltrials.gov/ct2/show/NCT03978520. Accessed December 12, 2020.

55. Study to evaluate safety and efficacy of filgotinib and lanraplenib in females with moderately-to-severely active cutaneous lupus erythematosus (CLE). Clinical-trials.gov Identifier: NCT03134222. Available at: https://clinicaltrials.gov/ct2/show/NCT03134222. Accessed December 12, 2020.

56. Baker M, Chaichian Y, Genovese M, et al. Phase II, randomised, double-blind, multicentre study evaluating the safety and efficacy of filgotinib and lanraplenib in patients with lupus membranous nephropathy. RMD Open 2020;6(3):e001490.

57. Sigurdsson S, Nordmark G, Goring HHH, et al. Polymorphisms in the tyrosine kinase 2 and interferon regulatory factor 5 genes are associated with systemic lupus erythematosus. Am J Hum Genet 2005;76(3):528–37.

58. A dose-ranging study to evaluate efficacy and safety of PF-06700841 in systemic lupus erythematosus (SLE). Clinicaltrials.gov Identifier: NCT03845517. Available at: https://clinicaltrials.gov/ct2/show/NCT03845517. Accessed December 12, 2020.

59. An investigational study to evaluate BMS-986165 in patients with systemic lupus erythematosus. Clinicaltrials.gov Identifier: NCT03252587. Available at: https://clinicaltrials.gov/ct2/show/NCT03252587. Accessed December 12, 2020.

60. Kim JM, Park SH, Kim HY, et al. A plasmacytoid dendritic cells-type I interferon axis is critically implicated in the pathogenesis of systemic lupus erythematosus. Int J Mol Sci 2015;16(6):14158–70.

61. Blomberg S, Eloranta ML, Magnusson M, et al. Expression of the markers BDCA-2 and BDCA-4 and production of interferon-alpha by plasmacytoid dendritic cells in systemic lupus erythematosus. Arthritis Rheum 2003;48(9): 2524–32.

62. Wu P, Wu J, Liu S, et al. TLR9/TLR7-triggered downregulation of BDCA2 expression on human plasmacytoid dendritic cells from healthy individuals and lupus patients. Clin Immunol 2008;129(1):40–8.

63. Furie R, van Vollenhoven R, Kalunian K, et al. Efficacy and safety results from a phase 2, randomized, double-blind trial of BIIB059, an anti- blood dendritic cell antigen 2 antibody, in SLE [abstract]. Arthritis Rheumatol 2020;72(suppl 10).

64. Werth V, Furie R, Romero-Diaz J, et al. BIIB059, a humanized monoclonal antibody targeting blood dendritic cell antigen 2 on plasmacytoid dendritic cells, shows dose-related efficacy in a phase 2 study in participants with active cutaneous lupus erythematosus [abstract]. Arthritis Rheumatol 2020;72(suppl 10).

65. Morel L. Immunometabolism in systemic lupus erythematosus. Nat Rev Rheumatol 2017;13:280–90.

66. Perl A. Mechanistic target of rapamycin pathway activation in rheumatic diseases. Nat Rev Rheumatol 2016;12:169–82.

67. Lai ZW, Kelly R, Winans T, et al. Sirolimus in patients with clinically active systemic lupus erythematosus resistant to, or intolerant of, conventional medications: a single-arm, open-label, phase 1/2 trial. Lancet 2018;391(10126): 1186–96.

68. Efficacy and safety of sirolimus in active systemic lupus erythematosus (SiroLupus). ClinicalTrials.gov Identifier: NCT04582136. Available at: https://clinicaltrials.gov/ct2/show/NCT04582136. Accessed December 12, 2020.

69. Suwannaroj S, Lagoo A, Keisler D, et al. Antioxidants suppress mortality in the female NZB x NZW F1 mouse model of systemic lupus erythematosus (SLE). Lupus 2001;10:258–65.

70. Banki K, Hutter E, Colombo E, et al. Glutathione levels and sensitivity to apoptosis are regulated by changes in transaldolase expression. J Biol Chem 1996;271:32994–3001.

71. O'Loghlen A, Perez-Morgado MI, Salinas M, et al. N-acetyl-cysteine abolishes hydrogen peroxide-induced modification of eukaryotic initiation factor 4F activity via distinct signalling pathways. Cell Signal 2006;18:21–31.

72. Lai ZW, Hanczko R, Bonilla E, et al. N-acetylcysteine reduces disease activity by blocking mammalian target of rapamycin in T cells from systemic lupus erythematosus patients: a randomized, double-blind, placebo-controlled trial. Arthritis Rheum 2012;64(9):2937–46.

73. Treatment of Systemic Lupus Erythematosus (SLE) With N-acetylcysteine (NAC). Clinicaltrials.gov Identifier: NCT00775476. Available at: https://clinicaltrials.gov/ct2/show/NCT00775476. Accessed December 12, 2020.

74. Gao S, Wang S, Song Y. Novel immunomodulatory drugs and neo-substrates. Biomark Res 2020;8:2.

75. Furie R, Werth VP, Gaudy A, et al. A randomized, placebo-controlled, double-blind, ascending-dose, safety, and pharmacokinetics study of CC-220 in subjects with systemic LUPUS erythematosus [abstract]. Arthritis Rheumatol 2017;69(suppl 10).

76. Merrill J, Werth V, Furie R, et al. Efficacy and safety of iberdomide in patients with active systemic lupus erythematosus: 24-week results of a phase 2, randomized, placebo-controlled study [abstract]. Arthritis Rheumatol 2020; 72(suppl 10).

77. Lipsky P, van Vollenhoven R, Dörner T, et al. Iberdomide decreases B cells and plasmacytoid dendritic cells, increases regulatory T cells and IL-2, and has enhanced clinical efficacy in active systemic lupus erythematosus patients with high Aiolos or the IFN gene expression signature [abstract]. Arthritis Rheumatol 2020;72(suppl 10).

78. Wallace DJ. Low-dose interleukin-2 for systemic lupus erythematosus? Lancet Rheumatol 2019;1(1):e7–8.

79. Lieberman LA, Tsokos GC. The IL-2 defect in systemic lupus erythematosus disease has an expansive effect on host immunity. J Biomed Biotechnol 2010;2010: 740619.

80. Langowski J, Kirk P, Addepalli M, et al. NKTR-38: A selective, first-in-class IL-2 pathway agonist which increases number and suppressive function of regulatory T cells for the treatment of immune inflammatory disorders [abstract]. Arthritis Rheumatol 2017;69(suppl 10).

81. Rosenzwajg M, Lorenzon R, Cacoub P, et al. Immunological and clinical effects of low-dose interleukin-2 across 11 autoimmune diseases in a single, open clinical trial. Ann Rheum Dis 2019;78(2):209–17.

82. Humrich JY, von Spee-Mayer C, Siegert E, et al. Low-dose interleukin-2 therapy in refractory systemic lupus erythematosus: an investigator-initiated, single-centre phase 1 and 2a clinical trial. Lancet Rheumatol 2019;1(1):e44–54.

83. He J, Zhang R, Shao M, et al. Efficacy and safety of low-dose IL-2 in the treatment of systemic lupus erythematosus: a randomised, double-blind, placebo-controlled trial. Ann Rheum Dis 2020;79(1):141–9.

84. Safety, tolerability, pharmacokinetics, pharmacodynamics, and immunogenicity of AMG 592 in participants with systemic lupus erythematosus. Clinicaltrials.gov Identifier: NCT03451422. Available at: https://clinicaltrials.gov/ct2/show/ NCT03451422. Accessed December 12, 2020.

85. A study of LY3471851 in adults with systemic lupus erythematosus (SLE) (IS-LAND-SLE). Clinicaltrials.gov Identifier: NCT04433585. Available at: https://clinicaltrials.gov/ct2/show/NCT04433585. Accessed December 12, 2020.

86. Merrill JT, Neuwelt CM, Wallace DJ, et al. Efficacy and safety of rituximab in moderately- to-severely active systemic lupus erythematosus: the randomized, double-blind, phase II/III systemic lupus erythematosus evaluation of rituximab trial. Arthritis Rheum 2010;62(1):222–33.

87. Rovin BH, Furie R, Latinis K, et al. Efficacy and safety of rituximab in patients with active proliferative lupus nephritis: the Lupus Nephritis Assessment with Rituximab study. Arthritis Rheum 2012;64(4):1215–26.

88. Beckwith H, Lightstone L. Rituximab in systemic lupus erythematosus and lupus nephritis. Nephron Clin Pract 2014;128(3–4):250–4.

89. Terrier B, Amoura Z, Ravaud P, et al. Safety and efficacy of rituximab in systemic lupus erythematosus: results from 136 patients from the French AutoImmunity and Rituximab registry. Arthritis Rheum 2010;62:2458–66.

90. Jonsdottir T, Gunnarsson I, Mourao AF, et al. Clinical improvements in proliferative vs membranous lupus nephritis following B-cell depletion: pooled data from two cohorts. Rheumatology (Oxford) 2010;49:1502–4.

91. Aguiar R, Araujo C, Martins-Coelho G, et al. Use of rituximab in systemic lupus erythematosus: a single center experience over 14 years. Arthritis Care Res (Hoboken) 2017;69(2):257–62.

92. McCarthy EM, Sutton E, Nesbit S, et al. Short-term efficacy and safety of rituximab therapy in refractory systemic lupus erythematosus: results from the British Isles Lupus Assessment Group Biologics Register. Rheumatology (Oxford) 2018;57(3):470–9.

93. Fernández-Nebro A, de la Fuente JL, Carreño L, et al. Multicenter longitudinal study of B-lymphocyte depletion in refractory systemic lupus erythematosus: the LESIMAB study. Lupus 2012;21:1063–76.

94. Md Yusof MY, Shaw D, El-Sherbiny YM, et al. Predicting and managing primary and secondary non-response to rituximab using B-cell biomarkers in systemic lupus erythematosus. Ann Rheum Dis 2017;76:1829–36.

95. Cassia MA, Alberici F, Jones RB, et al. Rituximab as maintenance treatment for systemic lupus erythematosus: a multicenter observational study of 147 patients. Arthritis Rheumatol 2019;71:1670–80.

96. Freitas S, Mozo Ruiz M, Costa Carneiro A, et al. Why do some patients with systemic lupus erythematosus fail to respond to B-cell depletion using rituximab? Clin Exp Rheumatol 2020;38:262–6.

97. Tani C, Elefante E, Signorini V, et al. Glucocorticoid withdrawal in systemic lupus erythematosus: are remission and low disease activity reliable starting points for stopping treatment? A real-life experience. RMD Open 2019;5:e000916.

98. Tselios K, Gladman D, Su J, et al. Gradual glucocorticoid withdrawal is safe in clinically quiescent systemic lupus erythematosus [abstract]. Arthritis Rheumatol 2020;72(Suppl 10).

99. Zen M, Gatto M, Benvenuti F, et al. SAT0163 Immunosuppressant withdrawal after remission achievement in lupus nephritis: effect on flare occurrence [abstract]. Ann Rheum Dis 2020;79(Suppl 1):1018.

100. Chakravarty E, Utset T, Kamen DL, et al. OP0167 Successful withdrawal of mycophenolate mofetil in quiescent SLE: results from a randomized trial [abstract]. Ann Rheum Dis 2020;79(Suppl 1):105.

101. Furie R, Parikh S, Harvey K, et al. Treatment of SLE with or without nephritis with the immunoproteasome inhibitor KZR-616: updated results of the MISSION study [abstract]. Arthritis Rheumatol 2020;72(suppl 10).

102. A study of KZR-616 in patients with SLE with and without lupus nephritis (MISSION). ClinicalTrials.gov Identifier: NCT03393013. Available at: https://clinicaltrials.gov/ct2/show/NCT03393013. Accessed December 12, 2020.

103. Study of EQ001 (itolizumab) in systemic lupus erythematosus with or without active proliferative nephritis (EQUALISE). ClinicalTrials.gov Identifier: NCT04128579. Available at: https://clinicaltrials.gov/ct2/show/NCT04128579. Accessed December 12, 2020.

104. Zhou T, Li HY, Liao C, et al. Clinical efficacy and safety of mesenchymal stem cells for systemic lupus erythematosus. Stem Cells Int 2020;2020:6518508.

105. Phase 2 trial of mesenchymal stem cells in systemic lupus erythematosus (MiSLE). ClinicalTrials.gov Identifier: NCT02633163. Available at: https://clinicaltrials.gov/ct2/show/NCT02633163. Accessed December 12, 2020.

106. Yang SK, Zhang HR, Shi SP, et al. The role of mitochondria in systemic lupus erythematosus: a glimpse of various pathogenetic mechanisms. Curr Med Chem 2019;26:1–15.

107. Lood C, Blanco LP, Purmalek MM, et al. Neutrophil extracellular traps enriched in oxidized mitochondrial DNA are interferogenic and contribute to lupus-like disease. Nat Med 2016;22:146–53.

108. Romo-Tena J, Kaplan MJ. Immunometabolism in the pathogenesis of systemic lupus erythematosus: an update. Curr Opin Rheumatol 2020;32(6):562–71.

109. El-Hattab AW, Zarante AM, Almannai M, et al. Therapies for mitochondrial diseases and current clinical trials. Mol Genet Metab 2017;122(3):1–9.

110. Blanco LP, Pedersen HL, Wang X, et al. Improved mitochondrial metabolism and reduced inflammation following attenuation of murine lupus with coenzyme Q10 analog idebenone. Arthritis Rheumatol 2020;72:454–64.

111. Karampetsou MP, Comte D, Suarez-Fueyo A, et al. Signaling lymphocytic activation molecule family member 1 engagement inhibits T cell-B cell interaction and diminishes interleukin-6 production and plasmablast differentiation in systemic lupus erythematosus. Arthritis Rheumatol 2019;71(1):99–108.

112. Linan-Rico L, Hernandez-Castro B, Doniz-Padilla L, et al. Analysis of expression and function of the co-stimulatory receptor SLAMF1 in immune cells from patients with systemic lupus erythematosus (SLE). Lupus 2015;24:1184–90.

113. Karampetsou MP, Comte D, Kis-Toth K, et al. Expression patterns of signaling lymphocytic activation molecule family members in peripheral blood mononuclear cell subsets in patients with systemic lupus erythematosus. PLoS One 2017;12:e0186073.

114. Cooper LJN, Topp MS, Serrano LM, et al. T-cell clones can be rendered specific for CD19: toward the selective augmentation of the graft-versus-B-lineage leukemia effect. Blood 2003;101(4):1637–44.

115. Brentjens RJ, Latouche JB, Santos E, et al. Eradication of systemic B-cell tumors by genetically targeted human T lymphocytes co-stimulated by CD80 and interleukin-15. Nat Med 2003;9(3):279–86.

116. Lim WA, June CH. The principles of engineering immune cells to treat cancer. Cell 2017;168(4):724–40.

117. Kansal R, Richardson N, Neeli I, et al. Sustained B cell depletion by CD19-targeted CAR T cells is a highly effective treatment for murine lupus. Sci Transl Med 2019;11(482):eaav1648.

Systemic Lupus Erythematosus Classification and Diagnosis

Martin Aringer, MD[a],*, Sindhu R. Johnson, MD, PhD[b]

KEYWORDS

- Systemic lupus erythematosus • Classification criteria
- Cutaneous lupus erythematosus • Neuropsychiatric SLE • Antinuclear antibodies
- Sensitivity • Specificity

KEY POINTS

- The European League against Rheumatism/American College of Rheumatology criteria have been externally validated in various systemic lupus erythematosus (SLE) populations, including patients with pediatric SLE.
- More than 95% of all SLE patients have (or at least had) positive antinuclear antibodies, but test quality may be an issue.
- For specificity, it is important to attribute symptoms and results to SLE only if there is no more likely alternative explanation.
- Uncommon mucocutaneous and neuropsychiatric lupus manifestations are more important for diagnostic than for classification purposes.
- Classification criteria are not designed as diagnostic tools and should never be used as an argument for withholding therapy.

The European League against Rheumatism/American College of Rheumatology (EULAR/ACR) classification criteria for systemic lupus erythematosus (SLE)[1,2] were externally validated by several studies in adult[3–12] and pediatric populations,[13–15] and more has been learned about their performance. Some investigators have referred to these classification criteria as diagnostic tools, but this is not appropriate and is highly discouraged by ACR and EULAR, given differences in methodology, statistical goals, and potentially adverse consequences for patients.[16,17] In this review, the authors highlight novel aspects of the EULAR/ACR SLE classification criteria and contrast their application with the diagnosis of SLE.

[a] Division of Rheumatology, Department of Medicine III, University Medical Center, Faculty of Medicine Carl Gustav Carus at the TU Dresden, Fetscherstrasse 74, Dresden 01037, Germany; [b] Division of Rheumatology, Department of Medicine, Toronto Western Hospital, Mount Sinai Hospital, Institute of Health Policy, Management and Evaluation, University of Toronto, Ground Floor, East Wing, 399 Bathurst Street, Toronto, Ontario M5T2S8, Canada
* Corresponding author.
E-mail address: martin.aringer@uniklinikum-dresden.de

Rheum Dis Clin N Am 47 (2021) 501–511
https://doi.org/10.1016/j.rdc.2021.04.011
0889-857X/21/© 2021 Elsevier Inc. All rights reserved.

rheumatic.theclinics.com

PERFORMANCE CHARACTERISTICS

The EULAR/ACR classification criteria project set out with the goal of preserving the excellent specificity of the ACR 1982 and 1997 classification criteria, while reaching better sensitivity, if possible, in the range of the Systemic Lupus International Collaborating Centers' (SLICC) 2012 criteria.[18] The validation cohort showed a specificity of 93%, on par with the ACR 1997 criteria, and a sensitivity of 96%, very close to the 97% of the SLICC criteria, with completely overlapping confidence intervals.[1,2]

Subgroup analyses found that the EULAR/ACR criteria work similarly well in women, in men, across ethnicities, and in early disease.[19] The overall performance with higher sensitivity than the ACR and higher specificity than the SLICC criteria was supported by cohort studies from China.[4,10] Importantly, the EULAR/ACR criteria also had excellent performance in pediatric SLE,[13–15] which had not been addressed in the EULAR/ACR classification criteria cohorts.

Regarding specificity, a review of the published literature on the EULAR/ACR 2019 criteria in various populations stresses the importance of following the EULAR/ACR attribution rule, according to which items should only be counted if there is no more likely alternative explanation.[20] Particularly in some of the articles published before the full publication of the EULAR/ACR criteria, there are indications that this rule was not followed, and this may explain a much lower specificity of the criteria than in all the other articles.[21]

WHEN DO YOU CONSIDER SYSTEMIC LUPUS ERYTHEMATOSUS?

Pretest probability is an important determinant of accurate diagnosis, which is particularly evident in situations whereby SLE is an uncommon cause. For example, in a recent study on 4766 patients with psychosis, 135 (15%) of the 911 patients tested for antinuclear antibodies (ANA) were ANA positive, but only 4 had SLE, and 2 of them had well-established disease diagnosed more than half a year earlier.[22] These numbers are less than 1 in 1000 of the total population and 0.4% of those tested for ANA.

Studies performed in the last few years highlight what symptoms and signs should cause such suspicion for SLE. In the international early SLE cohort study of 389 SLE patients, fever, weight loss, malar rash, discoid lesions, photosensitivity, oral ulcers, alopecia, inflammatory arthritis, pleuritis, pericarditis, leukopenia, and kidney involvement were all significantly more frequent in SLE patients than in those 227 patients with mimicking conditions, and were found in at least 5% of SLE patients.[23] Most common were arthritis (57.6%), malar rash (49.6%), fever (34.5%), photosensitivity (31.6%), and alopecia (30.6%). Of interest, fatigue (28.3 vs 37.0%), Raynaud (22.1% vs 48.5%), and arthralgias (20.3% vs 42.7%) were more common in the patients with mimicking conditions.[23] Still, in a patient survey performed with the German SLE patient association, 303 of 339 (89.4%) SLE patients reported fatigue as a symptom of their disease around the time of diagnosis, followed by joint pain (86.7%), photosensitivity (79.4%),[24] and fever (53.7%).

Similarly, in the 768 patients of the SLICC inception cohort, arthritis (75.9%) was most common, followed by hematologic disorder (66.8%), oral ulcers (38.3%), malar rash and photosensitivity (each 35.9%), and renal disorder (30.7%).[25] In their n = 199 early SLE cohort from China, Teng and colleagues[10] found leukopenia (63%), arthritis (52%), hemolytic anemia (44%), fever (38%), and proteinuria (31%) in more than 30% of their patients.

Therefore, arthritis, mucocutaneous features, noninfectious fever, leukopenia, and hemolytic anemia are certainly reasons to consider SLE. Because of their higher specificity, the same is true for serositis, and for unexplained proteinuria.[23] For unexplained proteinuria, biopsy usually will be indicated,[26] which will greatly increase specificity in case of typical findings of lupus nephritis.

ANTINUCLEAR ANTIBODIES

One of the strategic changes in the EULAR/ACR criteria was the repositioning of ANA to an obligatory entry criterion. This repositioning was also one of the hotly debated steps. The decision was made based on a metaregression of published data on 13,080 patients that found a sensitivity of 97.8%, with a 95% confidence of 96.8% to 98.5% at a titer of at least 1:80,[27] and supported by SLE expert consensus.[28]

Pisetsky and colleagues[29] presented data on differences in the performance of standard HEp-2 cell substrates. Serum samples from 103 SLE patients known to be previously ANA positive were tested with 3 different HEp-2 cell-based immunofluorescence kits, an enzyme-linked immunosorbent assay (ELISA), and a multiplex assay. These assays showed between 5% and 22% negative and an additional 2% to 9% indeterminate results. At rates of 14% (Multiplex) and 12% (ELISA) negative rates, the nonimmunofluorescence tests were in the range of the second best performing HEp-2 immunofluorescence assay (10% negative). The HEp-2000 substrate used for the immunofluorescence test with the worst performance might lead to a sensitivity as low as 78%, or 69%, if indeterminate results are treated as negative.

These issues are highly important and need to be resolved. Although they may play a role in some populations, most patients in recently published cohorts, namely 8648 of 8902 SLE patients (97.1%), were still positive (**Table 1**).

Frodlund and colleagues[35] investigated the ANA of 54 recently diagnosed SLE patients over 8 years. Of these 54 patients, 47 (87%) stayed constantly ANA positive, but 7 patients (13%) lost ANA positivity. Although anti-Ro-positive patients mostly stayed positive, half of the patients with antibodies to double-stranded DNA (dsDNA) and most of those with anti-histone antibodies lost ANA positivity. These effects are presumably due to therapeutic interventions and underscore the importance of accepting patients as fulfilling the obligatory entry criterion when ANA have ever been positive.

Conversely, negative ANA should not prevent an SLE diagnosis. The data presented in **Table 1** demonstrate that 254 individual SLE patients may have been truly and persistently ANA negative. Leaving them out of trials probably is not a major issue, whereas denying them appropriate therapy for their SLE would be. ANA may be (falsely negative) when patients have anti-Ro antibodies. Low complement proteins as an indication of immune complex disease may also be helpful, although this approach did not appear to cover most ANA-negative SLE patients. As mentioned above, ANA sensitivity is dependent on test quality, and retesting may be warranted.

For diagnostic considerations, dense fine-speckled anti-70 kDa (DFS-70) antibodies play a relevant role in that these antibodies make SLE and other connective tissue diseases unlikely.[36] There are occasional SLE patients with anti-DFS-70 antibodies, but then also there are other defined subsets and usually a relatively mild course.[37] Anti-DFS-70 antibodies also relate to a broader concept, namely, that ANA patterns often are useful for diagnostic purposes.[38]

THE EUROPEAN LEAGUE AGAINST RHEUMATISM/AMERICAN COLLEGE OF RHEUMATOLOGY CRITERIA RULES

Essential for correctly applying the EULAR/ACR SLE classification criteria are several rules (**Fig. 1**). First, SLE is a disease and should neither be classified nor diagnosed if there never were any clinical symptoms, including hematological symptoms, even in

Table 1
Antinuclear antibodies in cohorts of systemic lupus erythematosus patients related to systemic lupus erythematosus classification criteria

ANA Positive (n)	Total Population (n)	ANA Positive (%)	Cohort	Reference
499	501	99.6	EULAR/ACR derivation	Aringer et al,[1] 2019
691	696	99.3	EULAR/ACR validation	Aringer et al,[1] 2019
341	349	97.7	SLICC validation	Petri et al,[6] 2020
Σ 1531	Σ 1546	99.0	*Classification criteria cohorts*	
387	389	99.5	Early SLE cohort	Mosca et al,[23] 2019
1066	1137	93.8	SLICC inception	Choi et al,[30] 2019
646	690	93.6	Greek early SLE	Adamichou et al,[3] 2019
192	192	100.0	Chinese new onset	Teng et al,[31] 2020
Σ 2291	Σ 2408	95.1	*Early SLE*	
55	56	98.2	Swedish	Dahlström & Sjöwall,[32] 2019
332	336	98.8	Swedish	Elbagir et al,[33] 2020
95	98	96.9	Sudanese	Elbagir et al,[33] 2020
283	294	96.3	Dutch neuropsychiatric	Gegenava et al,[34] 2019
331	335	98.8	Korean	Lee et al,[5] 2020
1168	1217	96.0	GLADEL Latin American	Pons-Estel et al,[7] 2020
209	217	96.3	Beth Israel Deaconess United States	Rubio et al,[8] 2020
1830	1865	98.1	Chinese	Jin et al,[4] 2020
Σ 4303	Σ 4418	97.4	*Worldwide cohorts*	
156	156	100.0	Pediatric SLE	Ma et al,[15] 2020
108	112	96.4	Pediatric SLE	Aljaberi et al,[13] 2020
259	262	98.9	Pediatric SLE	Batu et al,[14] 2020
Σ 523	Σ 530	98.7	*Pediatric SLE cohorts*	
Total 8648	Total 8902	97.1	All data combined	

Studies were only included if not based on positive ANA as an inclusion criterion and if respecting the "ANA every positive" principle, that is, not reporting freshly done ANA tests at the current timepoint only.

Classification (ANA + ≥10)

Diagnostic considerations

Positive ANA (ever) required.	Truly **ANA negative SLE** possible.
≥1:80 on Hep-2 cells or an equivalent positive test	Consider antibodies to Ro, dsDNA, C1q, ribosomal P, and C3 activation

Do not consider items, if there is a more likely explanation other than SLE
occurrence once ever is sufficient, need not be simultaneous
Given associations, consider only one item (the highest weighted) in each domain

Nephritis		**Nephritis**
Class III/IV	10	Other forms (eg, IgA nephritis) are much
Class II/V	8	less common, but possible in SLE
Proteinuria >0.5 g/d	4	Hematuria/cylinders rare without protein

Musculoskeletal		**Musculoskeletal**
Joint involvement	6	Occasionally lupus myositis

Serositis		**Serositis**
Acute pericarditis	6	Sterile peritonitis possible
Pleural or pericardial effusion	5	Sterile meninigitis possible

Mucocutaneous		**Mucocutaneous**
ACLE (malar or generalized rash)	6	Consider also bullous lupus, toxic
SCLE or discoid lupus	4	epidermal necrolysis variant of SLE,
Oral ulcers	2	hypertrophic lupus, lupus panniculitis,
Non-scarring alopecia	2	Chillblains lupus, and nasal ulcers

Neuropsychiatric		**Neuropsychiatric**
Seizure	5	Rare manifestations include transverse
Psychosis	3	myelitis, chorea, mononeuritis multiplex,
Delirium	2	and cranial or peripheral neuropathy

Hematologic		**Hematologic**
Hemolytic anemia	4	Lymphopenia and anemia of chrionic
Thrombocytopenia <100,000	4	disease are common, but less specific
Leukopenia <4000	3	Consider also mild thrombocytopenia

Constitutional		**Constitutional**
Fever (>38.3°C)	2	Lymphadenopathy, weight loss possible

SLE-specific antibodies		**Less SLE-specific antibodies**
Anti-Sm(ith)	6	Consider antibodies to Ro,U1RNP, C1q,
Anti-dsDNA (≥90% specificity)	6	ribosomal P, nucleosomes, dsDNA (other)

Complement proteins		**Complement proteins**
C3 and C4 low	4	Where available, cell-bound complement
C3 or C4 low	3	split products are probably equivalent

Anti-phospholipid antibodies		**Anti-phospholipid antibodies**
LAC or ACLA or anti-β2-gpl IgG/M/A	2	Noncriteria antibodies may be considered

Fig. 1. Contrasting EULAR/ACR classification criteria features and diagnostic considerations.

the presence of impressive autoantibodies. Therefore, SLE classification still requires at least 1 clinical criterion, as with the previous classification criteria sets. Second, it is sufficient for any criterion to occur on at least 1 occasion, and criteria need not occur simultaneously.[39] When SLE is highly active in an individual patient, the disease may show the full array of organ symptoms this patient ever had, but this need not be the case. Only accounting for consecutive autoantibody-driven events will therefore take the full spectrum into account and display the character of SLE as a disease of multiple autoantibodies (and ensuing immune complexes).

Both the ACR and the SLICC criteria have treated the single criteria as independent. During the EULAR/ACR classification criteria project, it became evident that we did not have sufficient data to answer whether this was a correct assumption. Therefore, associations between criteria items were investigated in the early SLE cohort and validated in the Euro-Lupus cohort.[40] These analyses found relevant associations within organ domains. Such associations were present in mucocutaneous disease, as clinically suspected. Associations were also found in the hematological domain, between SLE-specific autoantibodies and between anti-phospholipid antibodies. Because these items were not independent, they were again grouped in domains. Therefore, within each domain only the highest weighted criterion is counted toward the total score.

Finally, a common attribution rule for the EULAR/ACR criteria replaced individual exceptions introduced into item definitions in the ACR[39] and the SLICC criteria.[41] Instead of defining "in the absence of offending drugs or known metabolic derangement; for example, uremia, ketoacidosis, or electrolyte imbalance" for seizures in the ACR criteria,[39] the attribution rule mandates to not count any criterion if there is a more likely explanation than SLE.

SYSTEMIC LUPUS ERYTHEMATOSUS ORGAN AND SEROLOGIC MANIFESTATIONS

The authors have also gained important insights about the individual criteria items[42]; this is of particular interest in areas where the EULAR/ACR criteria differ from the SLICC criteria, specifically among mucocutaneous and neuropsychiatric manifestations.

Mucocutaneous Manifestations

The EULAR/ACR and SLICC criteria overlap largely with regard to acute cutaneous lupus erythematosus (ACLE), subacute cutaneous lupus erythematosus (SCLE), and discoid lupus erythematosus, as well as nonscarring alopecia.[43] The differences are that bullous lupus, the toxic epidermal necrolysis variant, as well as other forms of photosensitive lupus rash are not part of the EULAR/ACR criteria, as are nasal ulcers. The chronic cutaneous LE items of the SLICC criteria also contain hypertrophic lupus, lupus panniculitis, mucosal lupus, LE tumidus, Chilblains lupus, and discoid LE/lichen planus overlap.[41] These manifestations were not included in the EULAR/ACR criteria, largely because they were considered SLE manifestations too uncommon for inclusion.

In their specialized Dermatology outpatient cohort, Zapata and Chong[44] found a total of 42 patients with forms of LE not included into the EULAR/ACR 2019 criteria. Of these, 17, namely 8 with LE tumidus, 5 with bullous lupus, and 2 each with lupus panniculitis and Chilblain lupus, met SLICC criteria for SLE, of whom 5 (2 with LE tumidus and one each with the 3 other LE forms) did not meet EULR/ACR criteria. Stec-Polak and colleagues[45] found the best specificity for the EULAR/ACR criteria in their 109 patients with SCLE and 75 patients with discoid LE, with the 15% of their cutaneous LE patients fulfilling the EULAR/ACR 2019 criteria still not developing severe organ disease. In their Chinese cohort, Jin and colleagues[4] found the EULAR/ACR criteria more specific than the SLICC criteria in distinguishing between cutaneous LE and

SLE. The ACR 1997 were more specific, but still at a level of only 69%. The true borderline between SLE and cutaneous LE remains somewhat unclear, with relevant proportions of patients diagnosed with cutaneous LE without SLE still having fever, arthritis, leukopenia, hemolytic anemia, or anti-Sm or anti-dsDNA antibodies.[4]

Neuropsychiatric Manifestations

Of the neuropsychiatric SLE (NPSLE) manifestations of the SLICC criteria,[41] seizure, psychosis, and delirium (termed acute confusional state in the SLICC criteria) remained in the EULAR/ACR criteria, but myelitis and mononeuritis multiplex were voted out in the definition stage[20] and cranial or peripheral neuropathy during the multicriteria decision analysis exercise of the EULAR/ACR criteria.[46] In the SLICC inception cohort, a total of 572 patients had 242 NPSLE events.[47] These events included 19 seizures (3% of 572), 12 acute confusional state (2%), 7 psychosis (1%), 8 polyneuropathy (1%), 5 cranial neuropathy (1%), 2 myelopathy, and 2 movement disorders.

In a cohort of 294 SLE patients and 66 non-SLE patients with neuropsychiatric symptoms, the EULAR/ACR criteria reached a sensitivity of 87%, as compared with 85% of the SLICC and 89% of the ACR 1997 criteria.[34] In this cohort, 28 (10%) had seizures versus 2 (3%) in the non-SLE group, 12 (4%) versus 2 (3%) psychosis, 9 (3%) versus 0 delirium, 10 (3%) versus 4 (6%) neuropathy, and 9 (3%) versus 2 (3%) myelitis. Thus, neuropathy and myelitis were not distinguishing between SLE and non-SE patients. Considerable groups of 31 and 30 patients, respectively, had cognitive dysfunction and cerebrovascular disease.

Complement Proteins

The SLICC group had included low complement, that is, low C3, low C4, and low CH50, into their criteria.[41] This definition was modified to either low C3 or C4 (3 points) or low C3 and C4 (4 points) in the EULAR/ACR 2019 criteria. Cell-bound complement activation products (CB-CAPs) had been considered during the expert Delphi exercise,[48] but had not reached sufficient support, based on insufficient test availability worldwide. Still, CB-CAPS are reflective of the same immune-complex-driven mechanisms reflected by low C3 (and low C4, unless genetically deficient). Although inclusion into classification criteria, as suggested,[49] would require worldwide availability, there are now data on a higher sensitivity of CB-CAPs,[50] which are of probable diagnostic value where the test is available.

SUMMARY

The EULAR/ACR 2019 classification criteria for SLE are a recent advance in the field, which reflects the current understanding of SLE. It is important to once more reiterate that classification criteria are not meant to be a diagnostic tool and should never be used as an argument for withholding appropriate treatment. The SLE diagnosis must rely on the experience of appropriately trained physicians. However, the data derived from the classification criteria process are helpful for educating physicians.

CLINICS CARE POINTS

- Most SLE patients are (or were) ANA positive, but ANA negative SLE occurs.
- Autoantibody test quality is essential for both ANA and antibodies to double-stranded DNA.
- While fever can be an early sign of SLE, infection needs to be excluded first. High CRP argues for infection.

- SLE symptoms can also be caused by other disease, count them for SLE only if not better explained otherwise.
- Within organ domains, associations of several symptoms are common.
- Never withhold appropriate SLE therapy because a patient does not meet classification criteria.

DISCLOSURE

The development of the SLE criteria was jointly funded by EULAR and ACR. M. Aringer and S.R. Johnson have acted as co-chairs of the EULAR/ACR classification criteria steering committee. No other conflicts of interest apply to this article.

REFERENCES

1. Aringer M, Costenbader K, Daikh D, et al. 2019 European League Against Rheumatism/American College of Rheumatology Classification Criteria for Systemic Lupus Erythematosus. Arthritis Rheumatol 2019;71(9):1400–12.
2. Aringer M, Costenbader K, Daikh D, et al. 2019 European League Against Rheumatism/American College of Rheumatology classification criteria for systemic lupus erythematosus. Ann Rheum Dis 2019;78(9):1151–9.
3. Adamichou C, Nikolopoulos D, Genitsaridi I, et al. In an early SLE cohort the ACR-1997, SLICC-2012 and EULAR/ACR-2019 criteria classify non-overlapping groups of patients: use of all three criteria ensures optimal capture for clinical studies while their modification earlier classification and treatment. Ann Rheum Dis 2020;79(2):232–41.
4. Jin H, Huang T, Wu R, et al. A comparison and review of three sets of classification criteria for systemic lupus erythematosus for distinguishing systemic lupus erythematosus from pure mucocutaneous manifestations in the lupus disease spectrum. Lupus 2020;29(14):1854–65.
5. Lee EE, Lee EB, Park JK, et al. Performance of the 2019 European League Against Rheumatism/American College of Rheumatology classification criteria for systemic lupus erythematosus in Asian patients: a single-centre retrospective cohort study in Korea. Clin Exp Rheumatol 2020;38(6):1075–9.
6. Petri M, Goldman DW, Alarcón GS, et al. A comparison of 2019 EULAR/ACR SLE classification criteria with two sets of earlier SLE classification criteria. Arthritis Care Res 2020. https://doi.org/10.1002/acr.24263.
7. Pons-Estel GJ, Ugarte-Gil MF, Harvey GB, et al. Applying the 2019 EULAR/ACR lupus criteria to patients from an established cohort: a Latin American perspective. RMD Open 2020;6(1):e001097.
8. Rubio J, Krishfield S, Kyttaris VC. Application of the 2019 European League Against Rheumatism/American College of Rheumatology systemic lupus erythematosus classification criteria in clinical practice: a single center experience. Lupus 2020;29(4):421–5.
9. Suda M, Kishimoto M, Ohde S, et al. Validation of the 2019 ACR/EULAR classification criteria of systemic lupus erythematosus in 100 Japanese patients: a real-world setting analysis. Clin Rheumatol 2020;39(6):1823–7.
10. Teng J, Zhou Z, Wang F, et al. Do 2019 European League Against Rheumatism/American College of Rheumatology classification criteria for systemic lupus erythematosus also indicate the disease activity? Ann Rheum Dis 2020;217017.

11. Ugarte-Gil MF, Pons-Estel GJ, Griffin R, et al. Patients who do not fulfill the 2019 EULAR/ACR criteria for systemic lupus erythematosus accrue less damage. Arthritis Care Res 2020. https://doi.org/10.1002/acr.24213.
12. Ugarte-Gil MF, Pons-Estel GJ, Harvey GB, et al. Applying the 2019 EULAR/ACR lupus criteria to patients from the LUMINA Cohort. Arthritis Care Res 2020. https://doi.org/10.1002/acr.24367.
13. Aljaberi N, Nguyen K, Strahle C, et al. The performance of the new 2019-EULAR/ACR classification criteria for systemic lupus erythematosus in children and young adults. Arthritis Care Res 2020;73(4):580–5.
14. Batu ED, Kaya Akca U, Pac Kısaarslan A, et al. The performances of the ACR 1997, SLICC 2012, and EULAR/ACR 2019 classification criteria in pediatric systemic lupus erythematosus. J Rheumatol 2020. https://doi.org/10.3899/jrheum.200871.
15. Ma M, Hui-Yuen JS, Cerise JE, et al. Validation of the 2017 weighted criteria compared to the 1997 ACR and the 2012 SLICC in pediatric systemic lupus erythematosus. Arthritis Care Res (Hoboken) 2020;72(11):1597–601.
16. Johnson SR, Goek ON, Singh-Grewal D, et al. Classification criteria in rheumatic diseases: a review of methodologic properties. Arthritis Rheum 2007;57(7):1119–33.
17. Aringer M, Costenbader KH, Dorner T, et al. Difference between SLE classification and diagnosis and importance of attribution. Response to: 'Do the 2019 EULAR/ACR SLE classification criteria close the door on certain groups of SLE patients?' by Chi et al. Ann Rheum Dis 2019. https://doi.org/10.1136/annrheumdis-2019-216338.
18. Aringer M, Dorner T, Leuchten N, et al. Toward new criteria for systemic lupus erythematosus-a standpoint. Lupus 2016;25(8):805–11.
19. Johnson SR, Brinks R, Costenbader KH, et al. Performance of the 2019 EULAR/ACR classification criteria for systemic lupus erythematosus in early disease, across sexes and ethnicities. Ann Rheum Dis 2020;79(10):1333–9.
20. Tedeschi SK, Johnson SR, Boumpas D, et al. Developing and refining new candidate criteria for systemic lupus erythematosus classification: an international collaboration. Arthritis Care Res(Hoboken) 2018;70(4):571–81.
21. Aringer M, Johnson SR. New lupus criteria: a critical view. Curr Opin Rheumatol 2021;33:205–10.
22. Spies MC, Gutjahr-Holland JA, Bertouch JV, et al. Prevalence of neuropsychiatric lupus in psychosis patients with a positive antinuclear antibody. Arthritis Care Res 2020. https://doi.org/10.1002/acr.24472.
23. Mosca M, Costenbader KH, Johnson SR, et al. Brief report: how do patients with newly diagnosed systemic lupus erythematosus present? A multicenter cohort of early systemic lupus erythematosus to inform the development of new classification criteria. Arthritis Rheumatol 2019;71(1):91–8.
24. Leuchten N, Milke B, Winkler-Rohlfing B, et al. Early symptoms of systemic lupus erythematosus as reported by members of the German Lupus Erythematosus Patient Association. Arthritis Rheumatol 2015;67(Suppl 10) (abstract 730).
25. Urowitz MB, Gladman DD, Ibañez D, et al. American College of Rheumatology criteria at inception, and accrual over 5 years in the SLICC inception cohort. J Rheumatol 2014;41(5):875–80.
26. Fanouriakis A, Kostopoulou M, Cheema K, et al. 2019 Update of the Joint European League Against Rheumatism and European Renal Association-European Dialysis and Transplant Association (EULAR/ERA-EDTA) recommendations for the management of lupus nephritis. Ann Rheum Dis 2020;79(6):713–23.

27. Leuchten N, Hoyer A, Brinks R, et al. Performance of antinuclear antibodies for classifying systemic lupus erythematosus: a systematic literature review and meta-regression of diagnostic data. Arthritis Care Res(Hoboken). 2018;70(3): 428–38.
28. Johnson SR, Khanna D, Daikh D, et al. Use of consensus methodology to determine candidate items for systemic lupus erythematosus classification criteria. J Rheumatol 2019;46(7):721–6.
29. Pisetsky DS, Spencer DM, Lipsky PE, et al. Assay variation in the detection of antinuclear antibodies in the sera of patients with established SLE. Ann Rheum Dis 2018;77(6):911–3.
30. Choi MY, Clarke AE, St Pierre Y, et al. Antinuclear antibody-negative systemic lupus erythematosus in an international inception cohort. Arthritis Care Res 2019;71(7):893–902.
31. Teng J, Ye J, Zhou Z, et al. A comparison of the performance of the 2019 European League Against Rheumatism/American College of Rheumatology criteria and the 2012 Systemic Lupus International Collaborating Clinics criteria with the 1997 American College of Rheumatology classification criteria for systemic lupus erythematous in new-onset Chinese patients. Lupus 2020;29(6):617–24.
32. Dahlström Ö, Sjöwall C. The diagnostic accuracies of the 2012 SLICC criteria and the proposed EULAR/ACR criteria for systemic lupus erythematosus classification are comparable. Lupus 2019;28(6):778–82.
33. Elbagir S, Elshafie AI, Elagib EM, et al. Sudanese and Swedish patients with systemic lupus erythematosus: immunological and clinical comparisons. Rheumatology (Oxford, England) 2020;59(5):968–78.
34. Gegenava M, Beaart HJL, Monahan RC, et al. Performance of the proposed ACR-EULAR classification criteria for systemic lupus erythematosus (SLE) in a cohort of patients with SLE with neuropsychiatric symptoms. RMD Open 2019; 5(1):e000895.
35. Frodlund M, Wetterö J, Dahle C, et al. Longitudinal anti-nuclear antibody (ANA) seroconversion in systemic lupus erythematosus: a prospective study of Swedish cases with recent-onset disease. Clin Exp Immunol 2020;199(3):245–54.
36. Mahler M, Andrade LE, Casiano CA, et al. Anti-DFS70 antibodies: an update on our current understanding and their clinical usefulness. Expert Rev Clin Immunol 2019;15(3):241–50.
37. Choi MY, Clarke AE, St PY, et al. The prevalence and determinants of anti-DFS70 autoantibodies in an international inception cohort of systemic lupus erythematosus patients. Lupus 2017;26(10):1051–9.
38. Damoiseaux J, Andrade LEC, Carballo OG, et al. Clinical relevance of HEp-2 indirect immunofluorescent patterns: the International Consensus on ANA Patterns (ICAP) perspective. Ann Rheum Dis 2019;78(7):879–89.
39. Tan EM, Cohen AS, Fries JF, et al. The 1982 revised criteria for the classification of systemic lupus erythematosus. Arthritis Rheum 1982;25(11):1271–7.
40. Touma Z, Cervera R, Brinks R, et al. Associations between classification criteria items in systemic lupus erythematosus. Arthritis Care Res 2020;72(12):1820–6.
41. Petri M, Orbai AM, Alarcon GS, et al. Derivation and validation of the Systemic Lupus International Collaborating Clinics classification criteria for systemic lupus erythematosus. Arthritis Rheum 2012;64(8):2677–86.
42. Aringer M, Johnson SR. Classifying and diagnosing systemic lupus erythematosus in the 21st century. Rheumatology (Oxford) 2020;59(Supplement_5):v4–11.
43. Aringer M, Petri M. New classification criteria for systemic lupus erythematosus. Curr Opin Rheumatol 2020;32(6):590–6.

44. Zapata L Jr, Chong BF. Exclusion of cutaneous lupus erythematosus subtypes from the 2019 European League Against Rheumatism/American College of Rheumatology classification criteria for systemic lupus erythematosus: comment on the article by Aringer et al. Arthritis Rheumatol 2020;72(8):1403.

45. Stec-Polak M, Matyja-Bednarczyk A, Wojas-Pelc A, et al. Higher specificity of the new EULAR/ACR 2019 criteria for diagnosing systemic lupus erythematosus in patients with biopsy-proven cutaneous lupus. Clin Exp Rheumatol 2020.

46. Tedeschi SK, Johnson SR, Boumpas DT, et al. Multicriteria decision analysis process to develop new classification criteria for systemic lupus erythematosus. Ann Rheum Dis 2019;78(5):634–40.

47. Hanly JG, Urowitz MB, Sanchez-Guerrero J, et al. Neuropsychiatric events at the time of diagnosis of systemic lupus erythematosus: an international inception cohort study. Arthritis Rheum 2007;56(1):265–73.

48. Schmajuk G, Hoyer BF, Aringer M, et al. Multicenter Delphi exercise to identify important key items for classifying systemic lupus erythematosus. Arthritis Care Res (Hoboken). 2018;70(10):1488–94.

49. Weinstein A. Cell-bound complement activation products are superior to serum complement C3 and C4 levels to detect complement activation in systemic lupus erythematosus: comment on the article by Aringer et al. Arthritis Rheumatol (Hoboken, NJ) 2020;72(5):860.

50. Ramsey-Goldman R, Alexander RV, Massarotti EM, et al. Complement activation in patients with probable systemic lupus erythematosus and ability to predict progression to American College of Rheumatology-classified systemic lupus erythematosus. Arthritis Rheumatol (Hoboken, NJ) 2020;72(1):78–88.

Treatment Update in Systemic Lupus Erythematous

Alberta Y. Hoi, MBBS, FRACP, PhD[a,b],
Eric F. Morand, MBBS, FRACP, PhD[a,b],*

KEYWORDS

- Lupus • Treatment target • Lupus low disease activity state • Lupus nephritis
- Mycophenolate • Euro-lupus • Anifrolumab • Belimumab

KEY POINTS

- The use of hydroxychloroquine in systemic lupus erythematosus has been recommended for all patients with attention paid to the dose threshold and appropriate monitoring for retinopathy.
- The potential harm with chronic glucocorticoid use has been highlighted with evidence to show that if daily dose is kept lower than 7.5 mg daily, irreversible harm is limited.
- Appropriate initiation of immunosuppressants, such as mycophenolate, azathioprine, and methotrexate, can facilitate steroid sparing.
- Novel biologic agents, such as belimumab and anifrolumab, based on sound understanding of immunopathogenesis, have now been shown to be effective in the treatment of SLE.
- Ongoing work to clarify the optimal treatment algorithm to incorporate existing drug and novel therapies, either as monotherapy or as combination, is needed.

INTRODUCTION

Systemic lupus erythematosus (SLE) is a prototypic chronic autoimmune disease characterized by multisystem manifestations, with organ-based pathology predominantly mediated by chronic inflammation in the context of a dysregulated immune system. Its clinical manifestations are diverse, but some manifestations, such as joint, skin, kidney, and hematologic, are more common than others.[1,2]

Significant advances have been seen in the understanding of the key pathogenetic pathways of SLE, involving the innate and adaptive immune systems. This has led to the development of novel therapeutics in the last decade. Nevertheless, the challenge of treating SLE remains high, even for lupus experts, because the breadth of its organ involvement can range from the central nervous system, to difficult-to-treat cutaneous

a Centre for Inflammatory Diseases, Monash University, Victoria, Australia; b Department of Rheumatology, Monash Health, 246 Clayton Road, Clayton, Victoria 3168, Australia
* Corresponding author. 246 Clayton Road, Clayton, Victoria 3168, Australia.
E-mail address: eric.morand@monash.edu

Rheum Dis Clin N Am 47 (2021) 513–530
https://doi.org/10.1016/j.rdc.2021.04.012
0889-857X/21/© 2021 Elsevier Inc. All rights reserved.

rheumatic.theclinics.com

disease, to organ-threatening renal disease. Good-quality studies are limited and frequently management of the disease is based on expert opinion. Nonetheless, there have been several recent publications from experts from around the world (eg, the European League Against Rheumatism [EULAR] and the Asia Pacific League of Associations for Rheumatology) that aimed to provide recommendations to guide clinicians in managing patients with SLE.[3] In 2012 there were also recommendations by the American College of Rheumatology published specifically for the management of lupus nephritis.[4]

Overarching Principles of Systemic Lupus Erythematosus Management

For a disease, such as SLE, with such wide spectrum of organ involvement and severity, it is easy to lose sight of the broader goals of management. The concept of overarching principles has been expressed by recent recommendations published by EULAR[3] and the Asia Pacific League of Associations for Rheumatology,[5] acknowledging the need to highlight common goals, before addressing the specific therapeutic challenges. These principles were first developed by the treat-to-target (T2T) SLE international taskforce, after extensive discussion and literature review, to bring clarity to the general approach toward managing patients with SLE and to put specific recommendations in context.[6] These principles are useful for all clinicians involved in delivering care to patients with SLE and serve as a practical paradigm that the specific recommendations are founded on.

The first of these statements reflect the importance of shared decision making between patients and physicians. Treatment plans should always involve a patent-centered process; many factors, not only clinical phenotypes and comorbidities, can influence therapeutic decisions. Some of these factors, for example, relate to access to health care, personal beliefs, individual medication tolerability, and circumstance, and are crucial in determining the final treatment plan.

The current treatment paradigm has its core goal to identify and control disease activity while seeking to minimize comorbidities and treatment-related toxicity. The goal is to ensure long-term survival, prevent organ damage, and to optimize quality of life. It is on this basis that different treatment strategies have been developed.

The treatment landscape for patients with SLE is also uniquely multidisciplinary given the breadth of organ involvement. Specialist involvement early in the course of the patient journey can facilitate early detection of organ involvement, particularly in the symptomatically silent organs, such as renal or pulmonary disease. Because SLE is an uncommon and complex multiorgan autoimmune disease, specialists who have expertise in SLE management are valuable in providing assessment of disease activity, severity, and prognosis, and therefore in guiding disease management.

The multidisciplinary nature of care should be emphasized because expertise may come from a variety of disciplines, such as rheumatology, nephrology, dermatology, or immunology. Primary care physicians often work with the treating specialist and play a key part in the monitoring and management of the disease and associated comorbidities. This is a model crucial for the successful and optimal management of chronic disease. The primary care physician has an important role in the management team, to help patients comprehend the complexity of disease pathogenesis and priorities in treatment. They play a key part in the monitoring and management of the disease and associated comorbidities. They also offer patients ongoing support and counseling, especially for those who may find coping with a chronic disease difficult.

Treat-to-Target Concept

As part of the general consideration of treatment goals is work toward defining an appropriate treatment target. Although remission is always the holy grail, sustained complete remission is uncommon and difficult to achieve in real-world SLE management.[7] The concept of lupus low disease activity state (LLDAS) has been put forward as an attainable treatment target, originally defined based on an expert consensus process among Asia Pacific lupus clinicians as a state of acceptable disease activity and low treatment burden. LLDAS consists of a disease activity threshold using SLEDAI-2K of 4 or less; without new or major organ involvement; physical global assessment of 1 or less on a 3-point scale; and allows for concomitant use of immunosuppressants, antimalarials, and prednisolone of no greater than 7.5 mg per day.[8] LLDAS has now been prospectively validated to be an important treatment target in SLE, because attainment of LLDAS was associated with protection from flare and damage accrual.[8–11] It has been evaluated in several large lupus cohorts and shown to be associated with favorable long-term outcomes, such as improved survival and quality of life.[12–15]

Studies examining low disease activity and different definitions of remission have shed some insights into what these targets mean and what their roles are in trials and in the clinic. LLDAS is certainly more attainable than remission, although still highly protective, and is now well-established as a T2T goal, whereas to date there have been a few definitions of remission with varying degree of stringency required.[16] These remission definitions, when applied to existing lupus cohorts, reveal that the prevalence changes depending on the definition used but they generally have a stepwise concentric relationship between different target state stringencies.

In everyday clinical management the choice of the treatment end point should be attainable and meaningful. The utility of LLDAS and remission in clinical practice supports a T2T strategy to SLE management, but the final treatment decision on escalation, de-escalation, or maintenance of immunosuppressant treatment is influenced by many factors beyond disease activity. Formal T2T strategy trials, such as using LLDAS nonattainment as a trigger for nonglucocorticoid treatment escalation, are needed to formally guide use of these targets.

UPDATE ON SPECIFIC PHARMACOTHERAPIES

Although there are many nonpharmacologic therapies and patient-centered strategies that are highly relevant to the overall management of SLE, this article focuses mostly on drug therapies. Currently many drugs used for the treatment of SLE were first used in other rheumatologic conditions, such as rheumatoid arthritis, and the understanding of these drugs and the specific way they work in SLE is still surprisingly limited and mostly based on observational studies. Many treatment recommendations therefore rely on studies that are of a low level of evidence, because there are few randomized controlled studies that compare one drug with placebo or a comparator, and even fewer to compare strategies.

On the horizon, there are many novel therapies that have been developed based on the improved understanding of lupus pathogenesis. Conceptually, four key pathways have been identified as dominant drivers for disease pathogenesis in SLE. They are broadly divided into dysregulation of the innate versus adaptive immune responses. These pathways include: (1) impaired regulation or clearance of "self" nucleic acid, (2) dysregulation of type 1 interferon (IFN) responses, (3) altered thresholds for immune cell activation and signaling, and (4) abnormal tissue response to injury. Although dysregulation of one pathway alone is often not sufficient for the development of clinical disease, future development of therapeutics is likely to target one or more of these pathways.

The next section provides an overview of the common drugs that are used in the treatment of SLE, and a few novel therapies that are at advanced stages of clinical development.

GLUCOCORTICOIDS

The practice of using glucocorticoids (GCs) in SLE as the mainstay of treatment has been increasingly challenged because of the known adverse effects related to its chronic use.[17] However, GCs are an effective anti-inflammatory therapy, and they will continue to play an important role in treatment of SLE. Consistent with the overall aim of therapy to control disease activity, GC use is well recognized to be able to rapidly control local and systemic inflammation, and thereby minimize organ damage in the short term.

The dose and route of administration of GC should depend on the type and severity of organ involvement. The anti-inflammatory effects of GC are largely mediated by the classic genomic pathways, through the binding of cytosolic GC receptor, which leads transactivation or transrepression of the expression of a variety of mediators. However, GCs also have a range of immunosuppressive, antiproliferative, and vasoconstrictive effects, some of which may also be mediated via a nongenomic mechanism. The rapid nongenomic immunosuppressive effect may be mediated by the membrane-bound GC receptor on monocytes and B cells, and generally thought to be part of the mechanism of actions of higher dosages of GC, such as with pulse intravenous doses.[18,19] GC doses of more than 30 mg prednisolone equivalent a day are considered high dose, because at these doses genomic receptor saturation begins to plateau and becomes almost completely saturated at a dose of appropriately 100 mg per day.

The adverse effects of GCs are dose-dependent and prolonged use can increase risk of infection, osteoporosis, avascular necrosis, diabetes, and accelerated atherosclerosis. These complications are part of the irreversible damage accrued during the patients' lupus journey. The current recommendation is to avoid using GC as monotherapy in patients with SLE. Where possible, when the treatment target (eg, low disease activity) is reached, GC treatment should be slowly reduced or, if possible, withdrawn. GC use can continue to contribute to damage accrual in SLE even in the absence of disease activity.[20] If GC cannot be stopped, then maintenance dose should be kept low, preferably less than 7.5 mg per day of prednisolone equivalent, a threshold established as protective in the LLDAS validation studies. Importantly, caution is needed in withdrawing GC even in patients without active disease, because the risk of flare remains.[21]

ANTIMALARIALS

The role of antimalarials, most often hydroxychloroquine (HCQ), in the treatment of SLE is considered in several different facets. It has long been used as an effective medication for the less severe symptoms of SLE, especially for arthritis and rash. Current treatment recommendation has suggested that in addition to symptom control, HCQ should be used in all patients with lupus unless contraindicated. Several cohort studies have demonstrated its protective effect in reducing flares and long-term damage accrual, and in conferring a survival benefit in patients with SLE.[22–24] Other antimalarials, such as chloroquine or quinacrine, are less often used because of their higher risk of adverse effects, but continue to be used in some countries because of access issues.

The anti-inflammatory effects of HCQ are mediated by its immunomodulatory actions on a range of immune cells, such as dendritic cells, macrophages, and lymphocytes. Pharmacologically HCQ is a weak base, and is known to increase lysosomal pH and decrease lysosomal protease activity. It can interfere with autophagy and the presentation of autoantigen to class II major histocompatibility complex. HCQ has been shown to inhibit Toll-like receptors 7 and 9 activity in vitro,[25] and therefore interfere with type 1 IFN and other cytokine production.[26]

HCQ also has other additional antithrombotic effects, such as interference with platelet aggregation.[27] In vitro studies have shown that HCQ can reverse the binding of antiphospholipid antibodies (APL) to beta 2 glycoprotein 1 and restore the annexin A5 shield in human endothelial cells and syncytiotrophoblasts.[28,29] It therefore may have additional benefits for patients with antiphospholipid syndrome (APLS).

The main concern of long-term HCQ therapy is its ocular adverse effects, and in particular the irreversible effects of cumulative exposure on the retina. In one study the cumulative risk of HCQ retinopathy may be 20% at 20 years.[30] The updated screening recommendation for HCQ retinopathy takes into account the relative rarity of this adverse event early in the exposure history. A baseline ophthalmologic examination that includes a thorough fundoscopy, automated 10 to 2 visual field testing, and spectrum domain optical coherence tomography is recommended, and it is further recommended to be repeated after 5 years treatment if the patient does not have symptoms. Certain risk groups may warrant an earlier review, such as those using doses higher than 5 mg/kg/d, or those with renal impairment, tamoxifen use, or preexisting macular disease.[30]

IMMUNOSUPPRESSANTS

Major SLE organ involvement should be treated with immunosuppression. Most of the earlier studies were done in lupus nephritis, but since then several immunosuppressive medications has been studied in nonrenal SLE, particularly as steroid-sparing agents. This include mycophenolate (MMF), azathioprine (AZA), and methotrexate; and for serious manifestations, cyclophosphamide (CYM). Calcineurin inhibitors, such as ciclosporin and tacrolimus, have been used in renal and nonrenal SLE cases, and newer calcineurin inhibitors, such as voclosporin, are under development to find new therapies for lupus nephritis with better efficacy and safety profiles. Occasionally drugs that are used for other rheumatic diseases, such as leflunomide, are used in patients with SLE particularly if they have prominent articular manifestations.

MMF has become the mainstay of induction and maintenance immunosuppressant for lupus nephritis. MMF was shown to be at least as effective as CYM by several studies, including the international randomized controlled Aspreva Lupus Management Study (ALMS).[30] The clinical decision between choosing MMF versus CYM depends on the shared patient-physician discussion, regional access considerations, and need for gonadal protection. A meta-analysis comparing the difference between MMF and CYM did not reveal superiority of one versus the other, and rates of adverse events were similar. One of the key reasons to use MMF often is for its potential benefit on gonadal protection, but in a Cochrane review, the data were less certain with a reduction in relative risk but a wide confidence interval (relative risk, 0.36; 95% confidence interval, 0.06–2.18), illustrating that there are many additional factors that determine gonadal function and success of future pregnancy for the individual with SLE.[31] The Euro-lupus CYM protocol has published favorable long-term outcomes, such as low rates of death and end-stage renal failure in a 10-year follow-up study, when compared with high-dose CYM.[32]

MMF is effective in nonrenal disease that is refractory to corticosteroids, and has been shown in a prospective open label randomized controlled trial (RCT) to be superior to AZA for nonrenal SLE.[33] The data supporting using MMF instead of AZA as maintenance therapy in lupus nephritis were first described in the MAINTAIN study, in which patients all received Euro-lupus CYM induction protocol and were then randomized between MMF and AZA. In this study there was a reduction in renal flares with MMF but it was not statistically significant.[34] In patients who completed the ALMS study, maintenance therapy with MMF was compared with AZA in a 36-month RCT, which showed that MMF was superior in maintaining renal response and preventing relapse.[35]

One adverse effect that sometimes leads to discontinuation of MMF is its gastrointestinal effects, particularly diarrhea. There is a suggestion that there may be ethnic differences in the tolerability of MMF with a higher proportion of Asian patients treated with MMF developed serious adverse events in ALMS.[36] Newer analogues, such as mycophenolic acid, may be better tolerated. MMF is also contraindicated in pregnancy and therefore not suitable for patients who are actively trying to conceive. AZA is useful in this setting, and is often used in young adult women with SLE as an alternative to MMF for this reason.

BIOLOGICS AND TARGETED THERAPIES

There has been considerable interest in pursuing the development of biologic therapies in the treatment of SLE but to date their exact roles are still to be determined. There have been several phase three studies, mostly on B-cell targeted therapies, such as rituximab (chimeric anti-CD20), belimumab (anti–B-cell activating factor [BAFF]), tabalumab (anti-BAFF, membrane and soluble bound), ocrelizumab (humanized anti-CD20), and epratuzumab (anti-CD22), for the treatment of SLE or lupus nephritis. Other non-B-cell targets that have been under investigation include costimulation inhibition with abatacept (CTLA4-Ig) as part of a way to modulate T-cell influence on disease, and various strategies to block the IFN pathway, such as anifrolumab. So far, the only positive phase 3 studies are those for belimumab and anifrolumab, and only belimumab has been approved.

Belimumab is a human monoclonal antibody against BAFF that inhibits the activation and proliferation of B cells. Based on two pivotal phase 3 studies (BLISS 52 and BLISS-76) the efficacy and safety of belimumab were demonstrated, and belimumab has since been approved by multiple agencies for treatment of moderately severe SLE.[37] Patients who received belimumab had consistent improvement in several other clinical outcome measures through the trials. The effect of belimumab on lupus nephritis was further explored by another RCT called BLISS-LN, in which patients were recruited based on active lupus nephritis within 6 months of screening. Induction immunosuppressant was allowed to start within 60 days and patients were randomized to belimumab versus placebo for the 2-year duration of the study. Patients received concurrent maintenance therapy of either MMF or AZA. The results showed that belimumab added to conventional therapy improved likelihood of a predefined renal response and this response was sustained from about Week 26 till the end of study of Week 104.[38]

As part of the emerging evidence that type 1 IFN drives and perpetuates disease pathogenesis in SLE, multiple strategies to block effects of IFN have been under investigation. There have been phase 2 trials of monoclonal antibodies against IFN-α and against the IFN-α receptor.[39–41] Anifrolumab, a human monoclonal antibody against type I IFN receptor, is the only compound that has efficacy data from phase 3 studies (TULIP1 and TULIP2). Even though the first of the phase 3 studies (TULIP1) failed to demonstrate benefit using its prespecified primary end point of SLE Responder Index 4 (SRI-4),[42] the results of several of its secondary measures were encouraging and results from the other phase 3 RCT (TULIP2) using a different primary end point were positive. Patients from the TULIP2 study had a higher rate of British Isles Lupus Assessment Group–based Composite Lupus Assessment response with anifrolumab compared with placebo,[43] and patients had significantly higher rates of GC tapering in TULIP 2 and TULIP1. Post hoc analyses from the combined TULIP1 and TULIP2 studies on skin disease, so far published only in abstract form, showed anifrolumab generated a rapid and durable response as measured by Cutaneous Lupus Erythematosus Disease Area and Severity Index–Activity. Subject to regulatory approval, anifrolumab will most likely be the first agent with this mechanism of action that will be available for clinicians. Several other novel agents that aim to interfere with the IFN pathway, such as anti-Blood Dendritic Cell Antigen-2 (BDCA2) monoclonal antibody (BIIB059), studied in active SLE and cutaneous lupus erythematosus (CLE), showed early promise (published in abstract form only).

Lupus trials continued to be plagued by difficult-to-use and poorly validated outcome measures, such that with current study design, the chosen end points can make or break the success of trials. The challenge remains to translate what these outcome measures mean for the patient. In the meantime, much is learnt from a range of secondary measures used in these RCTs. For example, there is a consistent observation that effective biologic agents can achieve a steroid-sparing effect.[44] Treatment targets, such as LLDAS, have been used in several clinical trials with success,[33,45] and this could also be an easier way to understand the effect of treatment, rather than a relative improvement from a heterogenous baseline used in SRI4 or British Isles Lupus Assessment Group–based Composite Lupus Assessment. Finally, carefully gathered real-world experience is needed to gain a sense of the type of patients and clinical manifestations that are most responsive to each drug, and specific treatment strategies, such as choice of concurrent or sequential therapies.

COMBINATION OR SEQUENTIAL THERAPY

Rheumatologists have long combined GC and HCQ with an immunosuppressant for patients with SLE, if the combination is well tolerated and can control disease activity adequately. There are several combination therapies that may be worth exploring, particularly in patients who fail to respond adequately. In lupus nephritis, in several open-labelled studies, multitarget therapy using MMF and tacrolimus has an increased likelihood of complete disease remission when compared with intravenous CYM.[46–49] It is not our practice to combine conventional immunosuppressants, such as MMF and AZA or methotrexate.

Alternatively, despite having only an off-label indication, rituximab is used as a second-line agent, in the setting of inadequate response, intolerance, or contraindication to first-line therapy. Rituximab is a chimeric B-cell-depleting antibody against CD20. In its pivotal RCTs, namely the Exploratory Phase II/III SLE Evaluation of Rituximab (EXPLORER) and the Lupus Nephritis Assessment with Rituximab (LUNAR) studies, it failed to show efficacy.[50,51] However it has continued being used in clinical practice for refractory disease, based on a reasonable body of evidence of observational studies[52] and the lack of alternatives. In most studies, rituximab is used as add-on treatment, so patients continue background immunosuppressants, such as MMF, AZA, or methotrexate.[50,51] Rituximab has also been used in combination with CYM, most notably in antineutrophil cytoplasmic antibody vasculitis, but has also been used in lupus in small studies.[53,54] Combination therapies such as these must be deployed with caution. Although there has been observation of greater efficacy with higher remission rate and few relapses, the risk of adverse effects, particularly infection, is not insubstantial. Ocrelizumab, a humanized anti-CD20 therapy trialed in combination with MMF and high-dose GC, had its trial prematurely terminated because of serious infections and mortality.[55]

The concept of sequential therapy has been studied in relation to limited response observed with treatment with either rituximab or belimumab monotherapy. The degree of B-cell depletion has been shown to predict response to rituximab in a post hoc analysis of the LUNAR study.[56] Relapse following rituximab seems to be associated with rising BAFF and anti-dsDNA levels.[57] A phase II study examining the combination of rituximab plus CYM followed by belimumab in lupus nephritis has demonstrated acceptable safety of this approach. In this study, called the Combination of Antibodies in Lupus Nephritis: Belimumab and Rituximab Assessment of Tolerance and Efficacy (CALIBRATE) trial, there was no improvement in the clinical efficacy end point, but the study showed there was a reduced percentage of naive B cells and an enhanced negative selection of autoreactive B cells.[58] In contrast, an open label study, called Synergetic B-cell Immodulation in SLE (SynBioSe), of sequential treatment with rituximab followed by belimumab on a background of MMF in lupus nephritis, has recently presented its preliminary results, which were promising in terms of overall response measured by LLDAS and renal response (Kraaij and colleagues, published in abstract form only).

Difficult-To-Treat Organ Involvement

Agreement on SLE treatment particularly in relation to specific organ manifestations has been lacking because of a lack of good-quality RCT data in these areas. However, most experts would agree that the use of an immunosuppressant is indicated when there is any major organ involvement, although the choice of immunosuppressant and pathways used are variable, and in some studies only a quarter of respondents agree on the treatment strategy.[59] In the absence of formal trial data, treatment algorithms are currently established according to consensus, and usually framed according to the specific target organ. It is worthwhile to consider some of these organs and particularly discuss therapies that are considered.

Constitutional

The management of constitutional symptoms in SLE is challenging, especially when this is not accompanied by significant other organ involvement. Symptoms, such as fatigue, are ranked much higher as priorities by patients than by physicians, highlighting a gap in expectations that should be addressed when discussing goals of care.[60] Low-grade fever is the only constitutional symptom that has a score on the most commonly used disease activity measure, SLEDAI, but when present it is generally associated with disease activity elsewhere and usually responds to treatment of those features. It is much more difficult to manage other constitutional symptoms, such as fatigue, weight loss, myalgia, or the presence of lymphadenopathy or splenomegaly. The emphasis in management is often around excluding other conditions that may also give rise to similar constitutional symptoms. When other conditions are excluded, there is poor consensus regarding what treatment should be used. Some rheumatologists use GC alone or combined with HCQ. Occasionally some may use methotrexate or other immunosuppressants.[59] Lifestyle recommendations relating to sleep hygiene and regular exercise are often suggested but there is to date but little evidence for their efficacy.

Mucocutaneous

To date, no drugs are approved specifically for the treatment of CLE. The treatment algorithm is generally a step-up approach, starting with topical therapy and then moving onto systemic agents if patients fail to respond. Topical GC and HCQ remain the first-line treatment.[61]

The choice of the strength of topical steroid is related to severity and site of involvement. The well-known cutaneous side effects of topical GC include atrophy, telangiectasis, and rosacea, and these are alleviated by correct intermittent dosing, and the adjunctive use of or replacement with a topical calcineurin inhibitor. Topical tacrolimus (0.1%) ointment has been used for several inflammatory skin conditions, such as atopic dermatitis, psoriasis, lichen planus, and cutaneous lupus. It has similar or superior potency to topical corticosteroid when studied in some of these conditions, with minimal side effects. Common side effects, such as burning sensation, tends to improve as treatment is continued, and it is not associated with skin atrophy because of a lack of effect on collagen synthesis.[62,63]

One aspect of the mucocutaneous manifestations in patients with SLE that is troublesome relates to refractory mouth ulcers. These aphthous ulcers are commonly experienced and are underrecognized as a source of morbidity. Topical steroid is applied directly to the lesion. An alternative includes the use of dexamethasone gargle (eg, at 0.5 mg in 5 mL oral solution), borrowing from the oncology literature.[64,65] This can sometimes increase the risk of oral candidiasis, and some would advocate to mix an antifungal to the steroid solution (eg, dexamethasone in solution).

Other immunosuppressants, such as methotrexate, AZA, cyclosporine, and MMF, have been all used in CLE but their use is primarily described in case reports, or as part of general SLE studies so the end points are generally global rather than specific skin outcomes. As a result, direct evidence of benefit of typical SLE immunosuppressant agents for CLE is limited.

Partly as a result of limited efficacy of standard approaches, several other agents have been used in CLE. Dapsone, an antibacterial sulfonamide, which has anti-inflammatory and immunomodulatory effects, has been suggested in a literature review to be 90% effective for bullous lupus.[66] Dapsone is able to inhibit neutrophil myeloperoxidase, and interfere with neutrophil chemotaxis in a dose-dependent manner. Another less commonly used agent is thalidomide, which has been reported to have beneficial effects in multiple subtypes of CLE.[67] The exact mechanisms of thalidomide in SLE are yet to be determined but it seems that it can bind to cereblon, which is a substrate adaptor molecule to the E3 ubiquitin ligase and is associated with significant immunomodulatory effects. The timely breakdown of key proteins through the ubiquitin-proteasome pathway is a major area of interest for drug development. The use of thalidomide has been limited by the high incidence of irreversible neurologic adverse effects and teratogenic risk. Lenalidomide, which is a related drug currently used for the treatment of multiple myeloma, has been suggested to be effective in CLE. This group of drugs, with such newcomers as iberdomide, is collectively called cereblon E3 ligase modulators, and their effects on SLE and CLE will be of great interest to clinicians.

Evidence for the role of targeted therapies in CLE is still limited. Even though rituximab and belimumab have some efficacy in patients with severe active CLE, the response is variable, and there certainly seem to be refractory cases that do not respond to B-cell depletion.[68,69] Recent advances in understanding of the pathogenesis of CLE has supported this to be a strongly IFN-driven disease.[70] Many of the IFN-regulated genes play a prominent pathogenic role in cutaneous lupus.[71,72] Recently both phase 3 trials of anifrolumab reported significant improvement in skin disease in response to IFN blockade and positive results in CLE of the pDC-targeting antibody BIIB059 have been reported in abstract forms. An alternative approach to block IFN may be via using a Janus kinase inhibitor, which depending on selectivity can block intracellular IFN signaling via the JAK-STAT pathway. Ruxolitinib, which is a JAK1/2 inhibitor used in myelofibrosis, has been studied in animal and laboratory models of cutaneous lupus with encouraging results.[73,74] Several JAK inhibitors, such as tofacitinib, baricitinib, and upadacitinib, are now being studied in SLE.

Neuropsychiatric lupus

Neuropsychiatric manifestations of SLE remain one of the most challenging areas to diagnose and manage, because of difficulty in determining a unifying pathogenesis. Although immune-mediated neuronal injury is the working hypothesis, involving humoral and cellular pathways, the spectrum of clinical syndromes is diverse and frequently coexists with other neurologic or psychiatric conditions. Symptomatic management plays a large part in the treatment of SLE neuropsychiatric syndrome, such as the use of antipsychotics, anxiolytics, antidepressants, and anticonvulsants.[75] The two main considerations in implementation of immunosuppression are whether local or systemic inflammation can be demonstrated. Using current clinical tools this may not be an easy process. Local inflammatory changes can be demonstrated by either neuroimaging or changes in the cerebrospinal fluid. Presence of serum or cerebrospinal fluid antineuronal autoantibodies may be helpful, but in most centers such tests are not routinely available. Systemic inflammation may manifest as presence of acute phase response or serologic activity (eg, a change in the complement or anti-dsDNA levels). In addition to excluding other comorbidities, especially infection in an immunosuppressed patient, other distinct immunopathogenic mechanisms, such as APLS or thrombotic microangiopathy, should be carefully considered and acted on. For example, an evidence-based algorithm to manage coagulopathy in APLS is available.

When it comes to empirical treatment with immunosuppression for neuropsychiatric lupus, the level of clinical evidence is frustratingly limited. Even though clinicians commonly use high-dose or intravenous pulse GC, there is little evidence from controlled studies to give guidance.[75] One small RCT of patients with incident severe neuropsychiatric manifestations compared monthly intravenous CYM with repeated intravenous methylprednisolone for 12 months and then tapering for another 12 months, and reported that the treatment arm using CYM had a much higher response rate.[76] There are other uncontrolled cohort studies that suggest patients treated with CYM have more stable response, compared with those treated with AZA.[77] As a result, many centers use CYM, usually combined with GC, as the drug of first choice in patients with severe neuropsychiatric lupus. Although uncommon, psychiatric adverse effects of GC should be borne in mind when assessing a patient with SLE with new-onset psychosis.

Antiphospholipid syndrome

Patients with SLE can experience clinical manifestations that are more to do with the thrombotic tendency brought on by the associated APL than with immune-mediated inflammation. The overlap between SLE and APLS is common enough to give special attention to this subgroup. The current classification criteria for APLS requires the demonstration of persistent and moderate to high titer APL, and a clinical event, such as an episode of venous or arterial thromboembolism or obstetric complication. However, whether patients present as full blown APLS or not, the APL profile can give additional information, such as risk prediction for the likelihood of future events. The APL profile is variable in patients with SLE in general, and therefore treatment algorithms should take into account the specific APL profile, and treatment options are also based on whether it is for primary or secondary prevention.

The APL profile consists of the type of APL (whether it is anticardiolipin antibody IgG or IgM, anti-beta 2 glycoprotein 1 IgG or IgM, or lupus anticoagulant), isolated or multiple (eg, triple positive), and their titer and the persistence. The threshold of moderately high titer is usually the 99th percentile, or greater than 40 international units measured by standardized enzyme-linked immunosorbent assay. A high-risk APL profile is defined as either persistence of lupus anticoagulant, or double or triple positivity, or very high and persistent titer APL.

Low-dose aspirin is recommended for those who carry a high-risk APL profile. For those who do not carry the high-risk APL profile, or the nonpregnant women with a history of obstetric APLS only, the role of using low-dose aspirin is more controversial and can be individualized, although low-dose aspirin is recommended in pregnancy in SLE because of the heightened risk of preeclampsia.

In patients who have definite APLS with a prior thrombotic event, treatment with a vitamin K antagonist with a target of international normalized ratio of 2 to 3 is recommended. There has been a recent EULAR updated recommendation published in 2019, highlighting some new evidence around the use of direct oral anticoagulant (DOAC) in patients with APLS. There are a few DOACs available, used in the prevention of thromboembolic events in the general population, but there has been limited evidence of their efficacy and safety in APLS. The RCT of rivaroxaban versus warfarin in patients for secondary prevention of triple-positive APLS was prematurely terminated because of an excess of thromboembolic events (mostly arterial) in the rivaroxaban arm.[78] Previously rivaroxaban was studied in a noninferiority study of patients with venous thrombotic APLS, and there were no differences in outcomes between the two arms. Criticisms for this study included a short-term follow-up period and an underrepresentation of high-risk patients.[79] As such, currently the recommendation is to use vitamin K antagonist rather than DOACs in the treatment of APLS unless patients are not able to achieve a target international normalized ratio of 2 to 3.

During pregnancy, the intensity of anticoagulation of the patients with APLS depends on prior events. In those who only have had obstetric events, heparin or low-molecular-weight heparin at prophylactic dose, and aspirin, are usually sufficient.[80] However, if the patient has had recurrent pregnancy loss, consideration is given for increasing the dose of heparin or low-molecular-weight heparin to the therapeutic dose. In those who have had a thrombotic history, therapeutic dose of heparin or low-molecular-weight heparin should be given throughout pregnancy. Regardless of the protocol during the pregnancy, anticoagulation should be continued for 6 weeks after delivery to reduce the risk of maternal thrombosis.

Currently there is no good-quality therapeutic trial examining the role of immunomodulatory agents for the treatment of APLS in SLE. Although GC can inhibit many of the known pathways implicated in APLS, currently they are only implemented for severe life-threatening cases of catastrophic APLS or in specific noncriteria manifestations.

Lupus nephritis

Lupus nephritis is a major cause of morbidity and mortality in SLE, but it can certainly present with a spectrum of clinical severity. The first-line treatment of proliferative forms of lupus nephritis is MMF or low-dose intravenous pulse CYM as reviewed previously.[3,81] MMF is at least comparable in terms of efficacy and may be superior to CYM as induction therapy because of high rates of complete remission.[31] The low-dose Euro-lupus CYM regimen is preferred over the high dose, because it has comparable efficacy and lower risk of gonadotoxicity.[32,82]

Tacrolimus is a potential alternative to MMF or CYM, with positive studies coming mostly from Asia, and smaller cohorts described from Europe; further studies to confirm the generalizability of the results are required to solidify a recommendation as an alternative first-line therapy.[83–85] The duration of the induction tacrolimus regimen in most trials is 6 months, and then patients were switched to AZA. The initial dose of tacrolimus used in these studies was 0.1 mg/kg/d in two divided doses. Therapeutic drug monitoring was not used consistently, but some advocated target level of 4 to 6 ng/mL.[85] Tacrolimus is also a reasonable option during pregnancy because it is not associated with known teratogenic effects.[86]

Most of the work on combination therapy for MMF with calcineurin inhibitors has been done on patients with lupus nephritis. EULAR has recommended that MMF be combined with low-dose calcineurin inhibitor in severe nephrotic syndrome or in those with inadequate renal response to MMF alone, provided clinicians monitor for the potential adverse effects, such as nephrotoxicity and neurotoxicity.[3,81] The alternative for poor response is to switch to high-dose CYM particularly in those with poor prognostic features.

There is still currently a bit of uncertainty regarding the rate of corticosteroid tapering and the timing of introduction of maintenance therapy. The general consensus has now advocated a lower starting dose of corticosteroid, such as 0.3 to 0.5 mg/kg/d, following pulse intravenous methylprednisolone.[81] The rate of corticosteroid reduction depends on individual patient responses, but a target to less than 7.5 mg/d by 3 to 6 months has been advocated by EULAR.[81]

Recently data from BLISS-LN, a phase 3 RCT of belimumab, added onto MMF or CYM standard of care in patients with active lupus nephritis, has shown efficacy over a 2-year study.[38] There seems to be a lag in the divergence between treatment arms of patients achieving the primary end point until after around 6 months, which may reflect the mechanism of action on B-cell activation that may have a slow effect on end-organ inflammation. Belimumab is considered as an add-on sequential therapy as discussed previously.[58] Ongoing studies are required to determine the optimal way to treat refractory lupus nephritis.

SUMMARY/FUTURE DIRECTIONS

Although there is no cure for SLE, therapies have come a long way in controlling the disease and its symptoms, and slowing the progression of any damage. New treatment recommendations have provided greater clarity in the way existing anti-inflammatory and immunomodulatory drugs are used, with a greater emphasis on treating to a target combining low disease activity and low GC exposure. It remains unsatisfactory that in many cases expert consensus guides treatment guidelines; formal strategy trials are still needed to provide evidence underpinning recommendations on the sequence and/or combination of agents for the treatment of SLE, including studies in individual organ manifestations. Based on improved understanding of the disease pathogenesis, novel biologic agents are anticipated to expand therapeutic options in the near future, but resolving SLE trial design and end point science also remains a major unmet need. Much work needs to be done thereafter in determining the optimal way to measure response in individual patients, and exploring ways to improve treatment algorithms for patients at large.

CLINICS CARE POINTS

- Monitoring of hydroxychloroquine retinopathy should include a baseline assessment of fundoscopy, automated visual field testing and spectrum domain optical coherence tomography, and then repeated after 5 years provided patient does not have any symptoms or risk factors.

- Mycophenolate mofetil is effective for both renal and non-renal disease.

- In refractory lupus nephritis or severe nephrotic syndrome due to lupus, mycophenolate mofetil can be combined with tacrolimus as an alternative to cyclophosphamide in some individuals.

DISCLOSURE

A.Y. Hoi has received research grants, consultancy fees, and honoraria from GSK, AstraZeneca, Merck Serono, UCB, and AbbVie. She was member of the Australian Benlysta Advisory Board in 2020, and is principal investigator for several phase 2 and 3 clinical trials in SLE. E.F. Morand has received research grants, consultancy fees, and honoraria from GSK, AstraZeneca, Merck Serono, UCB, Amgen, Eli Lilly, Biogen, Bristol Myers Squibb, and Janssen.

REFERENCES

1. Jakes RW, Bae S-C, Louthrenoo W, et al. Systematic review of the epidemiology of systemic lupus erythematosus in the Asia-Pacific region: prevalence, incidence, clinical features, and mortality. Arthritis Care Res 2012;64(2):159–68.
2. Chakravarty EF, Bush TM, Manzi S, et al. Prevalence of adult systemic lupus erythematosus in California and Pennsylvania in 2000: estimates obtained using hospitalization data. Arthritis Rheum 2007;56(6):2092–4.
3. Fanouriakis A, Kostopoulou M, Alunno A, et al. 2019 update of the EULAR recommendations for the management of systemic lupus erythematosus. Ann Rheum Dis 2019;78(6):736–45.
4. Hahn BH, McMahon MA, Wilkinson A, et al. American College of Rheumatology guidelines for screening, treatment, and management of lupus nephritis. Arthritis Care Res (Hoboken) 2012;64:797–808.
5. Chi Chiu Mok LH, Kasitanon N, Chen DY, et al. The Asia Pacific League of Associations for Rheumatology (APLAR) consensus statements on the management of systemic lupus erythematosus. Lancet Rheumatol 2021. https://doi.org/10.1016/S2665-9913(21)00009-6.
6. van Vollenhoven RF, Mosca M, Bertsias G, et al. Treat-to-target in systemic lupus erythematosus: recommendations from an international task force. Ann Rheum Dis 2014;73:958–67.
7. Golder V, Kandane-Rathnayake R, Huq M, et al. Evaluation of remission definitions for systemic lupus erythematosus: a prospective cohort study. Lancet Rheumatol 2019. https://doi.org/10.1016/S2665-9913(19)30048-7.
8. Franklyn K, Lau CS, Navarra SV, et al. Definition and initial validation of a Lupus Low Disease Activity State (LLDAS). Ann Rheum Dis 2016;75(9):1615–21.
9. Golder V, Kandane-Rathnayake R, Huq M, et al. Lupus low disease activity state as a treatment endpoint for systemic lupus erythematosus: a prospective validation study. 2019;1(2):E95–102. https://doi.org/10.1016/S2665-9913(19)30037-2.
10. Piga M, Floris A, Cappellazzo G, et al. Failure to achieve lupus low disease activity state (LLDAS) six months after diagnosis is associated with early damage accrual in caucasian patients with systemic lupus erythematosus. Arthritis Res Ther 2017;19(1):247.
11. Zen M, Iaccarino L, Gatto M, et al. Lupus low disease activity state is associated with a decrease in damage progression in caucasian patients with SLE, but overlaps with remission. Ann Rheum Dis 2018;77(1):104–10.
12. Alarcón GS, Ugarte-Gil MF, Pons-Estel G, et al. Remission and low disease activity state (LDAS) are protective of intermediate and long-term outcomes in SLE patients. Results from LUMINA (LXXVIII), a multiethnic, multicenter US cohort. Lupus 2019;28(3):423–6.
13. Mok CC, Ho LY, Tse SM, et al. Prevalence of remission and its effect on damage and quality of life in Chinese patients with systemic lupus erythematosus. Ann Rheum Dis 2017;76(8):1420–5.

14. Golder V, Kandane-Rathnayake R, Hoi AY, et al. Association of the lupus low disease activity state (LLDAS) with health-related quality of life in a multinational prospective study. Arthritis Res Ther 2017;19(1):62.

15. Sharma C, Raymond W, Eilertsen G, et al. Association of achieving lupus low disease activity state fifty percent of the time with both reduced damage accrual and mortality in patients with systemic lupus erythematosus. Arthritis Care Res (Hoboken) 2020;72(3):447–51.

16. Golder V, Tsang-A-Sjoe MWP. Treatment targets in SLE: remission and low disease activity state. Rheumatology (Oxford) 2020;59(Supplement_5):v19–28.

17. Zonana-Nacach A, Barr SG, Magder LS, et al. Damage in systemic lupus erythematosus and its association with corticosteroids. Arthritis Rheum 2000;43(8): 1801–8.

18. Buttgereit F, Straub RH, Wehling M, et al. Glucocorticoids in the treatment of rheumatic diseases: an update on the mechanisms of action. Arthritis Rheum 2004; 50(11):3408–17.

19. Buttgereit F, da Silva JA, Boers M, et al. Standardised nomenclature for glucocorticoid dosages and glucocorticoid treatment regimens: current questions and tentative answers in rheumatology. Ann Rheum Dis 2002;61(8):718–22.

20. Apostolopoulos D, Kandane-Rathnayake R, Louthrenoo W, et al. Factors associated with damage accrual in patients with systemic lupus erythematosus with no clinical or serological disease activity: a multicentre cohort study. Lancet Rheumatol 2019;1–7.

21. Mathian A, Mahevas M, Rohmer J, et al. Clinical course of coronavirus disease 2019 (COVID-19) in a series of 17 patients with systemic lupus erythematosus under long-term treatment with hydroxychloroquine. Ann Rheum Dis 2020;79(6): 837–9.

22. Mok CC, Penn HJ, Chan KL, et al. Hydroxychloroquine serum concentrations and flares of systemic lupus erythematosus: a longitudinal cohort analysis. Arthritis Care Res (Hoboken) 2016;68(9):1295–302.

23. Akhavan PS, Su J, Lou W, et al. The early protective effect of hydroxychloroquine on the risk of cumulative damage in patients with systemic lupus erythematosus. J Rheumatol 2013;40(6):831–41.

24. Alarcon GS, McGwin G, Bertoli AM, et al. Effect of hydroxychloroquine on the survival of patients with systemic lupus erythematosus: data from LUMINA, a multiethnic US cohort (LUMINA L). Ann Rheum Dis 2007;66(9):1168–72.

25. Kuznik A, Bencina M, Svajger U, et al. Mechanism of endosomal TLR inhibition by antimalarial drugs and imidazoquinolines. J Immunol 2011;186(8):4794–804.

26. Marmor MF, Kellner U, Lai TYY, et al, American Academy of Ophthalmology. Revised recommendations on screening for chloroquine and hydroxychloroquine retinopathy. Ophthalmology 2011;118:415–22.

27. Wallace DJ, Linker-Israeli M, Metzger AL, et al. The relevance of antimalarial therapy with regard to thrombosis, hypercholesterolemia and cytokines in SLE. Lupus 1993;2(Suppl 1):S13–5.

28. Rand JH, Wu XX, Quinn AS, et al. Hydroxychloroquine protects the annexin A5 anticoagulant shield from disruption by antiphospholipid antibodies: evidence for a novel effect for an old antimalarial drug. Blood 2010;115(11):2292–9.

29. Wu X-X, Guller S, Rand JH. Hydroxychloroquine reduces binding of antiphospholipid antibodies to syncytiotrophoblasts and restores annexin A5 expression. Am J Obstet Gynecol 2011;205(6):576.e7–14.

30. Marmor MF, Kellner U, Lai TYY, et al, American Academy of Ophthalmology. Recommendations on screening for chloroquine and hydroxychloroquine retinopathy (2016 revision). Ophthalmology 2016;123(6):1386–94.

31. Tunnicliffe DJ, Palmer SC, Henderson L, et al. Immunosuppressive treatment for proliferative lupus nephritis. Cochrane Database Syst Rev 2018;6:CD002922.

32. Houssiau FA, Vasconcelos C, D'Cruz D, et al. The 10-year follow-up data of the Euro-Lupus Nephritis Trial comparing low-dose and high-dose intravenous cyclophosphamide. Ann Rheum Dis 2010;69(1):61–4.

33. Ordi-Ros J, Sáez-Comet L, Pérez-Conesa M, et al. Enteric-coated mycophenolate sodium versus azathioprine in patients with active systemic lupus erythematosus: a randomised clinical trial. Ann Rheum Dis 2017;76(9):1575–82.

34. Houssiau FA, D'Cruz D, Sangle S, et al. Azathioprine versus mycophenolate mofetil for long-term immunosuppression in lupus nephritis: results from the MAINTAIN Nephritis Trial. Ann Rheum Dis 2010;69(12):2083–9.

35. Dooley MA, Jayne D, Ginzler EM, et al. Mycophenolate versus azathioprine as maintenance therapy for lupus nephritis. N Engl J Med 2011;365(20):1886–95.

36. Appel GB, Contreras G, Dooley MA, et al. Mycophenolate mofetil versus cyclophosphamide for induction treatment of lupus nephritis. J Am Soc Nephrol 2009;20(5):1103–12.

37. Hahn BH. Belimumab for systemic lupus erythematosus. N Engl J Med 2013; 368(16):1528–35.

38. Furie R, Rovin BH, Houssiau F, et al. Two-year, randomized, controlled trial of belimumab in lupus nephritis. N Engl J Med 2020;383(12):1117–28.

39. Khamashta M, Merrill JT, Werth VP, et al. Sifalimumab, an anti-interferon-α monoclonal antibody, in moderate to severe systemic lupus erythematosus: a randomised, double-blind, placebo-controlled study. Ann Rheum Dis 2016;75(11): 1909–16.

40. Furie R, Khamashta M, Merrill JT, et al. Anifrolumab, an anti-interferon-α receptor monoclonal antibody, in moderate-to-severe systemic lupus erythematosus. Arthritis Rheumatol 2017;69(2):376–86.

41. Kalunian KC, Merrill JT, Maciuca R, et al. A phase II study of the efficacy and safety of rontalizumab (rhuMAb interferon-α) in patients with systemic lupus erythematosus (ROSE). Ann Rheum Dis 2016;75(1):196–202.

42. Navarra SV, Guzmán RM, Gallacher AE, et al. Efficacy and safety of belimumab in patients with active systemic lupus erythematosus: a randomised, placebo-controlled, phase 3 trial. Lancet 2011;377(9767):721–31.

43. Morand EF, Furie R, Tanaka Y, et al. Trial of anifrolumab in active systemic lupus erythematosus. N Engl J Med 2020;382(3):211–21.

44. Oon S, Huq M, Godfrey T, et al. Systematic review, and meta-analysis of steroid-sparing effect, of biologic agents in randomized, placebo-controlled phase 3 trials for systemic lupus erythematosus. Semin Arthritis Rheum 2018;48(2):221–39.

45. Oon S, Huq M, Golder V, et al. Lupus Low Disease Activity State (LLDAS) discriminates responders in the BLISS-52 and BLISS-76 phase III trials of belimumab in systemic lupus erythematosus. Ann Rheum Dis 2019;78(5):629–33.

46. Choi CB, Won S, Bae SC. Outcomes of multitarget therapy using mycophenolate mofetil and tacrolimus for refractory or relapsing lupus nephritis. Lupus 2018; 27(6):1007–11.

47. Ikeuchi H, Hiromura K, Takahashi S, et al. Efficacy and safety of multi-target therapy using a combination of tacrolimus, mycophenolate mofetil and a steroid in patients with active lupus nephritis. Mod Rheumatol 2014;24(4):618–25.

48. Mok CC, To CH, Yu KL, et al. Combined low-dose mycophenolate mofetil and tacrolimus for lupus nephritis with suboptimal response to standard therapy: a 12-month prospective study. Lupus 2013;22(11):1135–41.

49. Liu Z, Zhang H, Liu Z, et al. Multitarget therapy for induction treatment of lupus nephritis: a randomized trial. Ann Intern Med 2015;162(1):18–26.

50. Merrill JT, Neuwelt CM, Wallace DJ, et al. Efficacy and safety of rituximab in moderately-to-severely active systemic lupus erythematosus: the randomized, double-blind, phase II/III systemic lupus erythematosus evaluation of rituximab trial. Arthritis Rheum 2010;62(1):222–33.

51. Rovin BH, Furie R, Latinis K, et al. Efficacy and safety of rituximab in patients with active proliferative lupus nephritis: the Lupus Nephritis Assessment with Rituximab study. Arthritis Rheum 2012;64(4):1215–26.

52. Mok CC. Current role of rituximab in systemic lupus erythematosus. Int J Rheum Dis 2015;18(2):154–63.

53. Li EK, Tam LS, Zhu TY, et al. Is combination rituximab with cyclophosphamide better than rituximab alone in the treatment of lupus nephritis? Rheumatology (Oxford) 2009;48(8):892–8.

54. McAdoo SP, Medjeral-Thomas N, Gopaluni S, et al. Long-term follow-up of a combined rituximab and cyclophosphamide regimen in renal anti-neutrophil cytoplasm antibody-associated vasculitis. Nephrol Dial Transplant 2018;33(5):899.

55. Mysler EF, Spindler AJ, Guzman R, et al. Efficacy and safety of ocrelizumab in active proliferative lupus nephritis: results from a randomized, double-blind, phase III study. Arthritis Rheum 2013;65(9):2368–79.

56. Gomez Mendez LM, Cascino MD, Garg J, et al. Peripheral blood B cell depletion after rituximab and complete response in lupus nephritis. Clin J Am Soc Nephrol 2018;13(10):1502–9.

57. Carter LM, Isenberg DA, Ehrenstein MR. Elevated serum BAFF levels are associated with rising anti-double-stranded DNA antibody levels and disease flare following B cell depletion therapy in systemic lupus erythematosus. Arthritis Rheum 2013;65(10):2672–9.

58. Atisha-Fregoso Y, Malkiel S, Harris KM, et al. Phase II randomized trial of rituximab plus cyclophosphamide followed by belimumab for the treatment of lupus nephritis. Arthritis Rheumatol 2020;73(1):121–31.

59. Muangchan C, van Vollenhoven RF, Bernatsky SR, et al. Treatment algorithms in systemic lupus erythematosus. Arthritis Care Res 2015;67(9):1237–45.

60. Golder V, Ooi JJY, Antony AS, et al. Discordance of patient and physician health status concerns in systemic lupus erythematosus. Lupus 2018;27(3):501–6.

61. Schrezenmeier E, Dörner T. Mechanisms of action of hydroxychloroquine and chloroquine: implications for rheumatology. Nat Rev Rheumatol 2020;16(3):155–66.

62. Bos JD. Non-steroidal topical immunomodulators provide skin-selective, self-limiting treatment in atopic dermatitis. Eur J Dermatol 2003;13(5):455–61.

63. Kuhn A, Landmann A, Wenzel J. Advances in the treatment of cutaneous lupus erythematosus. Lupus 2016;25(8):830–7.

64. Rugo HS, Seneviratne L, Beck JT, et al. Prevention of everolimus-related stomatitis in women with hormone receptor-positive, HER2-negative metastatic breast cancer using dexamethasone mouthwash (SWISH): a single-arm, phase 2 trial. Lancet Oncol 2017;18(5):654–62.

65. Jones VE, McIntyre KJ, Paul D, et al. Evaluation of miracle mouthwash plus hydrocortisone versus prednisolone mouth rinses as prophylaxis for everolimus-

associated stomatitis: a randomized phase II study. Oncologist 2019;24(9): 1153–8.

66. de Risi-Pugliese T, Cohen Aubart F, Haroche J, et al. Clinical, histological, immunological presentations and outcomes of bullous systemic lupus erythematosus: 10 new cases and a literature review of 118 cases. Semin Arthritis Rheum 2018; 48(1):83–9.

67. Chasset F, Tounsi T, Cesbron E, et al. Efficacy and tolerance profile of thalidomide in cutaneous lupus erythematosus: a systematic review and meta-analysis. J Am Acad Dermatol 2018;78(2):342–50.e4.

68. Md Yusof MY, Shaw D, El-Sherbiny YM, et al. Predicting and managing primary and secondary non-response to rituximab using B-cell biomarkers in systemic lupus erythematosus. Ann Rheum Dis 2017;76(11):1829–36.

69. Vital EM, Wittmann M, Edward S, et al. Brief report: responses to rituximab suggest B cell-independent inflammation in cutaneous systemic lupus erythematosus. Arthritis Rheumatol 2015;67(6):1586–91.

70. Kuhn A, Wenzel J, Bijl M. Lupus erythematosus revisited. Semin immunopathology 2016;38(1):97–112.

71. Tsoi LC, Gharaee-Kermani M, Berthier CC, et al. IL18-containing 5-gene signature distinguishes histologically identical dermatomyositis and lupus erythematosus skin lesions. JCI Insight 2020;5(16):e139558.

72. Fetter T, Smith P, Guel T, et al. Selective janus kinase 1 inhibition is a promising therapeutic approach for lupus erythematosus skin lesions. Front Immunol 2020;11:344.

73. Chan ES, Herlitz LC, Ali J. Ruxolitinib attenuates cutaneous lupus development in a mouse lupus model. J Invest Dermatol 2015;135(9):2338–9.

74. Klaeschen AS, Wolf D, Brossart P, et al. JAK inhibitor ruxolitinib inhibits the expression of cytokines characteristic of cutaneous lupus erythematosus. Exp Dermatol 2017;26(8):728–30.

75. Hanly JG, Harrison MJ. Management of neuropsychiatric lupus. Best Pract Res Clin Rheumatol 2005;19(5):799–821.

76. Barile-Fabris L, Ariza-Andraca R, Olguín-Ortega L, et al. Controlled clinical trial of IV cyclophosphamide versus IV methylprednisolone in severe neurological manifestations in systemic lupus erythematosus. Ann Rheum Dis 2005;64(4):620–5.

77. Lim LS, Lefebvre A, Benseler S, et al. Longterm outcomes and damage accrual in patients with childhood systemic lupus erythematosus with psychosis and severe cognitive dysfunction. J Rheumatol 2013;40(4):513–9.

78. Pengo V, Denas G, Zoppellaro G, et al. Rivaroxaban vs warfarin in high-risk patients with antiphospholipid syndrome. Blood 2018;132(13):1365–71.

79. Cohen H, Hunt BJ, Efthymiou M, et al. Rivaroxaban versus warfarin to treat patients with thrombotic antiphospholipid syndrome, with or without systemic lupus erythematosus (RAPS): a randomised, controlled, open-label, phase 2/3, non-inferiority trial. Lancet Haematol 2016;3(9):e426–36.

80. Tektonidou MG, Andreoli L, Limper M, et al. Management of thrombotic and obstetric antiphospholipid syndrome: a systematic literature review informing the EULAR recommendations for the management of antiphospholipid syndrome in adults. RMD Open 2019;5(1):e000924.

81. Fanouriakis A, Tziolos N, Bertsias G, et al. Update on the diagnosis and management of systemic lupus erythematosus. Ann Rheum Dis 2020;80(1):14–25.

82. Houssiau FA, Vasconcelos C, D'Cruz D, et al. Immunosuppressive therapy in lupus nephritis: the Euro-Lupus Nephritis Trial, a randomized trial of low-dose

versus high-dose intravenous cyclophosphamide. Arthritis Rheum 2002;46(8): 2121–31.

83. Miyasaka N, Kawai S, Hashimoto H. Efficacy and safety of tacrolimus for lupus nephritis: a placebo-controlled double-blind multicenter study. Mod Rheumatol 2009;19(6):606–15.

84. Mok CC, Ho LY, Ying SKY, et al. Long-term outcome of a randomised controlled trial comparing tacrolimus with mycophenolate mofetil as induction therapy for active lupus nephritis. Ann Rheum Dis 2020;79(8):1070–6.

85. Tani C, Elefante E, Martin-Cascón M, et al. Tacrolimus in non-Asian patients with SLE: a real-life experience from three European centres. Lupus Sci Med 2018; 5(1):e000274.

86. Baumgart DC, Pintoffl JP, Sturm A, et al. Tacrolimus is safe and effective in patients with severe steroid-refractory or steroid-dependent inflammatory bowel disease: a long-term follow-up. Am J Gastroenterol 2006;101(5):1048–56.

Moving?

Make sure your subscription moves with you!

To notify us of your new address, find your **Clinics Account Number** (located on your mailing label above your name), and contact customer service at:

Email: journalscustomerservice-usa@elsevier.com

800-654-2452 (subscribers in the U.S. & Canada)
314-447-8871 (subscribers outside of the U.S. & Canada)

Fax number: 314-447-8029

Elsevier Health Sciences Division
Subscription Customer Service
3251 Riverport Lane
Maryland Heights, MO 63043

*To ensure uninterrupted delivery of your subscription, please notify us at least 4 weeks in advance of move.

Moving?

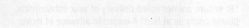

Printed and bound by CPI Group (UK) Ltd, Croydon, CR0 4YY

08/05/2025

01864700-0004